Practical Carotid Artery Stenting

Edited by

Sumaira Macdonald
The Northern Vascular Unit, Newcastle Upon Tyne, UK

Gerry Stansby
The Northern Vascular Unit, Newcastle Upon Tyne, UK

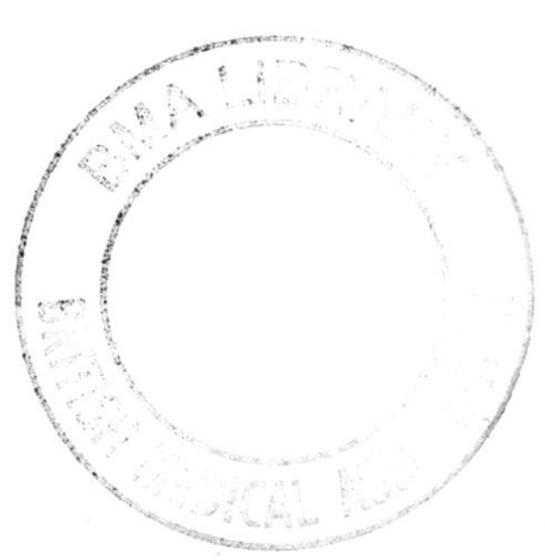

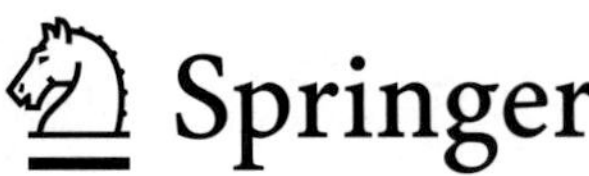

Editors
Sumaira Macdonald
The Northern Vascular Unit
The Freeman Hospital
Newcastle upon Tyne
UK

Gerry Stansby
The Northern Vascular Unit
The Freeman Hospital
Newcastle upon Tyne
UK

ISBN: 978-1-84800-298-2 e-ISBN: 978-1-84800-299-9
DOI: 10.1007/978-1-84800-299-9

British Library Cataloguing in Publication Data

Library of Congress Control Number: 2008939887

Printed on acid-free paper

Springer Science+Business Media
springer.com

Dedication

This book is dedicated to the memory of Dr. Bob Hobson, who contributed to the academic and professional development of countless faculty, fellows, and residents who have assumed leadership positions across America. He will be remembered by all those whom he mentored, and for his leadership in generating the next group of individuals to carry on his important missions.

Dr. Hobson graduated from the George Washington University School of Medicine in Washington, DC in 1963. After serving with the U.S. Army, he returned to complete a residency in General Surgery (1971) and a Fellowship in Vascular Surgery (1973) at the Walter Reed Army Medical Center. He was the founding Director of the Division of Vascular Surgery at the University of Medicine and Dentistry - New Jersey Medical School (1975-2003) and the institution's Vascular Disease Center.

Dr. Hobson enjoyed an illustrious career as an academic surgeon. He has been the President of numerous vascular societies in America, and was the president-elect of the International Vascular Society for the upcoming year. His major research interests included cerebrovascular physiology, carotid occlusive disease, and ischemia-reperfusion injury. He was a prolific author (over 375 manuscripts, over 100 book chapters, and 5 textbooks) and served on the Editorial Board of 8 journals. He was currently best known for a most successful multi-center NIH funded Clinical Trial, (carotid revascularization endarterectomy vs. stenting trial, CREST) comparing carotid artery stenting and endarterectomy.

Preface

He who studies medicine without books sails an uncharted sea (William Osler, 1849–1919)

In the management of vascular disease, there has been an inexorable drive toward less invasive endovascular treatment options. This has substantially altered the attitudes of patients, clinicians, and health care providers and has influenced service provision for these patients. Endovascular treatment of carotid disease is no exception. The aim of this book is to provide those taking up carotid stenting with an authoritative, practical, and contemporary guide to all aspects of the procedure.

When planning this book, we recognized at an early stage that carotid stenting is being performed by physicians from a variety of backgrounds including interventional radiologists, neurointerventional radiologists, vascular surgeons, interventional cardiologists, interventional neurologists, and angiologists. Because of that, we have deliberately asked a wide variety of authors to provide their expert contributions. Also, like any technically complex intervention, there are potential problems with respect to training and support. Inexperienced operators working on the steep part of their learning curves may find that their early complication rates are higher than they wish. Whilst this book cannot completely substitute for "hands-on" experience, we hope certain elements will help the novice carotid stenter to hasten their proficiency in the procedure and avoid some of the pitfalls others have encountered in the past.

We hope William Osler would have approved of this book. It is essentially a practical guide, tempered with advice about patient selection, the evidence for intervention, and warnings about difficult areas. Osler also said "*The practice of medicine is an art, not a trade; a calling, not a business.*" We think this remains true today.

S. Macdonald
G. Stansby

Editor's Biographies

Dr. Sumaira Macdonald is a consultant vascular/interventional radiologist, who has been responsible for setting up the carotid stenting program in Newcastle upon Tyne. She has published on carotid stenting and cerebral protection, is involved with several trials of carotid stenting, and regularly proctors and teaches the technique nationally and internationally.

Professor Gerry Stansby is a consultant vascular surgeon, experienced in carotid surgery and patient selection. He has published research on carotid surgery and is involved with several trials on carotid disease. He is a Cochrane Editor and a Council Member of the Vascular Society of Great Britain and Ireland.

Contents

Contributors

Babak Abai
Assistant Professor, Department of Vascular Surgery, UMDNJ-Robert Wood Johnson Medical School (Camden), Camden, NJ, USA

Alex Abou-Chebl
Associate Professor of Neurology and Neurosurgery, Director of Neurointerventional Services, University of Louisville School of Medicine, Louisville, KY, USA

David Beckett
Endovascular Fellow, Sheffield Vascular Institute, Sheffield, UK

Jos C. van den Berg
Head of the Service of Interventional Radiology Ospedale Regionale di Lugano, sede Civico, Lugano, Switzerland

Giancarlo Biamino
Interventional Cardio-Angiology Unit, Villa Maria Cecilia Hospital, Cotignola, Italy

Marc Bosiers
Department of Vascular Surgery, Dendermonde, Belgium

Martin M. Brown
Professor of Stroke Medicine, Stroke Research Group, Department of Brain Repair & Rehabilitation, UCL Institute of Neurology, London, UK

Fausto Castriota
Co-Director, Interventional Cardio-Angiology Unit, Villa Maria Cecilia Hospital, Cotignola, Italy

Alberto Cremonesi
Interventional Cardio-Angiology Unit, Villa Maria Cecilia Hospital, Cotignola, Italy

Jörg Ederle
Clinical Research Fellow, Stroke Research Group, Department of Brain Repair & Rehabilitation, UCL Institute of Neurology, London, UK

Robert Fathi
Interventional Cardiologist, Princess Alexandra Hospital, Brisbane, Australia

Peter A. Gaines
Professor of Radiology, Sheffield Vascular Institute, Sheffield, UK

Shane Gieowarsinghs
Fellow, Interventional Cardio-Angiology Unit, Villa Maria Cecilia Hospital, Cotignola, Italy

Robert W. Hobson II
Professor, Departments of Vascular Surgery and Physiology, UMDNJ-New Jersey Medical School, Newark, NJ, USA

Peter Humphrey
Consultant Neurologist, Walton Centre for Neurology & Neurosurgery, Liverpool, UK

Brajesh K. Lal
Associate Professor, Departments of Vascular Surgery and Physiology, UMDNJ-New Jersey Medical School, Newark, NJ
Associate Professor, Department of Biomedical Engineering, Stevens Institute of Technology, Hoboken, NJ, USA

Armando Liso
Interventional Cardio-Angiology Unit, Villa Maria Cecilia Hospital, Cotignola, Italy

Ridwan Lynn
Vascular Neurology Fellow, University of Pittsburgh, Pittsburgh, PA, USA

Sumaira Macdonald
Consultant Vascular/Interventional Radiologist, Freeman Hospital, Newcastle upon Tyne, UK

A. Ross Naylor
The Department of Vascular Surgery, Leicester Royal Infirmary, Leicester, UK

Juan C. Parodi
Department of Vascular Surgery, Jackson Memorial Hospital, University of Miami, Miami, FL, USA

Patrick Peeters
Department of Cardiovascular and Thoracic Surgery, Imelda Hospital, Bonheiden, Belgium

Peter A. Schneider
Division of Vascular Therapy, Department of Surgery, Hawaii Permanente Medical Group, Honolulu, HI, USA

Claudio Schönholz
Heart & Vascular Center, Medical University of South Carolina, Charleston, SC, USA

Gerard Stansby
Northern Vascular Centre, Freeman Hospital, Newcastle upon Tyne, UK

Luc Stockx
Vascular and Neurointerventional Radiologist, Ziekenhuis Oost Limburg, Genk, Belgium

Steve Thomas
Senior Lecturer and Consultant Vascular Radiologist, Academic Vascular Unit, The University of Sheffield, Sheffield, UK

Douglas Turner
Consultant Vascular Radiologist, Northern General Hospital, Sheffield, UK

Renan Uflacker
Heart & Vascular Center, Medical University of South Carolina, Charleston, SC, USA

Robin Williams
Consultant Interventional Radiologist, Freeman Hospital, Newcastle upon Tyne, UK
Department of Urology, Pelvic & Sexual Health Institute, Graduate Hospital, Philadelphia, PA, USA

1 Carotid Stenting: The Evidence Base

Jörg Ederle and Martin M. Brown

Introduction

Carotid artery stenosis accounts for a significant proportion of ischaemic strokes. With changes in life style and an aging population, it is likely that more and more people will be affected by carotid atherosclerosis and at risk of stroke. Not only can this have catastrophic consequences for the individual affected, but also it places a huge burden on society and the economy. Carotid stenosis is often only discovered after the patient has had a stroke. Research has for many years focused on treating symptomatic carotid stenosis to prevent further strokes. Carotid endarterectomy was introduced almost 50 years ago, and over the years many small reports suggested that it was an effective preventive treatment of symptomatic carotid stenosis. After two large trials, the North American Symptomatic Carotid Endarterectomy Trial (NASCET) [1] and the European Carotid Surgery Trial (ECST) [2], showed endarterectomy to be beneficial in preventing subsequent stroke in severe symptomatic carotid stenosis, surgery became the treatment of choice. In ECST, the risk of ipsilateral stroke at 3-year follow-up was reduced from 21.9 to 9.6% after carotid endarterectomy. NASCET showed a reduction from 26.6 to 12.6%. Within 30 days of treatment, the risk of death or stroke was 7.0% in ECST and 6.5% in NASCET. Attempts have also been made to demonstrate the value of treating asymptomatic patients to prevent stroke happening in the first place. However, the results from two large trials, the Asymptomatic Carotid Atherosclerosis Study (ACAS) [3] and the Asymptomatic Carotid Surgery Trial (ACST) [4], were less pronounced with a 5-year risk reduction of stroke or death from 11.5 to 5.1% in ACAS and 4.2 to 2.1% in ACST.

The results of the carotid endarterectomy vs. medicine trials provide the benchmark for endovascular treatment of carotid stenosis. To justify wide clinical use, endovascular treatment has to fulfill two objectives: it has to be as safe and as effective as carotid endarterectomy. By convention, events taking place within 30 days of treatment define the safety of the treatment. Analyzing events taking place further down the line allow us to make estimates of the efficacy of the treatment.

Endovascular treatment has been used as an alternative to carotid endarterectomy at some centers for 15 years or more, and numerous case series have been published reporting good results. However, these do not provide enough evidence to satisfy the current requirements of government control and clinical governance. Only randomized clinical trials provide sufficiently robust evidence. The first randomized trial, the Carotid and Vertebral Artery Transluminal Angioplasty Study (CAVATAS), was started in 1992 [5]. However, before CAVATAS was completed, a single-center study published in 1998, from Leicester, was stopped because of disastrous results in the stenting arm [6]. This sparked off controversy about the safety of carotid stenting, which continues to this day. There followed a whole series of randomized trials comparing endovascular treatment with surgery or medical treatment alone for both symptomatic and asymptomatic carotid

S. Macdonald and G. Stansby (eds.), *Practical Carotid Artery Stenting*,
DOI: 10.1007/978-1-84800-299-9_1,

stenosis [5]. Up to Spring 2007, ten more randomized clinical trials have been identified contributing over 3,000 patients [6–16] and a number of trials are still underway [17, 18].

It took only two trials each to establish carotid endarterectomy as treatment for symptomatic and asymptomatic stenosis. It is surprising that it should take more than six times as many trials to answer the question of safety and efficacy of endovascular treatment, but perhaps this is because not a single trial was able to recruit numbers similar to the surgery trials. While ECST and NASCET used slightly different measurements to establish the extent of stenosis, their outcome measures were similar, which allowed for a combined analysis of the results [19]. One of the problems of the many different endovascular studies is that they are difficult to analyze because of different inclusion criteria, outcome measures, and treatment modalities. But nonetheless, there are valuable conclusions to be drawn, and in this chapter we will try to guide you through the maze of these trials. For this purpose, one should look at symptomatic and asymptomatic patients separately. The surgery trials have shown that results are different in these patients and there is no reason to believe this is not equally true for endovascular treatment.

Symptomatic Carotid Stenosis: Endovascular Treatment vs. Surgery

Trial Characteristics

Before discussing the trial results in more detail, it is important to take a closer look at the characteristics of the trials. They can be broadly divided into trials that have been completed and those that have been stopped early for different reasons. Stopping a trial early always carries the risk of introducing bias. Trials can be stopped for different reasons with different impact on the results. A trial might be stopped because the investigators run out of money. This might lead to the trial not having enough power to answer the question it set out to resolve. But this has probably the least impact on the trial's results because the number of outcome events had not been taken into consideration and thus it is unlikely to introduce bias. Investigators might stop a trial early because they fail to meet their recruitment targets. This is a common problem encountered by trials running for a long time. This might again lead to the trial being underpowered but again it is unlikely to introduce a bias because outcome events have not been taken into account when the decision to stop the trial has been made. The most problematic reason to stop a trial is because of interim safety analysis. Randomized clinical trials have mechanisms in place that monitor trial safety. Usually, stopping rules are predefined and the trial can be stopped prematurely if the safety committee deems the trial to be too dangerous. This carries the risk of introducing bias because the accumulation of events might be due to chance, especially when the number of patients included in the trial is relatively small. The result of the stopped trial may then overestimate the risk of that procedure or underestimate the risk of the control procedure.

As far as trial design is concerned, four features are very important (1) the degree of stenosis required to be eligible for inclusion in the trial, (2) what defined "symptomatic," (3) what kind of endovascular treatment had been chosen, and (4) the experience and training of the investigators.

Completed Trials

Four completed trials have been identified comparing endovascular treatment with surgery in symptomatic patients [7, 9, 11, 12].

The Kentucky trial was a single-center study restricted to patients with symptoms confined to the carotid circulation within 3 months of randomization and only used stenting as endovascular treatment [7]. The cutoff level of stenosis was set at 70% as defined by NASCET criteria. The level of experience (i.e., the number of procedures performed before the study was started) was not specified in this trial.

CAVATAS was a multicenter trial undertaken in the 1990s. It was a family of three trials. One study compared endovascular treatment and surgery in symptomatic patients (CAVATAS–CEA) [9]. Three features characterized the trial. In CAVATAS–CEA, the trial was started before stenting was introduced and both stenting and angioplasty alone were used to treat carotid stenosis under the combined heading of "endovascular treatment." Roughly, a quarter of patients receiving endovascular treatment had a stent inserted. Second, the investigators included both symptomatic, and a small number (18%) of asymptomatic, patients. A patient was considered to be symptomatic if he/she had experienced "appropriate" symptoms within 6 months of randomization. Thirdly, patients were included in the trial with ipsilateral carotid stenosis greater than 50%. Since endovascular treatment for carotid stenosis was a relatively new technique at most centers, no previous experience was required, but inexperienced investigators received training and assistance from the more experienced centers.

The Basel Carotid Artery Stenting Study (BACASS) included only patients at a single center with at least 70% stenosis using the ECST criteria, roughly equivalent to 50% stenosis using the NASCET criteria [11]. All patients in this small trial were symptomatic but it was not specified how "symptomatic" was defined. Stenting was the sole endovascular treatment. Investigators in this study had a lot of experience with endovascular treatment having participated in CAVATAS.

The Trial of Endarterectomy vs. Stenting for the treatment of Carotid Atherosclerotic Stenosis in China (TESCAS-C) was only published in Chinese with only the abstract available in English [12]. It is therefore difficult to scrutinize this trial.

Stopped Trials

The first randomized trial of endovascular treatment compared with surgery to be stopped was conducted in Leicester [5]. Only symptomatic patients with carotid stenosis greater than 70% were included. The investigators did not specify their definition of "symptomatic" or the criteria used to define the degree of stenosis. Stenting was the sole endovascular treatment used. Although it had been planned for the data monitoring committee to perform an interim analysis after only 20 interventions, the investigators got cold feet after five consecutive stenting procedures out of seven led to treatment-related events and passed the results on to the data monitoring committee. The trial was terminated after treating only 17 patients.

The industry-sponsored WALLSTENT trial enrolled symptomatic patients with carotid stenosis greater than 60% without specifying the measurement technique or the definition of "symptomatic" [6]. Patients assigned to endovascular treatment were treated with stenting using a single device. The trial was stopped early, controversially not by an independent data monitoring committee but by the trial sponsor, well before the targeted sample size and the results have never been published in a peer-reviewed journal.

The Stenting and Angioplasty with Protection in Patients at High Risk for Endarterectomy study (SAPPHIRE) has several noteworthy characteristics [15]. It included only patients with a high surgical risk. Both symptomatic and asymptomatic patients were included and the majority of patients enrolled were asymptomatic. The level of stenosis depended on whether a patient was symptomatic (>60%) or asymptomatic (>80%). Making matters even more complicated, the trial used cerebral neuroprotection devices in the endovascular treatment arm. Interventional physicians had completed a median of 64 procedures before entering the trial. In the end, the trial was terminated early because of a slowdown in recruitment. Concern has also subsequently been expressed about the fact that the Chief Investigator of SAPPHIRE received undeclared royalties from sales of the protection device used in the trial.

The Endarterectomy vs. Angioplasty in patients with symptomatic severe carotid stenosis trial (EVA-3S) only included symptomatic patients. Symptoms had to be present within 120 days of randomization [13]. The level of stenosis was initially set at 70%, determined by NASCET criteria and later reduced to 60%. Endovascular treatment was by stenting. To join the trial, the interventional physician had to have performed at least 12 carotid stenting procedures or at least 35 stenting procedures in the supra-aortic trunks, of which five were in the carotid artery. The trial was briefly put on hold after an interim analysis suggested a much higher rate of stroke in patients stented without a protection device, and the mandatory use of cerebral neuroprotection devices was introduced. After a safety analysis by the data monitoring committee, the trial was suspended due to an excess number of events in one treatment arm.

The Stent-Protected Angioplasty vs. Carotid Endarterectomy trial (SPACE) enrolled symptomatic patients only [14]. Symptoms had to occur within 180 days before randomization and the degree of carotid stenosis had to be greater than 70% defined by NASCET criteria. Endovascular treatment was stenting, with or without a cerebral protection device. Roughly, one quarter of patients in the endovascular group was treated using such a device. Interventionalists had to show proof of at least 25 consecutive successful endovascular procedures in the carotid artery. The trial was designed as noninferiority study and after interim analysis revealed an insufficient sample size, the investigators terminated randomization because funds did not allow them to carry on randomizing.

Safety

One might argue that these striking differences in trial design described earlier forbid a combined analysis in the first place. However, combining the results and very cautiously interpreting the results still might be helpful in informing a decision on what route to take in treating patients with carotid stenosis and where we go next.

Firstly, is the treatment safe? Most commonly, the safety of endovascular treatment is assessed by a combined outcome of death and stroke within 30 days of procedure. The available evidence from the randomized trials is not clear at all and due to reasons laid out above, significant heterogeneity between the trials has to be assumed. The estimates of effect vary with the stopped trials favoring surgery and the completed trials neutral for major outcomes, but with wide confidence intervals. A combined estimate of effect with regard to death or stroke within 30 days of randomization reveals no significant difference between endovascular treatment and surgery. However, the odds ratio (OR) (endovascular:surgery) of 1.44, favours surgery, but with a wide 95% confidence interval (CI) of 0.91–2.26, $p = 0.12$, using the random effects model to combine the data (Fig. 1.1). This outcome measure excludes a common problem of carotid surgery, cranial nerve damage. This might be a minor event in some patients but can also lead to considerable disability with speech problems and difficulties swallowing. An analysis of this outcome strongly favors endovascular treatment with an OR (endovascular:surgery) of 0.09 (95% CI 0.04–0.25, $p < 0.00001$). Further analyses examining other combinations of outcome events show similar heterogeneity and can be found in our systematic Cochrane Review [20].

Efficacy

The safety of the procedure is only one side of the coin. Before it can be recommended for wider clinical use, endovascular treatment has to be shown to be effective in preventing long-term complications of carotid stenosis, i.e., subsequent stroke. Most trials used a combined endpoint of death or any stroke after a set time period, while some chose to report on rather obscure endpoints making it virtually impossible to compare their results. This question is even more difficult to answer than the safety question because fewer

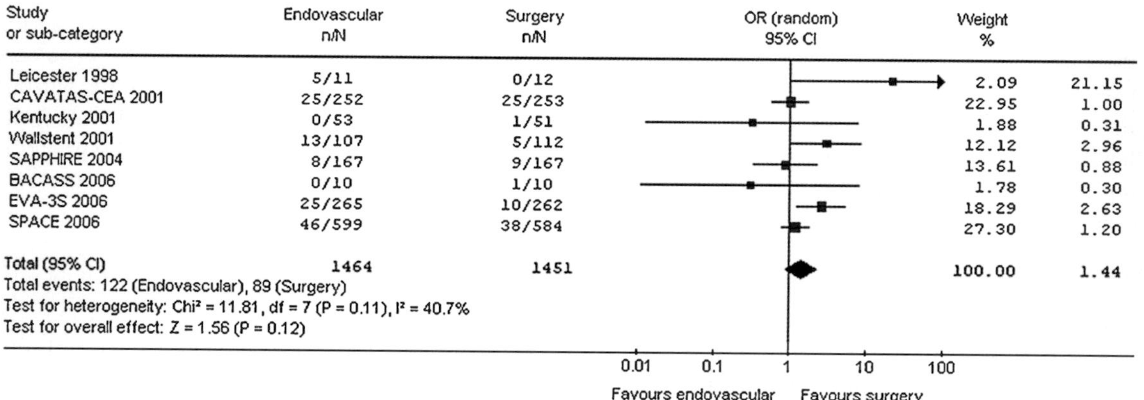

FIG. 1.1. Death or any stroke within 30 days of treatment of symptomatic carotid stenosis. *N* total number of patients, *n* number of events, *OR* odds ratio, *95% CI* 95% confidence interval, all calculations using a random effects model (from [20] with permission from the publisher)

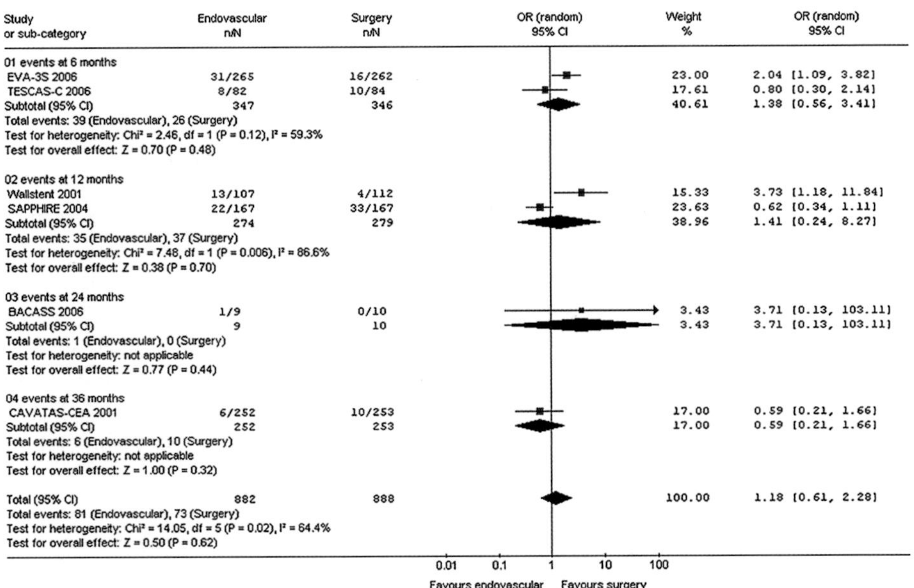

FIG. 1.2. Death or any stroke during follow-up of symptomatic carotid stenosis. *N* total number of patients, *n* number of events, *OR* odds ratio, *95% CI* 95% confidence interval, all calculations using a random effects model (from [20] with permission from the publisher)

trial results are available and different trials have reported on different lengths of follow-up. Overall, the combined estimate of effect suggests no difference between endovascular treatment and surgery. The OR (endovascular:surgery) was 1.18 (95% CI 0.61–2.28, $p = 0.62$; Fig. 1.2).

Symptomatic Carotid Stenosis: Endovascular vs. Medical Treatment

Because carotid endarterectomy is considered to be superior to medical treatment alone, most trials compared endovascular treatment with endarterectomy in patients suitable for surgery. Only in patients in whom surgery was not an option, endovascular treatment could be considered as a possible alternative to medical treatment.

Trial Characteristics

Only two trials compared endovascular with medical treatment and both trials were very small, contributing a total of 61 patients. Both trials were very underpowered to provide an answer for the question of safety and efficacy of endovascular treatment. The medical care study from the CAVATAS family (CAVATAS–MED) enrolled patients not suitable for surgery [10] and a number of patients who refused surgery. All other inclusion criteria were the same as in CAVATAS–CEA. Patients randomized to endovascular treatment could receive a stent or be treated by balloon angioplasty alone. Only 40 patients were enrolled in this trial. A trial conducted in China compared endovascular and medical treatment in patients with severe bilateral stenosis [16]. The report does not specify if these patients had been symptomatic. All patients allocated endovascular treatment received a stent. Neither trial specified "medical treatment" and it must be assumed that treatment differed considerably.

Safety

Only CAVATAS–MED reported results of the initial 30-day period. One patient in the endovascular group (5%) had a fatal stroke compared with no patient in the medical group.

Efficacy

Only 23 events were reported during follow-up of up to 10 years. Not surprisingly, there is no significant difference between medical and endovascular treatment in the combined analysis, perhaps because of the small numbers of patients randomized (OR (endovascular:medical) 0.28, 95% CI 0.02–3.23, $p = 0.30$).

Since the late 1990s when CAVATAS was conducted, medical treatment has changed considerably. This casts some doubt on the applicability of these results to today's clinical practice.

Asymptomatic Carotid Stenosis: Endovascular Treatment vs. Surgery

Endarterectomy has been shown to be effective in preventing stroke in asymptomatic patients although this effect is less pronounced than in the treatment of symptomatic carotid stenosis. There are many more subjects with asymptomatic stenosis than symptomatic patients with carotid stenosis. It is therefore understandable that endovascular treatment has been applied to asymptomatic carotid stenosis despite the lack of proof of benefit in symptomatic patients.

Trial Characteristics

Only one trial conducted in Kentucky enrolled only asymptomatic patients [8]. The trial was run by the same team as the symptomatic Kentucky trial. Persons with any cerebrovascular symptom were excluded from the trial and the degree of stenosis had to be greater than 80% applying the NASCET criteria. Endovascular treatment was stenting; no information about the stenting experience of the investigators was provided. SAPPHIRE included a large proportion of asymptomatic patients and CAVATAS–CEA also included a small number of asymptomatic patients randomized between endovascular treatment and surgery. SAPPHIRE reported a complex primary endpoint of cumulative incidence of death, stroke, or myocardial infarction within 30 days of the procedure and death or ipsilateral stroke between 31 days and 1 year. The outcome in CAVATAS–CEA was reported more conventionally as death or stroke within 30 days of procedure. This illustrates the difficulty of comparing trial results.

Results

The Kentucky trial reported a zero event rate for death or stroke within 30 days of treatment in both treatment groups. The risk of cranial nerve damage was, however, not totally avoided in the surgery group. The outcome in asymptomatic stenosis cannot be extracted from SAPPHIRE. In CAVATAS–CEA, there was no difference in death or stroke within 30 days of the procedure in asymptomatic patients.

Conclusions

It is impossible to draw any firm conclusions from the available evidence because of the marked variation in design and outcome in the various trials comparing endovascular treatment with carotid endarterectomy. The trials varied widely in many aspects. They used different definitions of what constitutes a symptomatic patient and some trials enrolled a mixture of symptomatic and asymptomatic patients. The method used to establish the degree of stenosis also varied and trials required different degrees of stenosis for enrollment. The chosen endovascular technique ranged from using balloon angioplasty alone in CAVATAS, to primary stenting with or without a neuroprotection device in later trials. It is likely that these differences influence outcome and, to make matters more difficult, different trials used different outcome measures. Another important point is the influence of the interventionalists' experience: the fact that the required experience for entering the study varied from trial to trial and that the experience of angioplasty and stenting of individual centers varied considerably within trials is likely to have had a major influence on the results.

The uncertainty generated by the results of the trials discussed in this chapter can only be resolved by data from larger, better designed randomized trials. Two trials are still underway recruiting symptomatic patients. The International Carotid Stenting Study (ICSS) [17] is restricted to symptomatic patients and the Carotid Revascularization Endarterectomy vs. Stenting Trial (CREST) [18] is also recruiting asymptomatic patients. Other trials are planned to assess endovascular treatment in asymptomatic patients. Even if the ongoing trial results finally show a slightly higher stroke risk at the time of treatment, the less invasive nature of stenting may lead patients and physicians to prefer stenting. It is notable that in coronary heart disease, stenting has all but replaced surgery as the treatment of first choice for coronary artery stenosis. This is despite the fact that the randomized trials have shown that coronary artery bypass grafting is superior to stenting in preventing long-term major cardiac adverse events [21]. It is therefore important that the endovascular treatment trials underway publish their results while they are still able to inform opinion before the medical community and patients have made up their minds. Ultimately, the choice of treatment may come down to the different departments' experience and patient perception of the risks and benefits of the two approaches.

Key Points

Symptomatic Stenosis

Endovascular Treatment vs. Surgery

- Various criteria to establish degree of stenosis.
- Definition of "symptomatic" varies between trials.
- Some trials included asymptomatic patients.
- Some trials were stopped early, possibly introducing bias.
- Combined analysis shows no significant difference between endovascular treatment and surgery with regard to death or stroke, but confidence interval wide and trend favours surgery.
- Endovascular treatment avoids the risk of cranial nerve damage.
- More data required from ongoing trials.

Endovascular vs. Medical Treatment

- Trials very much underpowered.
- Results not robust enough to draw firm conclusions.
- No clear difference between endovascular and medical treatment to date.
- Medical treatment has improved since the late 1990s.

Asymptomatic Stenosis

Endovascular Treatment vs. Surgery

- Trials very much underpowered.
- Results not robust enough to draw firm conclusions.
- Current trials will provide further data.
- A center's safety record should be considered in choosing treatments outside clinical trials.

Overall Conclusions

- The evidence base does not support a change in clinical practice away from recommending carotid endarterectomy as the treatment of choice.
- Ongoing trials will provide further data.
- A center's safety record should be considered in choosing treatments outside clinical trials.

References

1. Barnett, H.J., D.W. Taylor, M. Eliasziw, A.J. Fox, G.G. Ferguson, R.B. Haynes, R.N. Rankin, G.P. Clagett, V.C. Hachinski, D.L. Sackett, K.E. Thorpe, H.E. Meldrum, and J.D. Spence, Benefit of carotid endarterectomy in patients with symptomatic moderate or severe stenosis. North American Symptomatic Carotid Endarterectomy Trial Collaborators. N Engl J Med, 1998. 339(20): 1415–25.
2. Randomised trial of endarterectomy for recently symptomatic carotid stenosis: Final results of the MRC European Carotid Surgery Trial (ECST). Lancet, 1998. 351: (9113)1379–87.
3. Endarterectomy for asymptomatic carotid artery stenosis. Executive Committee for the Asymptomatic Carotid Atherosclerosis Study. JAMA, 1995. 273: (18)1421–8.
4. Halliday, A., A. Mansfield, J. Marro, C. Peto, R. Peto, J. Potter, and D. Thomas, Prevention of disabling and fatal strokes by successful carotid endarterectomy in patients without recent neurological symptoms: Randomised controlled trial. Lancet, 2004. 363(9420): 1491–502.
5. Naylor, A.R., A. Bolia, R.J. Abbott, I.F. Pye, J. Smith, N. Lennard, A.J. Lloyd, N.J.M. London, and P.R.F. Bell, Randomized study of carotid angioplasty and stenting versus carotid endarterectomy: A stopped trial. J Vasc Surg, 1998. 28(2): 326.
6. Alberts, M.J. Results of a multicenter prospective randomized trial of carotid artery stenting vs. carotid endarterectomy. Stroke, 2001. 32(1): 325.
7. Brooks, W.H., R.R. McClure, M.R. Jones, T.C. Coleman, and L. Breathitt, Carotid angioplasty and

stenting versus carotid endarterectomy: Randomized trial in a community hospital. J Am Coll Cardiol, 2001. 38(6): 1589.

8. Brooks, W.H., R.R. McClure, M.R. Jones, T.L. Coleman, and L. Breathitt, Carotid angioplasty and stenting versus carotid endarterectomy for treatment of asymptomatic carotid stenosis: A randomized trial in a community hospital. Neurosurgery, 2004. 54(2): 318–24; discussion 324–5.
9. Brown, M.M., J. Rogers, and J.M. Bland, Endovascular versus surgical treatment in patients with carotid stenosis in the Carotid and Vertebral Artery Transluminal Angioplasty Study (CAVATAS): A randomised trial. Lancet, 2001. 357(9270): 1729.
10. Ederle, J., R.L. Featherstone, J. Dobson, and M.M. Brown. Endovascular treatment versus medical care in patients with carotid artery stenosis not suitable for surgery: Long-term results from CAVATAS. In European Stroke Conference, Glasgow, 2007.
11. Hoffmann, A., C. Taschner, S.T. Engelter, P. Lyrer, J. Rem, E.W. Radue, and E.C. Kirsch, Carotid artery stenting versus carotid endarterectomy. A prospective, randomised trial with long term follow up (BACASS). In Annual meeting of the cerebrovascular working group of Switzerland, Bern. Schweiz Arch Neurol Psychiatr, 2006.
12. Ling, F. and L.Q. Jiao, Preliminary report of trial of endarterectomy versus stenting for the treatment of carotid atherosclerotic stenosis in China (TESCAS-C). Chin J Cerebrovasc Dis, 2006. 3(1): 4–8.
13. Mas, J.L., G. Chatellier, B. Beyssen, A. Branchereau, T. Moulin, J.P. Becquemin, V. Larrue, M. Lievre, D. Leys, J.F. Bonneville, J. Watelet, J.P. Pruvo, J.F. Albucher, A. Viguier, P. Piquet, P. Garnier, F. Viader, E. Touze, M. Giroud, H. Hosseini, J.C. Pillet, P. Favrole, J.P. Neau, and X. Ducrocq, Endarterectomy versus stenting in patients with symptomatic severe carotid stenosis. N Engl J Med, 2006. 355(16): 1660–71.
14. Ringleb, P.A., J. Allenberg, H. Bruckmann, H.H. Eckstein, G. Fraedrich, M. Hartmann, M. Hennerici, O. Jansen, G. Klein, A. Kunze, P. Marx, K. Niederkorn, W. Schmiedt, L. Solymosi, R. Stingele, H. Zeumer, and W. Hacke, 30 day results from the SPACE trial of stent-protected angioplasty versus carotid endarterectomy in symptomatic patients: A randomised non-inferiority trial. Lancet, 2006. 368(9543): 1239–47.
15. Yadav, J.S., M.H. Wholey, R.E. Kuntz, P. Fayad, B.T. Katzen, G.J. Mishkel, T.K. Bajwa, P. Whitlow, N.E. Strickman, M.R. Jaff, J.J. Popma, D.B. Snead, D.E. Cutlip, B.G. Firth, and K. Ouriel, Protected carotid-artery stenting versus endarterectomy in high-risk patients. N Engl J Med, 2004. 351(15): 1493.
16. Zhao, X.L., J.P. Jia, X.M. Ji, M. Peng, and F. Ling, A follow-up: Stroke in patients with bilateral severe carotid stenosis after intervention treatment. Zhongguo Linchuang Kangfu, 2003. 7(19): 2714.
17. Featherstone, R.L., M.M. Brown, and L.J. Coward, International carotid stenting study: Protocol for a randomised clinical trial comparing carotid stenting with endarterectomy in symptomatic carotid artery stenosis. Cerebrovasc Dis, 2004. 18(1): 69–74.
18. Hobson, R.W., II, CREST (Carotid Revascularization Endarterectomy versus Stent Trial): Background, design, and current status. Semin Vasc Surg, 2000. 13(2): 139–43.
19. Rothwell, P.M., M. Eliasziw, S.A. Gutnikov, A.J. Fox, D.W. Taylor, M.R. Mayberg, C.P. Warlow, and H.J. Barnett, Analysis of pooled data from the randomised controlled trials of endarterectomy for symptomatic carotid stenosis. Lancet, 2003. 361(9352): 107–16.
20. Ederle, J., R.L. Featherstone, and M.M. Brown, Percutaneous transluminal angioplasty and stenting for carotid artery stenosis. *Cochrane Database Syst Rev*, 2007. 4: CD000516.
21. Bakhai, A., R.A. Hill, Y. Dundar, R. Dickson, and T. Walley, Percutaneous transluminal coronary angioplasty with stents versus coronary artery bypass grafting for people with stable angina or acute coronary syndromes. Cochrane Database Syst Rev, 2005. 1: CD004588.

2 Patient Selection for Carotid Stenting

Peter Humphrey

Introduction

The clinical selection of patients for carotid artery stenting is largely similar to that for carotid endarterectomy which is the gold standard treatment for managing symptomatic internal carotid stenosis. This chapter will not consider criteria for treating asymptomatic stenoses as this will be covered by Ross Naylor in Chap. 3.

The place of carotid artery stenting in the management of cerebrovascular disease remains a major subject for research and debate. Martin Brown and Jörg Ederle (Chap. 1) have reviewed the evidence basis for stenting. While stenting is possible at most sites of carotid narrowing, the only rigorous trials have compared stenting with carotid endarterectomy to treat carotid stenosis at the origin of the internal carotid artery. There are other situations where stenting has been reported anecdotally but none of these other situations have been assessed with scientific rigor. It seems appropriate to first consider which patients should be selected for intervention when a symptomatic bifurcation internal carotid stenosis is found on investigation.

Internal carotid artery stenosis at the bifurcation of the common, external, and internal carotid arteries is a common cause of carotid transient ischemic attacks (TIAs) and stroke. The seminal publications of the European Carotid Surgery Trial (ECST) and the North American Symptomatic Carotid Endarterectomy Trial (NASCET) in 1991 proved the value of surgery in the prevention of stroke [1, 2]. ECST demonstrated that surgery was beneficial for those with stenoses of more than 70% while NASCET showed a similar benefit with stenoses of more than 50%. These trials used different methods to measure percentage stenosis [3]; because of these differences, a 70% ECST stenosis approximately equates to a 50% NASCET stenosis. The appreciation that different methods of measurement measure different things cannot be overemphasized. While this may seem obvious, it must be appreciated that newer imaging systems using doppler/duplex ultrasound, magnetic resonance angiography, and computer tomographic angiography are not measuring stenosis the same way as the NASCET and ECST trials which calculated a percentage stenosis from 2D images using either one, two, or occasionally three views of the carotid bifurcation derived by contrast carotid angiography.

Embolic TIAs

TIA or stroke following an internal carotid stenosis usually results, either from emboli passing distally into the intracerebral circulation or from the stenosis occluding at the carotid bifurcation. Embolic TIAs, if multiple, are often stereotyped. Sometimes, emboli enter different parts of the retinal and cerebral circulation but this is rare. Patients with both retinal and cerebral events often have more serious internal carotid atheroma. It is not surprising that TIAs are stereotyped as the symptoms are not coming from the stenosis per se

S. Macdonald and G. Stansby (eds.), *Practical Carotid Artery Stenting*,
DOI: 10.1007/978-1-84800-299-9_2,

but from a small ruptured plaque in the stenosis providing a focal source of emboli. Anyone who has played "Poohsticks" will know that if a stick is put into the river in the same place, whatever turbulence it experiences on the way it will end up in the same place, but put it in a different place upstream and it will end up in a different tributary of the river downstream [4].

Emboli may pass into the ipsilateral eye causing amaurosis fugax (transient monocular blindness) which is usually described as a sudden blackness or black shadow or curtain descending or ascending across the vision: all together patterns of transient visual loss are less likely to be associated with significant carotid stenosis [5]. Permanent retinal infarction results from retinal artery occlusion (RAO) which can be either complete (central RAO) or partial (branch RAO). Attacks of transient monocular visual loss may be difficult to differentiate from binocular visual loss unless the individual does a careful cover test at the time of the symptoms. Binocular visual loss, especially if hemianopic, usually arises from the occipital cortex but can occur with lesions of the optic tract or even occasionally the chiasm.

Emboli entering the cerebral circulation usually cause motor, sensory, or speech problems [6]. Isolated hemianopic visual symptoms may sometimes occur if the posterior cerebral artery is supplied by the internal carotid artery.

While symptoms may involve the complete face, arm, and leg, the shape of the homunculus with much larger representation for the hand and face than the leg means that motor or sensory TIAs frequently only affect a small part of one side of the body. TIAs or minor stroke affecting only one part (most commonly the hand) accounts for a third of all TIAs. While those affecting just the arm, hand, or face are quite common by the same analogy, isolated TIAs affecting the leg only are relatively uncommon. The latter, while making up only a small percentage of TIAs, frequently causes problems in diagnosis because it may not be appreciated that isolated episodes of leg paralysis or numbness arise centrally in the cerebral cortex.

Cortical weakness may be described as paralysis, but clumsiness and heaviness are also commonly used descriptions especially if the deficit is mild. Many patients misinterpret which side of the face is affected when facial paralysis occurs.

Isolated sensory symptoms, such as numbness or pins and needles, are less frequent and are usually associated with some motor symptoms. Isolated sensory symptoms restricted to the face or arm/hand are notoriously difficult to interpret and may be related to carpal tunnel syndrome or anxiety/hyperventilation, especially in younger patients with no risk factors.

Conversely, occasionally TIAs may have a radicular or peripheral nerve-like distribution and be restricted to certain fingers only, the significance of which is only appreciated when in subsequent attacks not only the first three fingers of the right hand are numb, but also speech is lost.

Hemi-phenomenon, both motor and sensory, can arise from both carotid and vertebrobasilar territory events. However, for practical purposes, all such attacks are investigated and managed as carotid events unless there are other symptoms such as double vision which strongly suggest a vertebrobasilar origin for the attacks.

Interpreting isolated speech deficits is difficult. A detailed description of the speech pattern especially when the individual is recovering may allow the examiner to decide if true dysphasia was present. Clearly, dysphasia localizes to the dominant hemisphere. A severe dysarthria can mimic dysphasia as far as the patient is concerned. A patient's description of "non-sense speech," or "can't get my words out" or "know what I want to say but can't get my words out" can still be dysarthric. Interpreting isolated dysarthria is difficult: while this may be a symptom of cortical weakness, it has very poor localizing value and occurs with both carotid and vertebrobasilar ischemia.

Embolic TIAs are usually abrupt in onset with a focal clear loss of function as described. They are maximal at onset. While by definition, TIAs can last up to 24 h, most last less than 30 min. TIAs lasting more than 1 h carry a higher risk of stroke. It is rare for recurrent TIAs to last more than 1 h; such attacks either cease or are followed by a stroke. Individuals with many attacks lasting several hours are usually suffering non-organic problems. Few people experience more than five attacks; indeed, most have only one or two episodes. Full investigation should follow a single episode. The "wait and see if it happens again" policy with regard to investigations is indefensible.

It is important to distinguish these types of focal symptoms from nonfocal symptoms which are frequently referred to *TIA clinics*. Focal symptoms from embolic TIAs are clear cut and usually affect vision, speech, or the motor or sensory cortex of the brain. Nonfocal symptoms are usually due to hypotension from whatever cause and results in symptoms of lightheadedness, general weakness, feelings of being faint, confusion, altered consciousness, pallor, sweating, change in heart rate, fading of vision or hearing, and eventually may lead to loss of consciousness.

The need for vigilant history taking in the assessment of TIAs cannot be overemphasized. Always ask the patients to describe the scene and let them describe the exact sequence and timing of the events. Do not interrupt and listen carefully to the words being used. At the end, it may be necessary to ask a lot of detailed questions but let the individual tell his story first.

Risk of Stroke

Rothwell and Warlow [7] have helped identify those patients with TIA or minor stroke who are at greatest risk of early stroke; while the initial ECST and NASCET crudely proved that those with stenoses of >70% (ECST method) benefited from carotid endarterectomy, it soon became clear that some individuals had a very low risk of stroke and therefore did not justify the small risk of endarterectomy whilst others had a much higher early risk of stroke. Overall, surgery is required for approximately 14 patients to prevent one ipsilateral carotid territory major ischemic stroke lasting longer than 7 days over the next 5 years.

Those at highest risk of stroke were more likely to have increasing stenosis (in the 70–99% range), have plaque surface irregularity, and have suffered cerebral rather than ocular events in the past 2 months. Interestingly, those with pseudo-occlusions (the stenosis is so tight that the distal internal carotid artery has collapsed) seemed to be at lower risk of stroke.

Furthermore, refinement of this scoring system leads to the development of the ABCD2 scoring system which identifies those at greatest risk of stroke in the first week after the initial ischemic event [8] (Table 2.1).

TABLE 2.1. ABCD2 risk scoring system [8].

			Points
A	AGE	≥60 years	1
B	BLOOD PRESSURE systolic	≥140	1
		Diastolic ≥90	1
C	CLINICAL	Unilateral motor weakness	2
		Speech disturbance	1
		Other	0
D	DURATION	≥60 min	2
		10–59 min	1
		<10 min	0
D2	DIABETES MELLITUS		1

Whilst most TIAs last less than 5–10 min, those that last more than 1 h are more likely to result in a stroke. Patients with pure ocular attacks have approximately half the stroke risk of those with hemisphere attacks.

A total score of 4 or more points helps identify those with the highest risk of stroke in the 7 days after the initial embolic event. Thus, a 65-year-old diabetic, hypertensive patient who presents with right arm weakness lasting more than 1 h has the highest risk of suffering a stroke in the next 7 days. Most of this high-risk group will have a tight internal carotid stenosis which should be assessed immediately and offered either carotid endarterectomy or stenting within less than 24 h of the clinical event.

Rothwell's data have done much to emphasize that the management of TIAs needs a complete rethink as regards the speed of investigation and treatment if the full benefit of stroke prevention is to be realized [9]. Seeing patients on the same day as their attack, instituting treatment immediately, and performing endarterectomy within 48 h if appropriate should be the aim of all units offering a TIA/Minor Stroke Service. The benefit of endarterectomy or stenting is largely lost if this whole process takes more than 1 month.

A major public education exercise needs to be undertaken to ensure that individuals with these symptoms act promptly. Most TIAs are embolic. These episodes are usually described as a sudden loss of function in a focal part of the brain without any associated symptoms. Most embolic TIAs last less than 10 min even though the TIAs with the poorest prognosis are those that last over 1 h.

During embolic TIAs, there are unlikely to be other more general symptoms such as headaches, dizziness, or any other nonfocal symptoms.

Hemodynamic and Low-Flow TIAs

A small percentage of TIAs are hemodynamic; it is difficult to quantify this figure as there is no gold standard to differentiate embolic and hemodynamic TIAs [10]. Hemodynamic TIAs are due to lack of blood flow – these patients often have severe widespread vascular disease with multiple stenoses and occlusions. Symptoms then occur when cerebral perfusion pressure falls transiently. Hemodynamic TIAs may thus be associated with symptoms of presyncope or syncope such as lightheadedness, pallor, generalized weakness, confusion, and arrhythmia or change in heart rate. They may occur at times when perfusion pressure falls, e.g., on standing, exercise, after taking hypotensive therapy, eating, or even when chewing or using a hair dryer; in the later situations, blood steals from the internal to the external circulation.

Hemodynamic amaurosis fugax often occurs when the individual enters a bright environment; the visual loss may be described as an enhancement of black/white contrast, a dimming of vision or loss of color vision before possibly progressing to a complete loss of vision. Hemodynamic attacks affecting the motor cortex may be associated with positive phenomenon such as involuntary movements or myoclonic jerking, so-called *jerking TIAs*. Hemodynamic TIAs tend to be less abrupt in onset than embolic TIAs and are much more variable in duration; they can also occur recurrently over prolonged periods of time, e.g., months or even years, without any serious sequelae.

The differentiation between embolic and hemodynamic TIAs is important when deciding on the most appropriate treatment. Hemodynamic TIAs will only be helped by improving cerebral blood flow, e.g., by avoiding too aggressive blood pressure treatment. However, it is often necessary to initiate a more definitive treatment aimed at improving cerebral blood flow by dealing with one of the intracranial or extracranial obstruction. This has led to a plethora of case reports of bypass operations to anastomose various extracranial arteries to improve flow to the brain if a standard endarterectomy was technically not possible. Angioplasty with stenting should reduce the need for such bypass procedures as it is technically more versatile than surgery and can be performed on the carotid, vertebrobasilar, subclavian, and innominate arteries. Furthermore, such patients tend to be less fit for any surgical procedure often because of coexisting cardiac disease or other comorbidities; they may however be candidates for angioplasty with stenting.

Ocular Ischemia

The chronic ocular ischemic syndromes may be a further situation appropriate for angioplasty and stenting. Retinal ischemia may be followed by rubeotic or neovascular glaucoma in which there is a very painful progressive loss of vision [6]. Due to carotid artery disease, there are usually both severe internal and external carotid artery stenoses and occlusions. Improving flow in either the internal or the external carotid artery may save vision provided it is performed before the rubeotic glaucoma progresses too far.

Lacunar TIAs/Stroke

Events arising in the cortical gray matter are much more likely to be embolic while lacunar events are associated with a low incidence of carotid stenosis [11]. Lacunar events are not "small" strokes except in pathological terms and it is better to use the term *subcortical TIAs* or *stroke* [12]. Pathologically, there is thrombosis in small perforating arteries with lipohyalinosis. The term *lacunar infarction* is used very loosely especially in radiological reports and can confuse the clinician about the pathophysiology of the stroke. For instance, infarcts in the striatocapsular/caudate region are often radiologically small and deep and can easily be labeled as lacunar lesion when a significant percentage of these lesions are due to thromboembolic disease and therefore need investigation for potential sources of emboli such as internal carotid stenosis.

Clinically, there are many different lacunar syndromes which arise from subcortical or brain stem ischemia or sometimes hemorrhage. The four classical lacunar syndromes comprise the pure motor syndrome with isolated weakness of face/

arm/leg, face/arm, or arm/leg, the pure sensory syndrome again with a similar distribution, the pure sensorimotor syndrome again with a similar distribution, and finally the ataxic hemiparesis syndrome. Clinical events restricted to just one part such as face, arm, or leg – while small clinically – are NOT lacunar and are much more likely to be cortical events. A lacunar or subcortical event must involve at least two or more of the three areas of face, arm, or leg with a deficit which affects the whole arm or leg and not just the hand or foot [12]. None of the classical lacunar syndromes should be associated with visual or cortical loss such as dysphasia.

While the differentiation of subcortical ischemic and cortical ischemia is useful in understanding mechanisms of disease, and valid for large clinical studies, it is not reliable enough in the individual patient to guide the pathogenesis of each event. A partial middle cerebral artery (MCA) cortical ischemic lesion can give a pure motor hemiplegia and thus mimic a subcortical event. In my view, clinical lacunar syndromes should be investigated for carotid stenosis and, if found, should be treated as the cause of the symptoms even though the yield from investigation is much lower than in those with definite cortical TIAs.

Differential Diagnosis

The diagnosis of TIA is largely clinical while the presence of a stroke can often be substantiated with radiological investigations [6, 10]. Studies have shown that the interobserver and intraobserver variability for the diagnosis of stroke is better than that for TIA, and it is highly likely that TIAs are considerably overdiagnosed [13, 14].

It is not possible to enter into a full discussion about the differential diagnoses, but migraine with aura, focal seizures, carpal tunnel syndrome, presyncope, and anxiety attacks (often via a combination of presyncope and hyperventilation) should be considered when the symptomatology bears some features of TIAs. A migraine aura usually builds up unlike an embolic TIA, tends to have positive features, and lasts 20–30 min (long for a TIA) and obviously may be followed by a headache. Focal seizures are often accompanied by some degree of altered consciousness, symptom march and may occur many times over a prolonged period (all uncommon in embolic TIAs); a witness description will usually suffice in making the diagnosis.

It is surprising how often attacks in which the predominant issue is syncope can be associated with focal symptoms especially sensory. Such patients often feel ill prior to the event, are lightheaded, may feel hot, cold, and clammy, be aware of heart rate change, and may even have headache or chest pain. A witness will nearly always describe pallor. All these features are rare in embolic TIA. Indeed, headache and simultaneous chest pain in someone thought to have had a TIA is virtually diagnostic of a nonorganic episode unless there is evidence of aortic or vertebral dissection or gross cardiac pathology.

Attacks more typical of TIAs or stroke may also be seen in patients with tumors, AVMs, giant aneurysms, carotid dissection, giant cell arteritis, chronic subdural hematomas, and metabolic disturbances, especially early morning hypoglycemia in patients with diabetes mellitus [6, 10].

In the UK TIA trial, there were a very small number of tumors whose attacks mimicked TIAs [15]. These patients had either sensory TIAs, speech arrest, jerking as part of the TIA, or some alteration in consciousness, all features which should alert the clinician.

Carotid dissection may be associated with neck pain, headache, or orbital pain; there may be a Horner's syndrome due to sympathetic nerve damage by the dilated carotid artery. Focal scalp tenderness overlying the temporal artery raises the possibility of giant cell arteritis in those over 50 years with ocular symptoms, especially ischemic optic neuropathy, although such patients can have no headache.

There is also a host of other nonatheromatous conditions which need to be considered in those with definite stroke and TIA [10, 16] which is beyond the scope of this chapter.

Summary

Carotid stenting is clearly possible not only at the bifurcation of the internal and external carotid artery in the neck, but also at the other sites of narrowing in the carotid artery and its tributaries. Other common sites include the common carotid artery (especially if the patient has had previous radiotherapy to the neck), the carotid siphon, and the MCA. The symptomatology associated with stenoses in these places will all be similar to those described except, of course, that retinal attacks will not occur with MCA stenoses; stenting for MCA disease was recently reviewed [17, 18].

This chapter has largely dealt with atheromatous disease at the carotid bifurcation. Other pathologies such as acute stroke, carotid dissection, fibromuscular disease, Moya Moya disease, and Takayasu's disease may also affect the large or medium size vessels but as yet there is no good evidence apart from anecdotal reports or small series that stenting has any part in the management of these diseases.

The recent results from CAVATAS comparing long-term outcome after angioplasty and stenting with medical treatment for vertebral artery stenosis show no added benefit from this intervention although the numbers were not large. Just because a treatment is technically possible, therefore one should not assume it supersedes conventional treatment without blinded randomized trials [19]. Such comparative studies will need to take into account the speed with which the intervention is implemented in view of the recent data from Rothwell et al. [7, 8].

Key Points

1. TIAs:
    - Most are embolic not hemodynamic.
    - Usually cause motor, sensory, or speech problems.
    - May result in ipsilateral amaurosis fugax (monocular).
    - Binocular visual loss usually arises from the occipital cortex.
    - Cortical weakness/paralysis may be described as clumsiness or heaviness.
    - Isolated TIAs involving the leg are rare.
    - Dysphasia localizes to the dominant hemisphere.
    - Most TIAs last less than 30 min.
    - TIAs lasting more than 1 h carry a higher risk of stroke.
2. Risk of stroke:
    - Can be quantified using the ABCD2 score.
    - Is less with ocular TIAs, which have half the risk of hemispheric TIAs.
    - Is bigger for 70–99% stenoses.
    - Retinal ischemia and loss of vision can be an indication for carotid intervention.
    - Lacunar TIAs/strokes can present with a variety of syndromes.
    - Lacunar TIAs/strokes are less often associated with carotid stenosis but it still needs to be excluded.

References

1. European Carotid Surgery Trialist's Collaborative Group. MRC European Carotid Surgery Trial: interim results for symptomatic patients with severe (70–99%) or with mild (0–29%) carotid stenosis. Lancet 1991; 337: 1235–1243.
2. North American Symptomatic Carotid Endarterectomy Trial Collaborators. Beneficial effect of carotid endarterectomy in symptomatic patients with high grade carotid stenosis. N. Engl. J. Med. 1991; 325: 445–453.
3. Rothwell PM, Gibson RJ, Slattery J, Sellar RJ, Warlow CP for the ECST Collaborative Group.Equivalence of measurements of carotid stenosis. A comparison of three methods on 1001 angiograms. Stroke 1994; 25: 2435–2439.
4. Knight R. The Poohsticks phenomenon. *Br. Med. J.* 2004; 329: 18–25.
5. Bruno A, Corbett JJ, Biller J, Adams HP, Qualls C. Transient monocular visual loss; patterns and associated vascular abnormalities. Stroke 1990; 21: 34–39.
6. Hankey GJ, Warlow CP. Clinical features and differential diagnosis. In Hankey GJ, Warlow CP (eds.) Transient Attacks of the Brain and Eye. Saunders, London, pp. 76–127, 1994 (ISBN 0-7020-1590-3).
7. Rothwell PM, Warlow CP on behalf of the ECST Collaborative Group. Prediction of benefit from carotid endarterectomy in individual patients: a risk modelling study. Lancet 1999; 353: 2105–2110.
8. Johnston SC, Rothwell PM, Nguyen-Hu Ynh MN et-al. The ABCD, California and unified ABCD2 risk scores predicted stroke within 2, 7 and 90 days after TIA. Lancet 2007; 369: 283–292.
9. Department of Health. Stroke: A Consultation on a National Strategy, 2007.
10. Warlow CP, Dennis MS, Van Gijn J, Hankey GJ, Sandercock PAG, Bamford JM, Wardlaw JM. Stroke – A Practical Guide to Management, 2nd edn. Blackwell, Oxford, pp. 223–300, 2003 (ISBN 0-632-05418-2).
11. Kappelle LJ, Koudstaal PJ, Van Gijn J, Ramos LMP, Keunen JEE. Carotid angiography in patients with lacunar infarction – prospective study. Stroke 1988; 19: 1093–1096.

12. Donnan G, Norrving B, Bamford J, Bogousslavsky J. (eds.) Subcortical Stroke.Oxford University Press, Oxford, 2002 (ISBN 019-263157-8).
13. Kraaijeveld CL, Van Gijn J, Schouten HJA, Staal A. Inter-observer agreement for the diagnosis of transient ischaemic attacks.Stroke 1984; 15: 723–725.
14. Martin PJ, Young G, Enevoldson TP,Humphrey PRD. Over-diagnosis of TIA and Minor Stroke: experience at a regional neurovascular clinic. Q. J. Med. 1999; 90: 759–763.
15. Coleman RJ, Bamford JM, Warlow CP for the UK TIA Study Group. Intracranial tumours that mimic transient cerebral ischaemia: lessons from a large multicentre trial. J. Neurol. Neurosurg. Psychiatry 1993; 56: 563–566.
16. Bogousslavsky J, Caplan L (eds.) Uncommon Causes of Stroke. Cambridge University Press, Cambridge, 2001 (ISBN 0-521-771455).
17. Donnan GA, Davis SM. Stenting for middle cerebral artery stenosis. Stroke 2007; 38: 1422.
18. Sacco RL, Adams R, Albers G, Alberts MJ et al. Guidelines for prevention of stroke in patients with ischaemic stroke of transient ischaemic attack – AHA/ASA guideline. Stroke 2006; 37: 577–617.
19. Coward LJ, McCabe DJH, Ederle J,Featherstone RL, Clifton A, Brown MM on behalf of the CAVATAS Investigators. Long term outcome after angioplasty and stenting for symptomatic vertebral artery stenosis compared with medical treatment in CAVATAS. Stroke 2007; 38: 1526–1530.

3 What Is the Evidence for Intervening in Asymptomatic Patients?

A. Ross Naylor

The truth is rarely pure and never simple
(Oscar Wilde, 1854–1900)

Introduction

The management of asymptomatic carotid artery disease remains one of the most enduring and controversial subjects in contemporary vascular practice. In the 1960s and 1970s, surgeons increasingly subscribed to the popular hypothesis that by intervening (prophylactically) on patients with asymptomatic carotid disease, large numbers of thromboembolic strokes would be prevented [1]. Because the rationale for intervention seemed very reasonable, the number of carotid endarterectomies (CEAs) performed annually increased dramatically [2] to the extent that, in some parts of the world, interventions in asymptomatic individuals far exceeded those on symptomatic patients.

By the early 1980s, however, concerns began to be expressed about the appropriateness of CEA in symptomatic patients. While these concerns were, for the most part, allayed by publication of the European Carotid Surgery Trial (ECST) and the North American Symptomatic Carotid Endarterectomy Trial (NASCET) [3, 4], it was inevitable that the management of asymptomatic patients would fall under similar scrutiny.

There have been five attempts at undertaking large-scale, randomized trials to determine the role of CEA in the management of asymptomatic disease [5–9]. Three (MACE, CASANOVA, and the VA study) have not really influenced practice [5–7]. However, only the Asymptomatic Carotid Atherosclerosis Study (ACAS) published in 1995 [8] and the Asymptomatic Carotid Surgery Trial (ACST) which reported in 2004 [9] have significantly contributed toward achieving (at least) some consensus on how best to develop international guidelines for practice.

The Asymptomatic Carotid Atherosclerosis Study [8]

Funding

- National Institute of Neurological Disorders and Stroke (NINDS)

Number Randomized

- One thousand six hundred sixty-two patients (derived from a screened population of 42,000) in 39 accredited centers involving 117 ACAS credentialed surgeons. ACAS recruited from 1987 to 1993

Inclusion Criteria

- Age 40–79 years with an asymptomatic unilateral or bilateral carotid stenosis ≥60%
- All patients to undergo formal angiography (NASCET measurement method)
- Independent Neurologist assessment
- Review of prior track record (surgeon)

S. Macdonald and G. Stansby (eds.), *Practical Carotid Artery Stenting*,
DOI: 10.1007/978-1-84800-299-9_3,

Exclusion Criteria

- Age ≥80 years
- Cerebrovascular events in the territory of the randomized artery at any time
- Any cerebrovascular symptoms referable to the contralateral carotid artery <45 days
- Contraindication to aspirin therapy
- "Any disorder that could seriously complicate surgery"
- "Any condition that could cause disability or death <5 years"

Medical Treatment

- Three hundred twenty-five milligram enteric-coated aspirin daily plus "risk factor modification" according to recommendations from the ACAS Risk Factor Reduction Committee

Surgical Treatment

Formal angiography had to be performed before surgery and the trial recommended that CEA should be performed within 2 weeks of randomization. Surgical patients with a postrandomization, presurgery angiogram showing (1) stenosis <60% or (2) a significant distal abnormality (aneurysm, AV malformation, or siphon stenosis exceeding the proximal stenosis) did not undergo surgery, but were retained in the surgical arm for "comparison analyses."

No attempt was made to standardize choice of anesthesia, shunt practice, or any other aspect of surgical technique in ACAS. These factors were left to the discretion of the surgeon.

Endpoint Analyses

Definition of "Stroke"

- Focal ischemic neurological deficit of abrupt onset lasting for >24 h

Procedural Risk

The surgeon, the ACAS Neurologist, and the ACAS Patient Coordinator examined each patient after 24 h. All strokes or deaths occurring within 30 days after randomization into the surgical arm (42 days in the medical group) were deemed as early, perioperative events.

Primary Endpoint

- Five-year ipsilateral stroke or any perioperative death/stroke

Secondary Endpoints

- Five-year "any" stroke or any perioperative death/stroke
- Five-year major ipsilateral stroke or any perioperative death/stroke
- Five-year major "any" stroke or any perioperative death/stroke
- Five-year ipsilateral TIA or stroke or any perioperative death/TIA/stroke

Subgroup Analyses

- Males vs. females
- Contralateral occlusion vs. patent contralateral carotid artery
- Age <68 vs. age ≥68 years
- Stenosis severity (60–69%, 70–79%, 80–99%)

Other Analyses of ACAS Data

- Selection process for surgeons
- Prevalence of baseline asymptomatic infarction
- Causes of perioperative morbidity and mortality
- Prevalence of recurrent stenosis

Results

This section deals with the primary and secondary analyses from ACAS involving a median of 2.7 years of follow-up (4,657 patient years).

General Observations

One hundred one out of eight hundred twenty five patients randomized to surgery did not undergo angiography or CEA, while 45 patients randomized to medical therapy underwent CEA during the course of follow-up without having become symptomatic. The principle reasons for not undergoing surgery were (1) patient refusal (n = 45), (2) severe cardiac disease (n = 12), (3) patient had a stroke or died before arteriography or surgery

($n = 3$), (4) ineligible after arteriography ($n = 33$) of whom 6 had intracranial abnormalities and 27 had an angiographic stenosis <60%, and (5) other reasons ($n = 8$).

Thirty-Day Death/Stroke

Nineteen surgical patients (2.3%) either suffered a stroke or died in the 30 days after randomization. As can be shown in Table 3.1, two surgical patients suffered nonfatal strokes and one died (etiology) in the postrandomization period, but before undergoing surgery. In addition, five surgical patients either died ($n = 1$) or suffered a nonfatal stroke ($n = 4$) as a direct consequence of angiography. In the "true" 30-day perioperative period after CEA, ten more patients suffered a nonfatal stroke, while another died following a myocardial infarction.

Only three patients in the medical group (0.4%) died (stroke) or suffered a nonfatal stroke during the comparable 42-day postrandomization period [8].

Principle Results

Table 3.2 summarizes the primary and secondary analyses from ACAS. As will subsequently become apparent, it is important to be sure that the same endpoint is being cited when looking at comparisons with ACST. In summary, ACAS demonstrated a *significant* reduction in the 5-year risk of ipsilateral death (including perioperative stroke/death) in patients randomized to surgery (from 11.0 to 5.1%) and *nonsignificant* reductions in (1) major ipsilateral stroke (including perioperative stroke/death), (2) any stroke (including perioperative stroke/death), and (3) any major stroke (including perioperative stroke/death), although each of the latter three endpoints were trending in favor of surgery.

Interestingly, the significant reduction in ipsilateral stroke at 5 years remained unchanged if one excluded the 146 "crossover" patients who did not receive their allocated treatment.

Accordingly, with a 2.3% procedural risk, CEA conferred a 5.9% absolute risk reduction (ARR) in late ipsilateral stroke (compared with medical therapy). This equates to a 54% relative risk reduction (RRR), 17 CEAs need to be performed to prevent one ipsilateral stroke at 5 years, and 59 strokes will be prevented at 5 years by performing 1,000 CEAs.

TABLE 3.1. Perioperative morbidity and mortality in ACAS [8, 19].

	Nonstroke death		Fatal stroke		Nonfatal stroke	
	CEA	BMT	CEA	BMT	CEA	BMT
Presurgery						
Preadmission	1				2	
Angiographic			1		4	
"Perioperative"	1 (MI)			1	10	2
Total	2	0	1	1	16	2

CEA patients randomized to carotid endarterectomy, *BMT* patients randomized to best medical therapy

TABLE 3.2. Common primary and secondary endpoints from ACAS and ACST.

	ACAS		ACST	
Five-year risk of	BMT (%)	CEA (%)	BMT (%)	CEA (%)
Ipsilateral stroke + any perioperative stroke/death	11.0	5.1 ($p = 0.004$)	No data published	
Major ipsilateral stroke + any perioperative stroke/death	6.0	3.4 ($p = 0.12$)	No data published	
Any stroke + any perioperative stroke/death	17.5	12.4 ($p = 0.09$)	11.8	6.4 ($p < 0.0001$)
Any major stroke + any perioperative stroke/death	9.1	6.4 ($p = 0.26$)	6.1	3.5 ($p = 0.004$)

BMT "best medical therapy," *CEA* carotid endarterectomy

Secondary Analyses

These will be presented in conjunction with the ACST findings.

Other Analyses

Surgeon Selection and Generalizability

During the 6-year period of study, 55 centers applied to randomize patients but only 39 were credentialed [10]. Twenty four centers contributed more than 30 patients, while 13 randomized more than 50 patients. During the period of trial recruitment (when 1,662 patients were randomized), the trial centers performed 12,080 CEAs. After review, 6% of these patients could have been randomized within ACAS, 6% were undertaken on patients already randomized within ACAS, while the remainder were (1) undertaken in symptomatic patients, (2) undertaken in ineligible patients, or (3) patients of surgeons not collaborating within ACAS. This suggests that the trial surgeons and centers were generally randomizing the majority of eligible patients.

To participate in ACAS, each surgeon had to submit (for central approval) a track record confirming the performance of >12 CEAs per annum. Thereafter, the surgeon had to demonstrate a combined 30-day death/stroke rate of <5% for all indications and a <3% complication rate in asymptomatic individuals [10]. One hundred sixty-four surgeons applied to be credentialed in order to randomize patients in ACAS. Seventeen (10%) were rejected (too few cases or excessive mortality/morbidity), while a further 30 were not reviewed at all (insufficient data or because the parent hospital was not approved). Six of seven rejected institutions failed to qualify as an ACAS randomizing center because they were unable to provide a surgeon who fulfilled the ACAS criteria [10].

Some Observations About ACAS

While ACAS was the first, high-quality randomized trial to demonstrate that CEA conferred a significant reduction in late stroke in asymptomatic individuals, there were a number of unexpected findings and some criticisms that merit documenting [11]:

- ACAS showed no evidence that CEA reduced the risk of disabling stroke. The reduction was only in nondisabling stroke.
- While men benefited significantly from surgery (ARR = 8%, RRR = 66%), women appeared to derive no advantage at all (ARR = 1.4% at 5 years, RRR = 17%). This difference is rarely commented upon when guidelines of practice are being reviewed (see later).
- You had to live 5 years to gain clinical benefit (the reduction in stroke only became significant in the fifth year of follow-up), but in some parts of the United States, the largest proportional increases in operation rates were observed in patients aged >84 years [12].
- The 5-year data in ACAS were projected. The median follow-up period was only 2.7 years and many felt that the trial had probably been stopped too soon.
- There were concerns over the surgeon selection process (see above) which only allowed highly experienced surgeons to randomize patients within the trial. Accordingly, the 2.3% operative risk was considered (by many neurologists) to be unlikely to be generalizable into routine clinical practice, i.e., in the "real world," the procedural risk would be much higher and so negate any long-term benefit.
- In ACAS, there was *no* association between stenosis severity and the long-term stroke risk (in fact this relationship was inverse). This will be discussed later.
- ACAS was unable to confirm the intuitively held belief that patients with bilateral severe carotid disease (especially contralateral occlusion) would face a higher risk of stroke than patients with unilateral disease if not subjected to CEA.

The Asymptomatic Carotid Surgery Trial [9]

Funding

- The UK Medical Research Council and the UK Stroke Association

Number Randomized

- Three thousand one hundred twenty patients from 126 hospitals in 30 countries. Recruitment into ACST continued from 1993 to 2003

Inclusion Criteria

- Asymptomatic unilateral or bilateral carotid stenosis ≥60% on ultrasound

- "Asymptomatic" defined as no ipsilateral symptoms within 6 months
- No age range specified
- No need for formal angiography
- Independent Neurologist assessment required
- Review of track record (surgeon)

Exclusion Criteria

- Any cerebrovascular events in the territory of the randomized artery <6 months
- Contraindication to aspirin therapy
- Likely cardioembolic source
- "Any expectation of poor surgical risk"
- "Any major life-threatening condition other than carotid stenosis"

Medical Treatment

Patients in both groups were to "receive appropriate medical care, which generally included antiplatelet therapy, antihypertensive treatment, and, increasingly, lipid lowering therapy" [9].

Surgical Treatment

Formal angiography was not required before CEA and surgeons were requested to perform surgery "as soon as possible" after randomization. No attempt was made to standardize choice of anesthesia, shunt practice, or any other aspect of surgical technique.

Endpoint Analyses

Definition of "Stroke"

ACST did not specify their definition of a "procedural" stroke, other than clarifying the definition of stroke severity. A nondisabling stroke was one where (at 6 months) the modified Rankin score [13] was 0–2 (ranging from "slight disability" through to "unable to carry out some previous activities but with no need for assistance in daily affairs"). A disabling stroke was where (at 6 months) the patient had a score of 3–5.

Procedural Risk

Patients undergoing CEA were assessed neurologically before discharge by the collaborating doctors, "many of whom were neurologists" [9].

Primary Endpoint

- Five-year "any stroke" including any perioperative death/stroke

Secondary Endpoints

- Five-year fatal or disabling stroke including any perioperative death/stroke
- Five-year any stroke *excluding* any perioperative stroke/death
- Five-year fatal or disabling stroke *excluding* any perioperative stroke/death
- Five-year ipsilateral stroke *excluding* any perioperative stroke/death
- Five-year fatal or disabling ipsilateral stroke *excluding* any perioperative stroke/death

Subgroup Analyses

- Five-year stroke in males and females *excluding* any perioperative stroke/death
- Five-year stroke in <65 years and 65–74 years *excluding* any perioperative stroke/death
- Five-year stroke in 60–79% and 80–99% *excluding* any perioperative stroke/death

Results

This section deals with the primary and secondary analyses from ACST involving a mean of 3.4 years of follow-up.

General Observations

The first observation to make is that the surgeons in ACST performed CEA with a commendably low procedural risk (2.8%). Among 1,560 patients randomized to "immediate" CEA, 50% underwent CEA within 1 month of randomization, 88% by 1 year, and 91% by 5 years. Among the 1,560 randomized to "deferred" CEA, approximately 4% (per year) underwent ipsilateral CEA. Overall, 201 "deferred" patients underwent ipsilateral CEA within 5 years [9]. Of these, only 61 were because the patient wished to undergo surgery, while the remainder were for "medical reasons."

ACST documented temporal changes in what constituted "best medical therapy" during the 11-year period of recruitment [9, 14]. Antiplatelet therapy remained fairly constant (1993–1996 = 88%, 2000–2003 = 91%), while the use of antihypertensive therapy increased during the same time periods from 61 to 72%, respectively. The most obvious change in practice, however, related to the use of lipid lowering therapy (LLT). Only 17% of ACST patients were on LLT between 1993 and 1996, increasing to 58% of patients in 2000–2003. Many observers will now consider the latter percentage to be still too low, but a 2004 survey of practice in ACST collaborators suggested that the proportion of trial patients now receiving LLT had increased to 90% [9, 14].

Thirty-Day Death/Stroke

The 30-day risk of death/stroke in patients randomized to "immediate" CEA was 2.8%. There were 15 deaths (stroke = 10, cardiac = 5), 9 disabling strokes, and 16 nondisabling strokes. The 30-day risk of death/stroke in the 229 patients undergoing 245 deferred CEAs (i.e., having been originally randomized to "best medical therapy") was 4.5%. Although some of the latter patients were still asymptomatic, the increased procedural risk in deferred patients will inevitably reflect the fact that many of these patients had become symptomatic during follow-up.

All 51 perioperative events occurring in patients undergoing "immediate" or "deferred" CEA were spread across 39 randomizing centers with no evidence of clustering of adverse outcomes [9].

Principle Results

Table 3.2 summarizes the primary and secondary analyses that were common for both ACAS and ACST. ACST reported a significant reduction in (1) the 5-year risk of "any" stroke (including any perioperative stroke/death) and (2) the 5-year risk of any fatal or disabling stroke (including any perioperative stroke/death). The latter statistic is one of the most important findings from the ACST trial as ACAS (probably because of the smaller number of patients) did not show any significant reduction in fatal or disabling stroke. Interestingly, most of the benefit from CEA (in terms of preventing "any" stroke) was largely confined to the >800 patients whose prerandomization cholesterol was >6.5 mmol L^{-1} [9].

Unlike ACAS, ACST has not published any data on the 5-year risk of *ipsilateral* stroke which also included the operative risk. However, the 5-year risk of ipsilateral stroke (*excluding* any perioperative events) was 9.5% for medically treated patients and 2.7% for those randomized to immediate CEA ($p < 0.0001$). Similar data for fatal or disabling ipsilateral stroke (*excluding* the operative risk) were 5.3% for medically treated patients compared with 1.6% in patients allocated to "immediate" CEA [9].

Accordingly, with a 2.8% procedural risk, "immediate" CEA conferred a 5.4% ARR in "any" stroke at 5 years (compared with medical therapy), a calculation which does take account of the operative risk. This equates to a 46% RRR, 19 CEAs would need to be performed to prevent one stroke at 5 years, and 53 strokes (of all types) will be prevented at 5 years by performing 1,000 CEAs. Using the same procedural risk, 40 CEAs would need to be performed to prevent one disabling or fatal stroke at 5 years, increasing to 70 if the 30-day risk of death/stroke increased to 4%.

Secondary Analyses

These will be presented in combination with the parallel ACAS findings.

Some Observations About ACST

ACST was unusual (compared with ECST, NASCET, and ACAS) in that most of the published cumulative analyses *excluded* the perioperative risk. Accordingly, the reader should bear this in mind when interpreting ACST data. As will be seen, this is particularly relevant in the controversy as to whether women gain as much benefit as men.

The second discrepancy was the absence of any cumulative data on the 5-year risk of ipsilateral stroke (including the perioperative risk). While ACST had every right to select their own primary endpoint, it would have been very useful to have been able to compare the ACST outcomes with ACAS, especially as almost 10 years had elapsed between the two publications. Finally, and on a similar theme, no one has been able to explain the glaring anomaly in Table 3.2. The two common endpoints that ACAS and ACST did publish were the 5-year risk of "any" stroke (including the perioperative risk). In ACAS, the 5-year risk of "any" stroke in medically treated patients was 17.5%, falling to 12% in surgically treated patients. Contrast that with ACST where the 5-year risk of "any" stroke in medically treated patients was now 12%, falling to 6% after CEA. Readers will be aware that most presentations and commentaries on the asymptomatic trials generally state that ACAS and ACST published similar findings (i.e., surgery reduced the risk of stroke by 50% from approximately 12% at 5 years to approximately 6%). While this is, to an extent true (yes, both showed an approximate 50% RRR), but it omits clarification that the "12%" in ACAS refers to ipsilateral stroke, while the "12%" in ACST refers to "any" stroke.

What Were the Recommendations from the Two Trials?

ACAS [8]

Patients with an asymptomatic carotid artery stenosis of 60–99% and whose general health makes them good candidates for elective surgery will have a reduced 5-year risk of ipsilateral stroke if CEA (performed with a ≤3% perioperative morbidity and mortality) is added to aggressive management of modifiable risk factors.

ACAS [9]

In asymptomatic patients aged <75 with a carotid diameter reduction of about 70% or more on ultrasound, immediate CEA halved the net 5-year stroke risk from about 12% to about 6% (including the 3% perioperative hazard). Half this 5-year benefit involved disabling or fatal strokes. But, outside trials, poor patient selection or bad surgery could obviate such benefits.

Secondary Analyses from ACAS and ACST

There is no doubt that the appropriateness and relevance of "subgroup analyses" arouses considerable hostility in certain "statistical" quarters. This is largely because of the potential for inappropriate interpretation of outcomes in smaller cohorts of patients from multiple trials that may have not been powered to make these conclusions.

Notwithstanding this caveat, ACAS and ACST (themselves) have published a number of secondary analyses, several of which have important implications for practice. These relate to (1) the impact of age on benefit from "immediate" CEA, (2) the relevance of gender on benefit from "immediate" CEA, (3) the impact of contralateral occlusion on benefit, and (4) does stenosis severity affect overall benefit. A fifth should have been the impact of performing CEA with unacceptably high complication rates (and will therefore be included in this review).

Why are these particular subgroup analyses of relevance? The answer is largely because many of them were independent predictors of enhanced benefit (for surgery) in *symptomatic* patients [15, 16].

Age and Benefit from CEA

In NASCET, symptomatic patients aged >75 years gained more benefit from CEA than any other age group [17]. It was, therefore, not unreasonable to assume that the same might also be true for asymptomatic patients.

In their original publication, ACAS presented outcomes for patients stratified for age [8]. However, because ACAS did not randomize patients aged ≥80 years, the published data (regarding age) were somewhat biased and difficult to interpret meaningfully. ACAS observed that in patients aged ≤68 years, CEA reduced the 5-year risk of ipsilateral stroke from 11.8 to 4.7% [8]. Parallel data for patients aged >68 years were 9.7% (on medical therapy), decreasing to 5.5% in those randomized to surgery. The difference in overall benefit (with regard to age) was not statistically significant, but one does have to recognize the fact that the "older" analyzed cohort in ACAS was not particularly elderly. It would not, therefore, be reasonable to cite this ACAS subgroup analysis to justify intervening on all elderly patients.

By contrast, ACST was able to perform a more meaningful analysis, primarily because it was a much larger study with no upper age limit for randomization [9, 14, 18]. ACST observed significant benefits for surgery in patients aged <65 years and those aged between 65 and 74, but failed to demonstrate any significant benefit in patients aged over

75 years (Table 3.3). When interpreting Table 3.3, it is important to remember that the data presented are the 5-year risk of "any" stroke, *excluding* the perioperative risk. Accordingly, the 30-day risk of death/stroke for each age group (available online [14, 18]) has been included in Table 3.3 for completeness.

In summary, there is evidence of significant benefit (for CEA) in the younger patient (<75 years of age). However, the *nonsignificant* ARR of +3.3% at 5 years conferred by CEA in the >75-year-old group is further nullified by the 3.7% procedural risk.

Gender and Benefit from CEA

As was highlighted in the section on "Some Observations About ACAS," the principle investigators conceded (from the outset) that women did not appear to gain significant benefit from prophylactic CEA [8]. The observed 5-year risks and ARR/RRR relating to gender in ACAS are summarized in Table 3.4. At the time, many surgeons felt that this "lack of apparent benefit" in women might be due to a statistical error and most continued to treat males and females as being of equivalent risk, while awaiting the outcome of ACST. However, what is often not mentioned in debates on this subject is that even when the ACAS data were reanalyzed having *excluded* all women who died or suffered a stroke within 30 days, CEA *still* did not confer significant benefit in women [19].

When ACST reported in 2004, its "banner headlines" suggested that any concerns about surgery conferring less benefit in women were premature. Unlike its sister trial, ACST reported that immediate CEA conferred significant benefit in males *and* females and this conclusion was (uncritically) accepted by a great many observers [11]. Rothwell [20] was the first to question the trial's conclusion regarding women. He observed that unlike the primary endpoint, the published ACST data regarding gender *did not* include the operative risk. When the operative risks were later included (2.7% for males, 3.8% for females), all evidence of *significant* benefit for women disappeared [20].

These seemingly discordant interpretations of the same data were analyzed in the 2005 Cochrane Review (Fig. 3.1). Repeating Rothwell's analyses, the Cochrane Group combined the ACAS and ACST data, having included the operative risk and then stratified for gender. Figure 3.1 shows a very clear benefit for males in both trials. In males, "best medical therapy" was associated with a twofold increase in the 5-year risk of stroke (odds ratio 2.0; 95% CI 1.5–2.8). However, the benefit for women was much less certain. Figure 3.1 indicates that *both* trials (individually) demonstrated reduced benefit in women as compared with men (i.e., both were reporting the same trend). When the data for females were combined (involving some 1,640 patients), medical therapy was associated with no excess risk of stroke (odds ratio 1.04; 95% CI 0.7–1.6) [21].

TABLE 3.3. Five-year risk of "any" stroke in ACST (*excluding the perioperative risk*): impact of age [9, 14, 18].

	<65 years	65–74 years	≥75 years
Medical treatment	9.6%	9.7%	8.8%
Immediate CEA	1.8%	2.2%	5.5%
ARR (95% CI)	7.8% (4.3 to 11.3)	7.5% (4.7 to 10.3)	3.3% (−1.9 to 8.4)
p Value	<0.0001	<0.0001	0.21
Thirty-day death/stroke after CEA	2.6%	2.6%	3.7%

TABLE. 3.4. Five-year risk of ipsilateral stroke (including the perioperative risk) in ACAS stratified for gender [8].

	Five-year risk of ipsilateral stroke				
Gender	*n*	Medical (%)	Surgery (%)	ARR at 5 years (%)	RRR at 5 years (%)
Males	1,091	12.1	4.1	8.0	66
Females	568	8.7	7.3	1.4	16

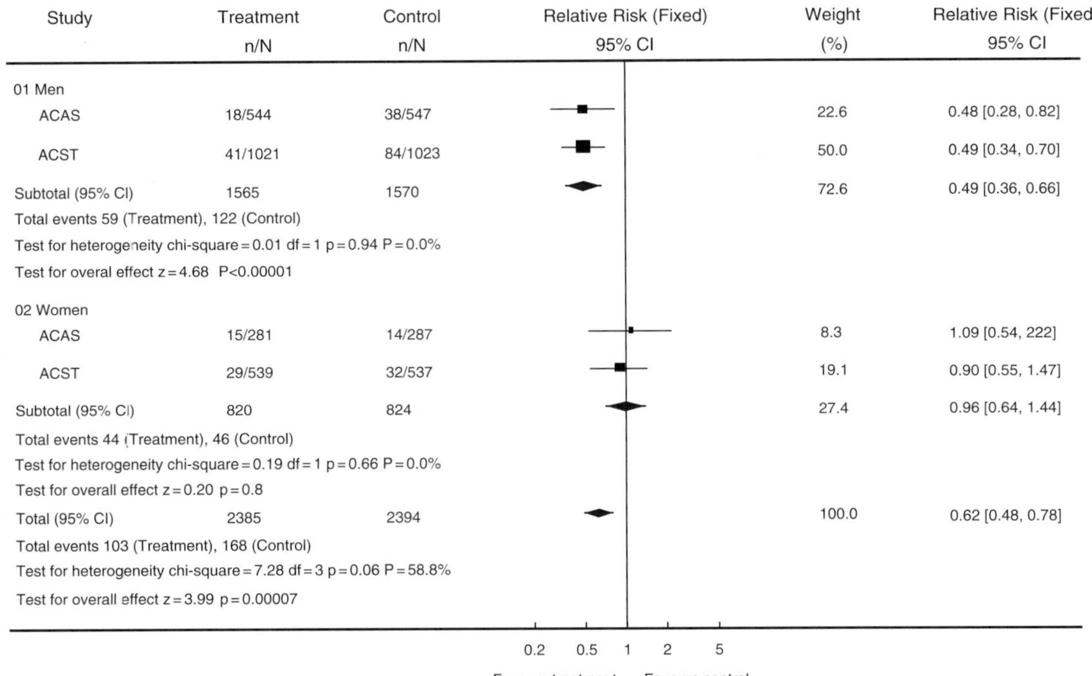

FIG. 3.1. Cochrane Review of the effect of "immediate" CEA on the 5-year risk of stroke (including the operative risk) stratified for gender. From [21]. Copyright Cochrane Collaboration reproduced with permission

The ACST responded to Rothwell's comments by publishing updated 6-year results (Table 3.5) which now included the operative risk [22]. At 6 years, the ARR in "any" stroke conferred in males by CEA was 6.6% (average 1.1% per annum). This was highly statistically significant ($p < 0.0001$). Conversely, in women, the ARR in stroke at 6 years conferred by surgery was only 4.0% (i.e., averaging 0.6% per annum). While there was now a clear trend (favoring intervention) in females, this was still not statistically significant ($p = 0.07$).

Accordingly, it is an indisputable fact that both trials reported the same trends and, when combined, there is evidence that the magnitude of benefit in women is clearly much less than that observed in males. It is, therefore, inappropriate to continue treating *all* female, asymptomatic patients as if they have an equivalent stroke risk to their male counterparts.

TABLE 3.5. Updated ACST 6-year risks of "any" stroke (*including perioperative risk*) in males and females [22].

	Males	Females
Medical treatment	13.9%	11.8%
Immediate CEA	7.4%	7.8%
ARR	6.6% at 6 years	4.0% at 6 years
Average ARR per annum	1.1%	0.6%
p Value	<0.0001	0.07

Does Contralateral Occlusion Increase the Benefit from Intervention?

In the symptomatic trials, the presence of a contralateral occlusion was one of the biggest predictors of benefit from CEA [16]. Not surprisingly, ACAS performed a subgroup analysis of the effect of the status of the contralateral artery [23] to see whether the same applied to the asymptomatic patient (Table 3.6).

TABLE 3.6. Five-year risk of stroke (including perioperative risk) stratified for status of contralateral carotid artery [23].

	Five-year risk of stroke			
	Surgery (%)	Medical (%)	ARR (%)	Operative risk (%)
60–99% stenosis with contralateral occlusion	5.5	3.5	−2.0	2.3
60–99% stenosis with no contralateral occlusion	5.0	11.7	+6.7	2.2

Table 3.6 summarizes their findings. Contrary to expectation, the presence of a contralateral occlusion was *not* associated with increased benefit following surgery. Indeed, it may have been associated with harm (ARR = -2.0% at 5 years). This apparent lack of benefit was not due to an excess procedural risk, which was only 2.3% in patients with contralateral occlusion as compared with 2.2% in patients with a patent contralateral carotid [23].

Does Increasing Stenosis Severity Increase the Benefit from Intervention?

Subgroup analyses in the symptomatic trials showed very clearly that as stenosis severity increased so too did the benefit conferred by CEA [16]. However, once again, this association was not demonstrated (individually) in either ACAS or ACST or following the Cochrane Review of both trials [21].

Is the Surgeon a "Risk Factor" for an Adverse Outcome?

It is an uncomfortable observation that the surgeon can be an important risk factor for an adverse outcome following carotid surgery. Both ACAS and ACST concluded that CEA conferred long-term benefit, but *only* if the 30-day risk of stroke/death was ≤3%. This "risk threshold" in the asymptomatic patient is now one of the cornerstones of the American Heart Association Guidelines [24]. More importantly, if the procedural risk exceeds 4%, all long-term benefit (in terms of stroke prevention) ceases [25].

Unfortunately, published reports from the "real world" suggest that this guideline is not being adhered to. The available evidence suggests that many hospitals and surgeons are performing CEA (and more recently carotid angioplasty with stenting – CAS) in asymptomatic patients with procedural risks well in excess of 3%, with little evidence that practice is being changed, i.e., audit does not seem to be happening in the true sense of its definition.

Table 3.7 presents a selection of published outcomes following both CEA and CAS in asymptomatic patients. The intention of Table 3.7 is *not* to suggest that practitioners of either CAS or CEA publish worse outcomes, but simply to highlight the worrying discrepancies between what is recommended in guidelines [24] and what is happening "in the real world" by practitioners of both treatment options. Interestingly, none of the constituent studies detailed in Table 3.7 ever considered that their published risks might be in excess of accepted standards.

Is There Such a Thing as a "High-Risk" Asymptomatic Patient?

Inevitably, the answer will be "yes," but (for the moment) we just do not know who they are.

The question, however, is now very topical because of the emergence of "high-risk" CAS registries which were a direct consequence of the SAPPHIRE trial [26]. SAPPHIRE chose to randomize patients deemed "high risk" for CEA. A cohort of 307 patients (derived from an eligible pool of 723) was randomized between CAS using a protection device and CEA. Notwithstanding the many criticisms of this trial [27], the key issue to have emerged in the ensuing debate regarding "how best to treat asymptomatic patients" was the crucial importance of differentiating between being "high risk" for CEA and "high risk" for stroke.

SAPPHIRE [27] reported a 30-day death/stroke rate of 5.8% following CAS in their asymptomatic patients (who made up >70% of the overall trial cohort) compared with 6.1% following surgery

TABLE 3.7. Evidence that CEA and CAS may be being performed out with recommended "risk thresholds".

Study	Intervention	Thirty-day death/stroke (%)
Global registry [28]	CAS	1.8[a]
ACAS [8]	CEA	2.3
ACST [9]	CEA	2.8
USA: Multistate audit 2004 [30]	CEA	3.8
Global registry [28]	CAS	4.0[b]
Canada: Toronto [31]	CEA	4.0
USA: Multistate audit 2001 [32]	CEA	4.1
Twelve audited series [33]	CEA	4.6[c]
Canada: Edmonton [34]	CEA	5.2
ARCHeR [29]	CAS	6.6[a,d]
SAPPHIRE [26]	CAS	5.8[a,d]
SAPPHIRE [26]	CEA	6.1[d]
PASCAL (unpublished data)	CAS	7.5[a]
AHA guidelines [24] for recurrent carotid stenosis	CEA	<10 acceptable

[a]Protected CAS
[b]Unprotected CAS
[c]Systematic review of 12 published series where all CEA patients were independently reviewed by neurologists
[d]Trials including patients deemed "high risk" for CEA

(Table 3.7). While their main conclusion was that "CAS was not inferior to CEA," nowhere in this debate did anyone concede that at these levels of risk, *none* of their patients (CAS or CEA) would ever achieve any long-term benefit in terms of stroke prevention [28].

SAPPHIRE spawned a proliferation of "high-risk" stent registries whose aim was to demonstrate that outcomes using a different corporate stent or protection device were comparable to those achieved in SAPPHIRE. Few registries have published in peer-reviewed journals, most preferring to release their data via a variety of internet-based Web sites. One registry which did submit its data to peer review was ARCHeR [29]. In the concluding sentence of the abstract, the authors state that "the ARCHeR results demonstrated that extracranial carotid artery stenting with embolic filter protection is not inferior to historical results of endarterectomy and suggest that carotid artery stenting is a safe, durable and effective alternative in high surgical risk patients." When you actually read the chapter, this statement is somewhat difficult to reconcile with the fact that the 30-day death/stroke rate in their asymptomatic cohort was 5.4%. To this observer, ARCHeR and many of its sister publications have shown little in the way of evidence that any of these so-called "high risk for CEA" patients benefited from any sort of intervention at all. Moreover, how can it remain acceptable for the American Heart Association to allow surgery (and thus by implication CAS) to be performed for an asymptomatic restenosis after CEA with a recommended threshold of procedural risk of <10% [24]?

Not least because of the current intensity of the debate, the concept of the "high-risk" patient is very important to resolve. One day, we will learn what biochemical, imaging, and other associated markers can reliably identify a patient/plaque as being "high risk for stroke." When that day dawns, it may then become perfectly reasonable to "raise the threshold" of acceptable risk in patients undergoing CEA and CAS. But not until then!

Key Points: How Have the Asymptomatic Trials Influenced My *Own* Practice?

- The first priority (for *any* service) has to be the rapid treatment of *symptomatic* patients.
- If it takes >4 weeks to schedule CEA/CAS in otherwise fit, symptomatic patients, it is difficult to justify treating myriads of lower-risk asymptomatic patients. Many more strokes will occur in your symptomatic patients while they wait for their intervention.
- I am happy to undertake prophylactic CEA in "standard-risk" asymptomatic males if they are aged <75 years, or females <70 years, provided our audited procedural risks remain ≤3%.
- I am unconvinced that the older (>75 years) asymptomatic patient requires any intervention other than "best medical therapy." I would, however, be happy to concede that this may be a "gray area" and hence would be happy to randomize these patients in a trial.
- I also remain cautious about submitting any other "high risk for CEA" asymptomatic patients to any intervention (e.g., those with radiation arteritis, restenosis after CEA, severe pulmonary/cardiac disease, etc.), although it is conceded that

each case has to be considered on its individual merits.

- However, surgeons or interventionists who do advocate treatment of "high risk" for CEA patients still have to adhere to the guideline that their procedural risks should not exceed 3%. Unlike in the symptomatic patient, there is currently no evidence that this risk threshold should be increased in asymptomatic patients.
- I remain uncertain about the conflicting data regarding whether asymptomatic patients with contralateral occlusion are at higher risk of stroke if treated medically. Intuitively, one feels that they should face a higher risk of stroke if left on "best medical therapy." At present, this author still considers them for surgery.
- ACAS and ACST showed that the predictors of benefit were very different compared with ECST and NASCET. Predictors of maximum benefit in the symptomatic trials were (1) age >75 years, (2) contralateral occlusion, and (3) incremental stenosis severity but not subocclusion. None of these were predictive of significant benefit in asymptomatic patients.
- Some authorities view ACAS and ACST as being "out of date" and that advances in CAS and CEA render them obsolete. I would counter that if these trials were to be repeated today, with the major advances in "best medical therapy," it is likely that the benefit conferred by surgery (and thus by implication CAS) will be very much less and possibly nonexistent.
- Finally, it should be clear that there are many more unresolved issues regarding the management of the asymptomatic patient than their symptomatic counterparts. The author urges colleagues and readers to randomize patients into one of the four ongoing asymptomatic trials, so that science (rather than dogma or intuition) finally determines practice regarding effects due to age, gender, and contralateral occlusion and whether CAS is superior/equivalent to CEA.

References

1. Thompson J.E., Patman R.D., Talkington C.M. Asymptomatic carotid bruit: Long term outcome of patients having endarterectomy compared with unoperated controls. Ann Surg 1978;188:308–316.
2. Hsai D.C., Krushat W.M., Moscoe L.M. Epidemiology of carotid endarterectomy among Medicare beneficiaries: 1985–1996 update. Stroke 1998;29:346–350.
3. European Carotid Surgery Trialists' Collaborative Group. MRC European Carotid Surgery Trial: Interim results for symptomatic patients with severe (70–99%) or with mild (0–29%) stenosis. Lancet 1991;337:1235–1241.
4. North American Symptomatic Carotid Endarterectomy Trial Collaborators. Beneficial effect of carotid endarterectomy in symptomatic patients with high grade stenosis. N Engl J Med 1991;325:445–453.
5. Mayo Asymptomatic Carotid Endarterectomy Study Group. Effectiveness of CEA for asymptomatic carotid stenosis: Design of a clinical trial. Mayo Clin Proc 1989;64:897–904.
6. The Casanova Study Group. Carotid surgery versus medical therapy in asymptomatic carotid stenosis. Stroke 1991;22:1229–1235.
7. Hobson R.W., Weiss D.G., Fields W.S., The VA Co-operative Study Group. Efficacy of carotid endarterectomy for asymptomatic carotid stenosis. *N Engl J Med* 1993;328:221–227.
8. Executive Committee for the Asymptomatic Carotid Atherosclerosis Study. Endarterectomy for asymptomatic carotid artery stenosis. JAMA 1995;273: 1421–1461.
9. Asymptomatic Carotid Surgery Trial Collaborators. The MRC asymptomatic carotid surgery trial (ACST): Carotid endarterectomy prevents disabling and fatal carotid territory strokes. Lancet 2004;363:1491–1502.
10. Moore W.S., Vescera C.L., Robertson J.T., Baker W.H., Howard V.J., Toole J.F. Selection process for surgeons in the asymptomatic carotid atherosclerosis study. Stroke 1991;22:1353–1357.
11. Naylor A.R. The asymptomatic carotid surgery trial: Bigger study, better evidence. Br J Surg 2004:91:787–789.
12. Huber T.S., Wheeler K.G., Cuddeback J.K., Dame D.A., Flynn T.C., Seeger J.M. Effect of the asymptomatic carotid atherosclerosis study on carotid endarterectomy in Florida. *Stroke* 1998;29:1099–1105.
13. Van Swieten J.C., Koudstaal P.J., Visser M.C., Schouten H.J., van Gijn J. Inter-observer agreement for the assessment of handicap in stroke patients. Stroke 1988;19:604–607.
14 ACST Web site. http://www.sgul.ac.uk/static/survey/acst.
15. Naylor A.R., Rothwell P.M., Bell P.R.F. Overview of the principal results and secondary analyses from the European and the North American randomised trials of carotid endarterectomy. Eur J Vasc Endovasc Surg 2003;26:115–129.
16. Naylor A.R. An update on the randomised trials of interventions for symptomatic and asymptomatic

carotid artery disease. *I*tal J Vasc Endovasc Surg 2006;13:111–120.

17. Alamowitch S., Eliasziw M., Algra A., Meldrum H., Barnett H.J.M. for the NASCET Trial. Risk, causes and prevention of ischaemic stroke in elderly patients with symptomatic internal carotid artery stenosis. Lancet 2001;357:1154–1160.
18. http://image.thelancet.com/extras/04art3083webtable.pdf.
19. Young B., Moore W.S., Robertson J.T., Toole J.F., Ernst C.B., Cohen S.N. et al. An analysis of perioperative surgical mortality and morbidity in the asymptomatic carotid atherosclerosis study. Stroke 1996;27:2216–2224.
20. Rothwell P.M. ACST: Which subgroups will benefit most from carotid endarterectomy. *Lancet* 2004;364:1122–1123.
21. Chambers B.R., Donnan G.A. Carotid endarterectomy for asymptomatic carotid stenosis. Cochrane Database of Systematic Reviews 2005, Issue 4. Art. No.: CD001923. DOI 10.1002/14651858.CD001923.pub2.
22. ACST Writing Committee. Authors reply. Lancet 2004;364:1125–1126.
23. Baker W.H., Howard V.J., Howard G., Toole J.F., for the ACAS Investigators. Effect of contralateral occlusion on long term efficacy of endarterectomy in the asymptomatic carotid atherosclerosis study. Stroke 2000;31:2330–2334.
24. Biller J., Feinberg W.M., Castaldo J.E., Whittemore A.D., Harbaugh R.E., Dempsey R.J. et al. Guidelines for carotid endarterectomy: A statement for healthcare professionals from a special writing group of the Stroke Council, American Heart Association. Stroke 1998;29:554–562.
25. Barnett H.J., Eliasziw M., Meldrum H.E., Taylor D. Do the facts and figures warrant a 10-fold increase in the performance of carotid endarterectomy on asymptomatic patients? Neurology 1996;46(3):603–608.
26. Yadav J.S., Wholey M.H., Kuntz R.E., Fayad P., Katzen B., Mishkel M.R. et al. for the SAPPHIRE Investigators. Protected carotid artery stenting versus endarterectomy in high-risk patients. N Engl J Med 2004;351:1493–1501.
27. Naylor A.R. SAPPHIRE: Precious gem or fool's gold? Vasc Dis Manage 2006;3:346–349.
28. Wholey M.H., Al-Mubarak N., Wholey M.H. Updated review of the Global carotid artery stent registry. Catheter Cardiovasc Interv 2003;60:259–266.
29. Gray W.A., Hopkins L.N., Yadav S., Davis T., Wholey M., Atkinson R. et al. Protected carotid stenting in high surgical risk patients: The ARCHeR results. J Vasc Surg 2006;44:258–269.
30. Kresowik T.F., Bratzler D.W., Kresowik R.A., Hendel M.E., Grund S.L., Brown K.R. et al. Multistate improvement in process and outcomes of carotid endarterectomy. J Vasc Surg 2004;39:372–380.
31. Kucey D.S., Bowyer B., Iron K., Austin P., Anderson G., Tu J.V. Determinants of outcome after carotid endarterectomy. J Vasc Surg 1998;28:1051–1058.
32. Kresowik T.F., Bratzler D.W., Karp H.R., Hemann R.A., Hendel M.E., Kresowik R.A. et al. Multistate utilization processes and outcomes of carotid endarterectomy. J Vasc Surg 2001;33:227–235.
33. Bond R., Rerkasem K., Rothwell P.M. High morbidity due to endarterectomy for asymptomatic carotid stenosis. Cerebrovasc Dis 2003;16(Suppl):65.
34. Wong J.H., Findlay J.M., Suarez-Almazor M.E. Regional performance of carotid endarterectomy: Appropriateness, outcomes and risk factors for complications. Stroke 1997;28:891–898.

4 Carotid Artery Stenting. First Steps: Training, Support, and Proctorship

Gerard Stansby and Sumaira Macdonald

Introduction

Percutaneous carotid interventions are a rapidly emerging treatment modality, accompanied by rapid technological and methodological development. There is now a large evidence base for the procedure, by which individual results can be compared and judged, in relation to acceptability of outcome measures and complications. In the contemporary setting, in most countries, it is no longer acceptable for practitioners to start on new procedures without some form of training and, ideally, accreditation.

For carotid interventions, the debate has been further complicated by the fact that several disciplines have been involved with its development to date – vascular surgeons, neurosurgeons, interventional radiologists, and cardiologists. When regarded as an experimental procedure, it was perhaps acceptable for individuals to construct their own training and move into the field when they felt it appropriate. This may not now be the case in many countries. An experimental procedure (also sometimes referred to as an investigational procedure) is usually considered to be one which has not been accepted into clinical practice and has not been critically assessed in peer-reviewed medical literature or academic meetings. A procedure is not experimental if sufficient studies are available to prove its efficacy and safety. Carotid artery stenting (CAS) in general, by these definitions, can no longer be regarded as experimental. A procedure cannot be classified as "experimental" or "investigational" simply because of the inexperience of the practitioner or institution.

An additional factor to be considered is whether training in percutaneous carotid interventions should be solely consultant based or whether, in some form, it should be included in junior training programs. The transferable skills will differ considerably depending on the background speciality of the operator concerned. As CAS continues to expand, it seems likely that an integrated training program across specialities leading to accreditation will be essential.

General Principles

Prior to developing a training program in CAS, the aims of the program must be clear. The key questions/options are:

1. Is the aim to produce a practitioner able to independently deliver safe and effective therapy at the end of the training period?
2. Is the aim to give a solid grounding to the practitioner such that they can subsequently develop to the point of being a safe independent operator? Such training may only involve some aspect of the procedure, either theoretical or practical.

In our view, no standalone program can offer option 1 unless it is accompanied by a system of subsequent mentoring or proctorship. These and other terms are used with variable meanings on occasion and so, for the purposes of this chapter we now include some definitions of relevant terms.

S. Macdonald and G. Stansby (eds.), *Practical Carotid Artery Stenting*,
DOI: 10.1007/978-1-84800-299-9_4, © Springer-Verlag London Limited 2009

Key Definitions

Competence. Competence is the minimum level of skill, knowledge, and/or expertise, derived through training and experience, required to safely and proficiently perform a task or procedure. Successful completion of any one or more training components or objectives does not necessarily signify an individual's overall clinical competence in a specific procedure or technique.

Credentials. Credentials are documents provided following successful completion of a period of education or training. When acceptable for recognition of competence, this is often referred to as *accreditation*. In some countries such as the USA, this may lead to the awarding of Clinical Privileges, which is authorization by a local institution (usually a hospital) to perform a particular procedure. In other countries, accreditation at a local level (or even national) may not exist.

Courses. A course is a limited period of instruction with defined objectives designed to educate participants in clinical skills, techniques, or procedures. Course structure and duration will necessarily vary according to the course objectives which should be stated. Ideally, the successful completion of the objectives can be quantitatively and/or qualitatively assessed. The faculty (teachers) must be appropriately clinically trained and experienced themselves. Sponsorship or links with the industry must be clearly declared.

Training program. This is a longer-term approach to training which may include attendance at courses, but also follows a curriculum which includes stated learning components and outcomes and includes assessment and feedback. The duration of training should be sufficient for an individual to acquire the desired level of performance, preferably based on objective measures. A training program should regularly evaluate the degree to which its goals are being met through a formal assessment process. Such evaluation should be ongoing and systematically documented and include faculty evaluation by trainees.

Mentoring. This is a form of teaching that includes working alongside the person concerned, allowing them to learn from your example. It is about giving help and support in a nonthreatening way, in a manner that the recipient will appreciate and value which will empower them to move forward with confidence toward what they want to achieve. It is an important adjunct to most clinical training programs.

Proctorship. Traditionally, a proctor is a person who supervises or monitors students. In the context of CAS, training a proctor differs from a mentor or a preceptor in that they act as an observer and evaluator rather than directly participate in patient care. A proctor should be free of perceived or actual conflicts of interest and should be prepared to confidentially document their opinions including the number and type of procedures observed. The issue of whether and to what extent a proctor should intervene in a procedure is a complex issue. Certain clinical situations, or ethical concerns, may dictate that the proctor feels obliged to intervene or assist directly in a procedure which is going badly. However, such involvement will necessarily result in a duty of care to the patient and may have medicolegal implications.

Preceptor. This is an expert who undertakes to impart his/her clinical knowledge and skills in a defined setting to a preceptee. The relationship over a period of time is often referred to as a *preceptorship*. To serve as a preceptor in a specific procedure or technique, the individual should be a recognized authority in the particular field of expertise. The preceptorship must have stated objectives and is usually more intensive than simple clinical supervision. The objectives must include a program outline and a proposed list of tasks and skills to be addressed during the training period. The preceptor must document in writing both qualitative and quantitative descriptions of the trainee's experiences. Some of the roles of a preceptor may overlap with those of a mentor. In general, the relationship with a mentor is over a longer time period and involves aspects of personal development as well as the development of professional or technical skills.

The Skill Requirements for Training in CAS

Training physicians from multiple specialities in the necessary cognitive and technical skills for carotid angiography and CAS present specific challenges, because vascular surgeons, interventional radiologists, and interventional cardiologists all have acquired very different skill sets in prior training.

Schneider [1] has defined five cognitive areas required for successful training in CAS. These are:

1. Understanding the behavior of atherosclerotic lesions of the carotid arteries
2. A broad understanding of the management options and long-term outcomes of various medical, endovascular, and surgical treatments
3. Experience with angioplasty and stenting of other arteries
4. Experience with assessment and management of arch anatomy, selective carotid catheterization, and carotid angiography
5. The ability to evaluate cerebral vasculature and use a cerebral protection device

In addition, we feel that an important additional requirement is the ability to work within a multidisciplinary team structure, and to possess adequate mechanisms for follow-up and audit. Brooks et al. [2] have suggested that the low number of neurologic complications observed in their series was partially a result of the presence of a "cerebral endovascular team" comprised of neurosurgeons possessing skills in endarterectomy and catheter techniques, experienced interventional cardiologists and neurologists. In terms of training programs, a unit must have sufficient throughput to enable training to proceed in a timely and seamless way.

The recent (2005) SCAI/SVMB/SVS clinical competence statement described requirements for CAS training in terms of cognitive, technical, and clinical requirements [3]. Cognitive aspects included clinical knowledge of cerebrovascular diseases, natural history, diagnostic methods, and treatment alternatives. It also includes case selection, knowledge of anatomy, and role of follow-up. Technical requirements hinge around minimum numbers of procedures required to achieve competence. This is stated as 30 cervicocerebral angiograms and 25 CAS procedures, half as primary operator. Clinical requirements include the ability to manage inpatient and outpatient care and to obtain appropriate consent [3]. Ideally, individuals should be adequately trained in all these areas before undertaking CAS.

The Learning Curve

The concept of a learning curve for CAS procedures is an important one for training and accreditation. It may also influence the interpretation of clinical trial results. Clearly, those participating in clinical trials should not be in the earlier stages of a learning curve. But how many cases does this require? Indeed, one common criticism of CAS trials is that they are performed by expert participants and the results may not be applicable to a "real-world" setting. Of course, the same arguments were leveled at carotid endarterectomy when it was evaluated in "landmark" trials. For example, surgeons operating within the ACAS trial were carefully selected; 40% of surgeon applicants were turned down on the basis of their adverse event rate or poor throughput [4]. Alberts and Smith [5] were the first to report that learning curves might present problems in CAS trial design. Others have also suggested that complications are worse with less experienced operators [6–8]. However, in a recent Cochrane Review of CAS, it was not possible for the authors to analyze specifically whether there was a learning curve, because individual patient data were not available [9]. To date, clinical trials such as the ICSS have influenced training requirements and methodologies in some countries [9].

Clearly, for training purposes, a minimum numbers of procedures "required" would be a useful concept. To be robust, however, the number would need to be based on evidence.

The risk of stroke and death was analyzed by center experience within the original trial comparing endovascular carotid intervention (at that time carotid *angioplasty*) with CEA and CAVATAS [10]. The stroke rate fell significantly with increasing center experience, in both limbs of the trial.

An early paper from angiologists reported the impact of learning curve success rate and complications of carotid stenting in a single center, with one physician performing unprotected CAS with routine predilatation and stents adapted from peripheral platforms (i.e., the rolling membrane Wallstent, a nondedicated carotid stent) [11]. Three hundred twenty internal carotid arteries were treated in 301 patients with carotid stenoses ≥70%. Four groups of 80 consecutive interventions were compared with regard to primary technical success and periprocedural complications. Stenting was successful in 298 (93%) arteries. The combined neurological complications (transient ischemic attacks and all strokes) and 30-day death rate were 8.2% ($n = 25$), but the all stroke and 30-day death rate were 3.0% ($n = 9$). A significant reduction in the frequency of neurological complications after the initial 80 interventions was observed ($p = 0.03$), but technical success was not appreciably improved with increasing experience thereafter. It was concluded that a relatively large number of interventions (i.e., 80) should be performed to overcome the negative effects of the initial learning phase.

Lin et al. [12] (vascular and endovascular surgeons) described their experience in 200 more contemporary consecutive cases undergoing protected CAS cases (182 patients). Technical success and postprocedure complications were the main outcome measures, compared in four sequential groups of 50 procedures. Demographics, clinical indications, and risk factors were similar between the groups. Contrast load and procedures times decreased and complications were lower in the latter three cohorts. The 30-day stroke and death rate was 8% in the first cohort, 2% in the second, and zero in cohorts 3 and 4. This would suggest a learning curve of 50 procedures and it is somewhat surprising that the number of patients comprising the learning curve for CAS would be lower for unprotected than that for protected CAS, as protection devices come in many shapes and forms and each has its own specific learning curve.

Learning curve for CAS may be influenced by the speciality of the operator. In a recent publication, two periods of CAS experience were analyzed by vascular surgeons performing CAS: 2001–2003 in which 195 procedures were performed and 2004–2006 in which 432 procedures were performed [13]. The authors stated that the "significant decrease in the overall stroke/death rate between the first and the last interval of the study period enhances the importance of an appropriate learning curve that involves a caseload larger than that generally accepted for credentialing." It is not clear whether the very lengthy learning curve here reflects the fact that these were "classically trained" vascular surgeons, presumably without prior formal training in catheter/guidewire techniques.

The CASES–PMS study (Carotid Artery Stenting with Emboli Protection Surveillance–Postmarketing Study) which included 73 different clinical sites examined whether physicians with varying carotid stent experience could obtain comparable efficacy and safety to those obtained within the SAPPHIRE trial [14, 15]. One thousand four hundred ninety-three patients were enrolled; 78.2% were asymptomatic. Centers were included with low (<30), medium (30–100), and high (>100) annual carotid stent volumes. Physicians were also classified into training levels based on number of procedures previously completed and completion of the CASES (Carotid Artery Stenting Education System) program. Level 1 was exempt from training having performed >25 CAS procedures and >10 with the AngioGuard XP protection device, level 2 had also performed >25 CAS but <10 with the AngioGuard XP protection device, and level 3 had performed <25 CAS procedures and underwent full CASES training. There were no differences in technical- or device-related success by training level. Major adverse events were similar to those in the SAPPHIRE trial (3.5% combined death, stroke, and myocardial infarction). Again, these were similar across training levels, carotid stent volumes, and type of institution (academic vs. nonacademic) [14].

The CAPTURE registry was a requirement for the FDA approval of the RX Acculink Carotid Stent and Accunet Embolic Protection System (then Guidant, now Abbott Vascular) [16–18]. Three thousand five hundred patients were enrolled at 144 sites by 353 physicians with varying backgrounds and experience. One third of the operators had no prior carotid stenting experience and underwent certification training before participating in the study. Interestingly, only 13.8% of patients were symptomatic. The overall 30-day stroke and death rate was 5.7% (10.6% symptomatic patients, 4.9% asymptomatic patients). Physicians were classified as levels I, II, and III [18]:

- *Level I.* Previous CAS experience including 5 as primary operator using RX Acculink CAS system
- *Level II.* Ten carotid stent procedures as primary operator
- *Level III.* Adequate interventional experience (25 carotid angiograms and 10 peripheral stent procedures and 10 procedures with 0.014″ systems).

8.1% of patients were enrolled by a level I physician, 67.9% by a level II physician, and 24.0% by a level III physician.

All participants underwent training organized by the manufacturer, including hands-on practice with the device. Less experienced operators underwent a structured 2-day carotid training program of didactic sessions, case reviews, and hands-on and simulator training focused on clinical management, imaging, and procedural education [15]. After training, clinical specialists (from Abbott Vascular) supported the first three cases. The availability of proctoring by an experienced physician was also addressed as needed or requested [18].

In terms of the main outcome of 30-day death and stroke rate, there was a trend for better results in more experienced physicians (levels I = 4.6%, II = 5.4%, and III = 6.9%) but this did not reach statistical significance [18]. One major confounding variable was the difference in patient population treated; less experienced physicians treated fewer symptomatic patients. However, the authors' conclusions were that the training program used was effective [15].

The educational programs arranged for the CASES–PMS study and CAPTURE registry highlight the potential impact of dedicated training programs on outcomes for CAS.

In our view, the published data do not allow a precise quantification of the length of the CAS learning curve. This is particularly because much of the data available to date are from randomized trials which inevitably involve senior and more experienced operators rather than trainees, and also because of the need to consider prior experience in trainees from different backgrounds. However, the data do perhaps support the cautious statement that 25–50 procedures seem to represent the entry requirement for CAS within randomized trials. Notably, 85% of operators performing CAS within EVA3S had performed ≤50 cases [19].

Simulators in CAS Training

Virtual reality (VR) simulation has been extensively used as a training method in fields such as aviation and laparoscopic surgery [20]. In procedures such as CAS where basic skills, such as the manipulation of a wire in three dimensions, are required, it may be possible to acquire these skills more rapidly using simulators of various sorts. These may be particularly appropriate for those, such as surgical trainees, without prior experience in endovascular skills [21]. The essential aim is to reduce the learning curve when the techniques are applied to real patients [22]. Traditional clinical teaching may be too time consuming to be considered feasible in many units, especially with a reduction in the number of diagnostic procedures being performed. There are also ethical issues concerned with letting inexperienced physicians "practice" on patients in an area such as CAS where there may be a narrow margin of benefit (asymptomatic patients) and potentially catastrophic outcomes.

In addition, a simple quantification of the number of procedures performed and the duration of training is only a crude measure of operator proficiency. VR simulators may provide a standardized mechanism to assess post-training skills. Such systems may also allow an objective measurement of the attainment of such skills over time [21]. The options for simulation include live animal operating, cadaver-based procedures, mechanical models, and computer-based VR models. Animal models and cadaver-based training do not appear to have been widely used in CAS training courses to date and mechanical models probably lack the sophistication required. However, VR simulators are expensive and access to them has also not been widespread to date in many units.

Chaer et al. [21] compare two groups of surgical trainees with and without exposure to training on a VR simulator. They used the Procedicus VIST system (Mentice Corporation, Gothenburg, Sweden) which utilizes software producing a three-dimensional representation of the arterial system coupled to a module utilizing a force feedback system allowing the use of standard catheters and guidewires, injection of contrast, deployment of stents, etc., with a simulated fluoroscopic display. Simulation led to improvement in almost all measures of individual performance. Aggarwal et al. [23] have described the performance of the VIST simulator in allowing surgeons with minimal endovascular experience to improve catheter skills. The authors suggest that such a VR system could be useful in reducing the early part of the learning curve. It was also seen to differentiate between different levels of prior experience and its use may result in lower fluoroscopic time [24].

The importance of such systems has been highlighted by the approval of CAS by the US Food and Drug Administration (FDA), leading to an increased number of physicians from different disciplines wishing to be trained in the procedure. The FDA has subsequently endorsed the use of VR simulators as part of training.

A learning curve can also be demonstrated in VR simulators [22]. Patel et al. used the VIST simulator (Mentice Corporation, Gothenburg, Sweden) to study performance in 20 cardiologists in a carotid angiography training program. After training, five simulated procedures were performed, with measurable improvements in procedure time, contrast load, and catheter-handling errors. However, similar studies are needed with trainees from other specialities.

Finally, as well as allowing basic training, VR simulators may also allow case planning and take even experienced operators through some of the less common scenarios which can potentially lead to complications in advance of a real case [25]. In the future, it is likely that the sophistication of simulators will increase. In the very near future, they will be able to provide ongoing monitoring of performance, and simulate rarer but important anatomical variants and technical mishaps. It is likely that they will become essential components of most training programs.

Published Guidelines on Training and Accreditation in CAS

In 2005, the AAN/AANS/ASITN/ASNR/CNS/SIR guidelines gave guidance on training requirements before the independent performance of CAS [26]. It defined 100 supervised cerebral angiograms and either 25 noncarotid stents, 4 supervised CAS procedures, and 16 h of CME, or 10 supervised CAS procedures with acceptable results as the minimum requirement. The CME was a mixture of didactic teaching and hands-on training. The message was clearly stated that there was a requirement for training in both the cognitive and technical aspects of CAS. As a neuroscience-based statement, it also required a minimum of 6 months of formal cognitive neuroscience training in an approved program in radiology, neuroradiology, neurosurgery, neurology, or vascular radiology.

The clinical competence statement from the SCAI/SVMB/SVS Writing Committee was also issued in 2005 [3]. As mentioned earlier, the technical requirements hinge around minimum numbers of procedures required to achieve competence. This is stated as 30 cervicocerebral angiograms and 25 CAS procedures, half as primary operator. Clinical requirements include the ability to manage inpatient and outpatient care and to obtain appropriate consent [3].

In 2006, a joint consensus statement was coordinated and issued by the American College of Cardiology Foundation Task Force on carotid stenting which contained recommendations for training [27]. It states that operators should previously (to performing CAS) have achieved a high level of proficiency in catheter-based interventions, completed dedicated training in CAS, and be credentialed at their hospital [27]. It included consideration of the previous statements/consensus documents from the SCAI/SVMB/SVS and the AAN/AANS/ASITN/ASNR/CNS/SIR but was not able to unify them [3, 26]. It set out requirements for training, proctoring, and use of simulators. It also stated that the FDA has approved industry training programs for CAS which should augment, not supplant, professional society training and volume requirements [27].

The Royal College of Radiologists (UK) has also issued guidance about training in CAS [28]. It highlights the currently very different training requirements between interventional radiology, cardiology, and vascular surgery in the UK and also the fact that most diagnostic carotid imaging is now noninvasive in the UK making training problematic. Recommendations were that prior to training in the technical aspects of CAS, the physician should have primary operator experience of:

1. A minimum of 30 diagnostic cervicocerebral angiograms
2. One hundred diagnostic angiograms from a percutaneous puncture
3. Fifty non-neurological selective angiograms from a percutaneous puncture
4. Twenty-five peripheral or coronary stents from a percutaneous puncture
5. Microcatheter techniques and snares from a percutaneous puncture

6. Experience in neuroimaging, both noninvasive (carotid ultrasound, MRI, MRA, CT, CTA, etc.) and invasive (cervicocerebral angiography), to select and manage patients

It also states that the current training program in the UK was designed for the ICSS trial which assumed appropriate prior diagnostic and endovascular skills. The program consists of a structured day of lectures and live cases attended by the entire team, a visit by the team to observe in an experienced center, and a proctor to attend (from an experienced center) to progressively teach the procedure in the new center. The advantage is that the proctor can determine the endpoint of training rather than it be predetermined by a specific number of procedures as the learning curve is likely to vary between individuals. The minimum number of cases per year for a center to be viable is stated as being 15 [28]. There is currently no mechanism in the UK to specifically accredit the successful participant in any CAS training program.

The ICCS–SPREAD (Italian Consensus Carotid Stenting) consensus statement discusses the importance of teams of expertise and the need for independent external audit [29]. It recommends for minimum competence 150 procedures on supra-aortic vessels within 2 years with 100 as the primary operator and at least 75 CAS stenting procedures with 50 as the primary operator. Subsequently, 50 procedures are required per year.

Maintenance of Competence

There is a significant relationship between volume and outcome for CEA [30] and there is no reason to believe that this is not also the case for CAS. Arguably, any complex intervention with a small margin of error is unsafe in low volume. For CEA, there is a significant reduction in procedural complications when annual center volume is ≥85 cases per annum.

The Royal College of Radiologists suggests that 15 CAS procedures are performed per year per interventionist [28], whilst the ICCS–SPREAD Joint Committee suggested 50 CAS procedures per year per interventionist [29].

It may be argued that it is unethical to embark on a CAS program unless one can guarantee sufficient throughput to maintain competence.

Conclusions

Currently, there are still no well-defined pathways for training in CAS. However, certain key themes are emerging. Training needs to be tailored to the background of the individual and that a significant learning curve exists must be taken into account when designing training programs and granting accreditation. The use of VR simulators holds enormous promise for training in the future and the use of proctorship and mentoring also seem essential to enable the transition into safe practice. As CAS continues to expand, it seems likely that an integrated training program across specialities leading to accreditation will be essential. Ideally, such a program will be endorsed by both National Societies and Governmental organizations.

Key Points

Training

- Training should be both cognitive (clinical decision making) and practical (skills based).
- Trainees from different background will require different approaches to training.
- Trainees from different backgrounds should be trained to the same ultimate standards.
- Teams and their training needs should be considered in addition to those of individuals.
- Virtual reality models are likely to play an important role in future training.
- Mentoring and proctoring are essential before "solo" practice.
- Societies are attempting to define how many cases, and what experience, are required before solo practice.

Advice to Someone Wishing to Train in CAS

- Aim to have developed catheter skills by attachment to a busy unit.
- Aim for a thorough understanding of clinical decision making/investigation of neurovascular patients – attend MDTs where possible.
- Identify an appropriate mentor.
- Attend workshops/courses to improve knowledge base.

- Attend workshops/courses which enable teaching on simulators.
- Keep an accurate logbook of all relevant training.

Advice to Someone Setting Up a CAS Training Course/Program

- At an early stage, decide on the "aims" of the course/program.
- Be very clear about what the course/program qualifies the candidate to do subsequently.
- Develop a clearly defined curriculum.
- Decide on entry level requirements for participants.
- Recruit appropriately experienced individuals who are also good teachers.
- Develop assessment mechanisms which are objective whenever possible.
- Consider use of simulators.
- Consider use of live demonstrations.
- Consider involvement of industry.
- Consider getting approval from specialist societies.
- If providing proctorship subsequently, define mechanisms for this and avoid conflicts of interest.

References

1. Schneider PA. Optimal training strategies for carotid stenting. Semin Vasc Surg 2005;18(2):69–74.
2. Brooks WH, McClure RR, Jones MR, Coleman TC, Breathitt L. Carotid angioplasty and stenting versus carotid endarterectomy: Randomized trial in a community hospital. J Am Coll Cardiol 2001;38(6):1589–1595.
3. Rosenfield K, Babb JD, Cates CU, Cowley MJ, Feldman T, Gallagher A, et al. Clinical competence statement on carotid stenting: Training and credentialing for carotid stenting – multispecialty consensus recommendations: A report of the SCAI/SVMB/SVS Writing Committee to develop a clinical competence statement on carotid interventions. J Am Coll Cardiol 2005;45(1):165–174.
4. Moore WS, Young B, Baker WH, et al. Surgical results: A justification of the surgeon selection process for the ACAS trial: The ACAS investigators. J Vasc Surg 1996;23:323–328.
5. Alberts MJ, McCann R, Smith TP. A randomized trial: Carotid stenting versus endarterectomy in patients with symptomatic carotid stenosis: Study designs. J Neurovasc Dis 1997;2:228–234.
6. Roubin GS, New G, Iyer SS, Vitek JJ, Al-Mubarak N, Liu MW, et al. Immediate and late clinical outcomes of carotid artery stenting in patients with symptomatic and asymptomatic carotid artery stenosis: A 5-year prospective analysis. Circulation 2001;103(4): 532–537.
7. Wholey MH, Al-Mubarek N, Wholey MH. Updated review of the global carotid artery stent registry. Catheter Cardiovasc Interv 2003;60(2):259–266.
8. Wholey MH, Wholey M, Bergeron P, Diethrich EB, Henry M, Laborde JC, et al. Current global status of carotid artery stent placement. Cathet Cardiovasc Diagn 1998;44(1):1–6.
9. Ederle J, Featherstone RL, Brown MM. Percutaneous transluminal angioplasty and stenting for carotid artery stenosis. Cochrane Database Syst Rev 2007;4:CD000515.
10. CAVATAS Investigators. Endovascular versus surgical treatment in patients with carotid stenosis in the Carotid and Vertebral Artery Transluminal Angioplasty Study (CAVATAS): A randomized trial. Lancet 2001;357:1729–1737.
11. Ahmadi R, Willfort A, Lang W, Schillinger M, Alt E, Gschwandtner ME et al., Carotid artery stenting: Effect of learning curve and intermediate-term morphological outcome. J Endovasc Ther 2001;8: 539–546.
12. Lin PH, Bush RL, Peden E, Zhou W, Kougias P, Henao E, et al. What is the learning curve for carotid artery stenting with neuroprotection? Analysis of 200 consecutive cases at an academic institution. Perspect Vasc Surg Endovasc Ther 2005;17(2):1 13–123.
13. Verzini F, Cao P, De Rango P, Parlani G, Maselli A, Romano L et al., Appropriateness of learning curve for carotid artery stenting: An analysis of periprocedural complications. J Vasc Surg 2006;44: 1205–1211.
14. Katzen BT, Criado FJ, Ramee SR, Massop DW, Hopkins LN, Donohoe D, et al. Carotid artery stenting with emboli protection surveillance study: Thirty-day results of the CASES–PMS study. Catheter Cardiovasc Interv 2007;70(2):316–323.
15. Yadav JS, Wholey MH, Kuntz RE, Fayad P, Katzen BT, Mishkel GJ, et al. Protected carotid-artery stenting versus endarterectomy in high-risk patients. N Engl J Med 2004;351(15):1493–1501.
16. Fairman R, Gray WA, Scicli AP, Wilburn O, Verta P, Atkinson R, et al. The CAPTURE registry: Analysis of strokes resulting from carotid artery stenting in the post approval setting: Timing, location, severity, and type. Ann Surg 2007;246(4):551–556; discussion 556–558.
17. Gray WA, Yadav JS, Verta P, Scicli A, Fairman R, Wholey M, et al. The CAPTURE registry: Predictors

of outcomes in carotid artery stenting with embolic protection for high surgical risk patients in the early post-approval setting. Catheter Cardiovasc Interv 2007;70(7):1025–1033.

18. Gray WA, Yadav JS, Verta P, Scicli A, Fairman R, Wholey M, et al. The CAPTURE registry: Results of carotid stenting with embolic protection in the post approval setting. Catheter Cardiovasc Interv 2007;69(3):341–348.
19. Mas JL, Chatellier G, Beyssen B et al., Endarterectomy versus stenting in patients with symptomatic severe carotid stenosis. N Engl J Med 2006;355:1660–1671.
20. Seymour NE, Gallagher AG, Roman SA, O'Brien MK, Bansal VK, Andersen DK, et al. Virtual reality training improves operating room performance: Results of a randomized, double-blinded study. Ann Surg 2002;236(4):458–463; discussion 463–464.
21. Chaer RA, Derubertis BG, Lin SC, Bush HL, Karwowski JK, Birk D, et al. Simulation improves resident performance in catheter-based intervention: Results of a randomized, controlled study. Ann Surg 2006;244(3):343–352.
22. Patel AD, Gallagher AG, Nicholson WJ, Cates CU. Learning curves and reliability measures for virtual reality simulation in the performance assessment of carotid angiography. J Am Coll Cardiol 2006;47(9):1796–1802.
23. Aggarwal R, Black SA, Hance JR, Darzi A, Cheshire NJ. Virtual reality simulation training can improve inexperienced surgeons' endovascular skills. Eur J Vasc Endovasc Surg 2006;31(6):588–593.
24. Van Herzeele I, Aggarwal R, Choong A, Brightwell R, Vermassen FE, Cheshire NJ. Virtual reality simulation objectively differentiates level of carotid stent experience in experienced interventionalists. J Vasc Surg 2007;46(5):855–863.
25. Cates CU, Patel AD, Nicholson WJ. Use of virtual reality simulation for mission rehearsal for carotid stenting. JAMA 2007;297(3):265–266.
26. Connors JJ, III, Sacks D, Furlan AJ, Selman WR, Russell EJ, Stieg PE, et al. Training, competency, and credentialing standards for diagnostic cervicocerebral angiography, carotid stenting, and cerebrovascular intervention: A joint statement from the American Academy of Neurology, American Association of Neurological Surgeons, American Society of Interventional and Therapeutic Radiology, American Society of Neuroradiology, Congress of Neurological Surgeons, AANS/CNS Cerebrovascular Section, and Society of Interventional Radiology. Radiology 2005;234(1):26–34.
27. Bates ER, Babb JD, Casey DE, Jr., Cates CU, Duckwiler GR, Feldman TE, et al. ACCF/SCAI/SVMB/SIR/ASITN 2007 Clinical Expert Consensus Document on carotid stenting. Vasc Med 2007;12(1):35–83.
28. The Royal College of Radiologists. Advice from the Royal College of Radiologists Concerning Training for Carotid Artery Stenting (CAS). London: The Royal College of Radiologists (2006).
29. Cremonesi A, Setacci C, Bignamini A et al., Carotid artery stenting: First consensus document of the ICCS–SPREAD Joint Committee. Stroke 2006;37(9):2400–2409; Epub 2006 Aug 10.
30. Holt PJ, Poloniecki JD, Loftus IM et al., The relationship between hospital case volume and outcome from carotid endartectomy in England from 2000 to 2005. Eur J Vasc Endovasc Surg 2007;34:646–654.

5 Preprocedure Imaging

Jos C. van den Berg

Introduction

In the past, the treatment of carotid artery disease has been either conservative with medical therapy, or surgical, using carotid endarterectomy. Traditionally, diagnosis was made using duplex ultrasound and additional imaging consisting of selective carotid arteriography has been considered necessary to confirm the duplex findings, to clarify equivocal or unreliable duplex findings [1] (Table 5.1), to demonstrate or exclude tandem lesions (that may occur in up to 10% of cases [2]), and finally to obtain additional anatomical information (e.g., relation of carotid bifurcation and mandibular angle) (Fig. 5.1). Duplex ultrasound is used as the sole imaging test before carotid endarterectomy in some institutions, but in most instances there is a requirement for a less operator-dependent, reliable confirmatory noninvasive diagnostic test to improve confidence in correct patient selection [2, 3].

With the advent of carotid artery stenting (CAS) as an alternative to surgical treatment of stenotic internal carotid artery disease, additional imaging has become even more important and considered mandatory to evaluate the anatomy of the access vessels, the configuration of the aortic arch, the tortuosity and length of the common carotid artery and internal carotid artery, and to demonstrate the presence of disease of the external carotid artery. Additional imaging should also allow for evaluation of the intracranial circulation, since concomitant disease of the intracranial vessels can influence the outcome of treatment.

Evaluation of patency of access vessels (common femoral artery and common and external iliac artery) is not routinely performed but occasionally access problems may arise. Duplex ultrasound can be used as an alternative to screen for disease of the access vessels.

Arch configuration is of importance in deciding upon suitability of an endovascular procedure, and additional imaging is needed for classification of aortic arch morphology, and for visualization of anatomical variants (Fig. 5.2). Knowledge of the length and degree of tortuosity of the common carotid artery is of importance to evaluate the possibility of safe placement of the guiding catheter or long introduction sheath. Evaluation of plaque calcification and ulceration and intimal thickening is of importance in determining the optimal (endovascular) approach (choice of protection device). Plaques that are more prone to disruption, fracture, or fissuring may be associated with a higher risk of embolization, occlusion, and consequent ischemic neurological events [4]. The absence of (occlusive) disease of the external carotid artery is essential to allow for placement of a long guidewire in the external carotid artery to perform an exchange of the diagnostic catheter for a long introduction sheath or guiding catheter (Fig. 5.3). Suitability for carotid stenting may be as low as 36% as judged by anatomical criteria (mainly due to carotid tortuosity and proximal arch disease) [5].

S. Macdonald and G. Stansby (eds.), *Practical Carotid Artery Stenting*,
DOI: 10.1007/978-1-84800-299-9_5, © Springer-Verlag London Limited 2009

TABLE 5.1. Specific anatomic criteria and categories defining inadequate or indeterminate carotid duplex scan (adapted from [1]).

Incomplete imaging of carotid bifurcation and cervical region
– Deep anatomy
– Extensive calcific shadowing
– High carotid bifurcation
– Long internal carotid artery plaque
– Small internal carotid artery diameter
– Internal carotid artery redundancy (kinking, coiling)
Suspected extracervical occlusive disease
– Proximal commson carotid artery or innominate artery disease
– Posterior circulation disease
– Distal or intracranial internal carotid artery disease
Borderline or equivocal internal carotid artery disease severity
Carotid near-occlusion ("trickle flow")
Diffuse, recurrent carotid stenosis

In this chapter, the various alternative imaging modalities that can be used in the preprocedural assessment related to internal CAS stenting will be dealt with. Advantages and disadvantages as well as diagnostic accuracy will be discussed. A glimpse toward future developments will be given.

Imaging Modalities

Imaging modalities currently used in routine practice are digital subtraction angiography (DSA), CT angiography (CTA), MR angiography (MRA), and less frequently three-dimensional rotational angiography (3D-RA) with or without application of soft tissue imaging techniques that offer the capability of rendering CT-like images.

Digital Subtraction Angiography

DSA has been considered the gold standard in carotid artery imaging for many years. It typically involves selective catheterization of the common carotid artery and has an inherent risk of bleeding complications at the level of the puncture site, and risk of transient ischemic attack, stroke, and mortality. In patients with symptomatic ischemic cerebrovascular disease, the risk for disabling stroke and death can be as high as 4 and 1%, respectively [6]. Awareness of local angiographic complication rates is important in the selection process of diagnostic

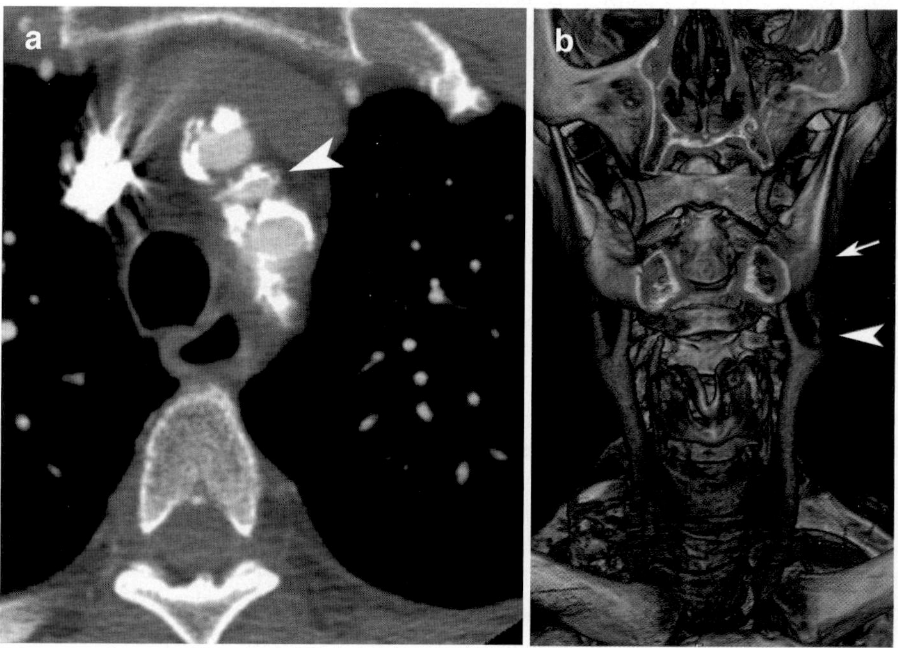

FIG. 5.1. Axial CTA image (**a**) at the level of the origin of the supra-aortic arteries: severe concomitant disease of all branches is seen (patient with severe internal carotid artery stenosis). VRT image (**b**) demonstrating anatomical relationship between carotid artery bifurcation, stenosis of the internal carotid artery (*arrowhead*), and mandibular angle (*arrow*)

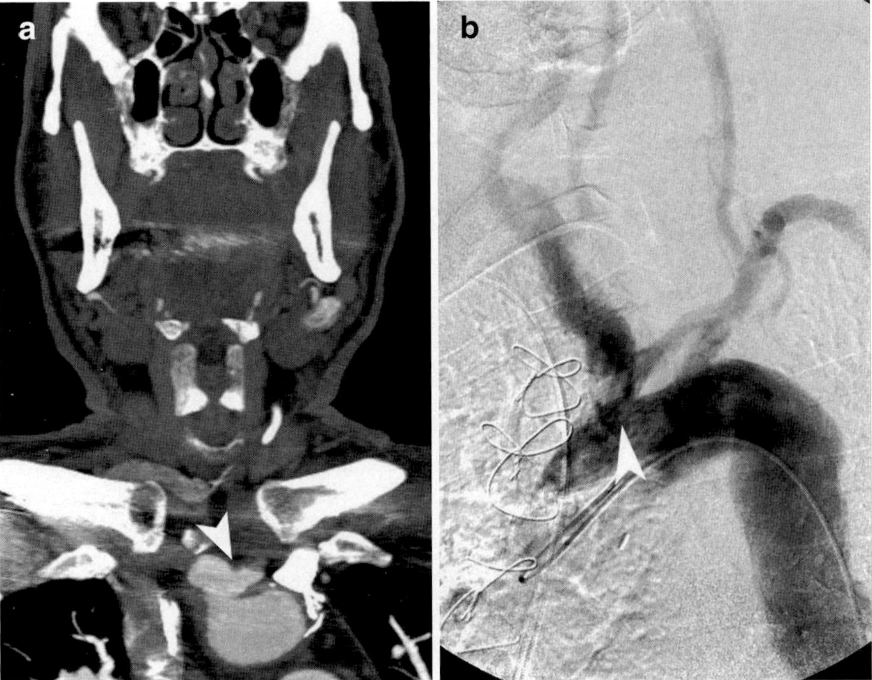

FIG. 5.2. Coronal CTA image (**a**) and angiographic image during aortography (**b**) demonstrating presence of a common origin of the brachiocephalic trunk and left common carotid artery (bovine trunk)

tests to be performed [7]. Minor adverse reactions, including TIA, groin hematoma, unstable angina, need for blood transfusion, leg ischemia, and iliac artery dissection, can occur in up to 10% of procedures [6].

The morbidity and mortality of angiography can significantly be reduced by performing nonselective angiography in multiple projections, with contrast being injected into the aortic arch using a pigtail catheter [8]. Arch aortography is associated with a much lower neurological complication rate. The major advantage of angiography is its high resolution, and ability to demonstrate flow dynamics, both of the diseased artery and collateral circulation (circle of Willis and external carotid artery; Fig. 5.4).

CT Angiography

Major progress in imaging has been made with the advent of multidetector row CT (MDCT). As compared to single-slice CT scanning speed of MDCT has increased 40-fold, which makes it possible to scan a large volume within a short breath-hold. The present generation of multidetector row or multislice CT scanners allows for a simultaneous acquisition of up to 64-slices, while in the near future systems with over 64 detectors will become available. With an MDCT, a single acquisition yields a volume of data, instead of a number of slices (as when using helical CT). Thus, far resolution in the z-axis ("slice thickness") was still a limiting factor in image quality for multiplanar reconstruction (MPR). With an increase of the number of detectors, resolution increases as well, and thus (near) isotropic imaging becomes possible (i.e., imaging with a resolution that is equally high in all directions). For example, a 16-slice detector typically yields a slice thickness of 0.75 mm, while a 64-row detector yields 0.6-mm thick slices.

It has been demonstrated that to get optimal enhancement of the aortic arch and supra-aortic vessels, preferably high-concentration contrast should be used (>300 mg I mL^{-1}), followed by flushing with a saline bolus [9–11]. Scan delay can be optimized, and contrast medium dosage can be reduced by using a test bolus technique or using

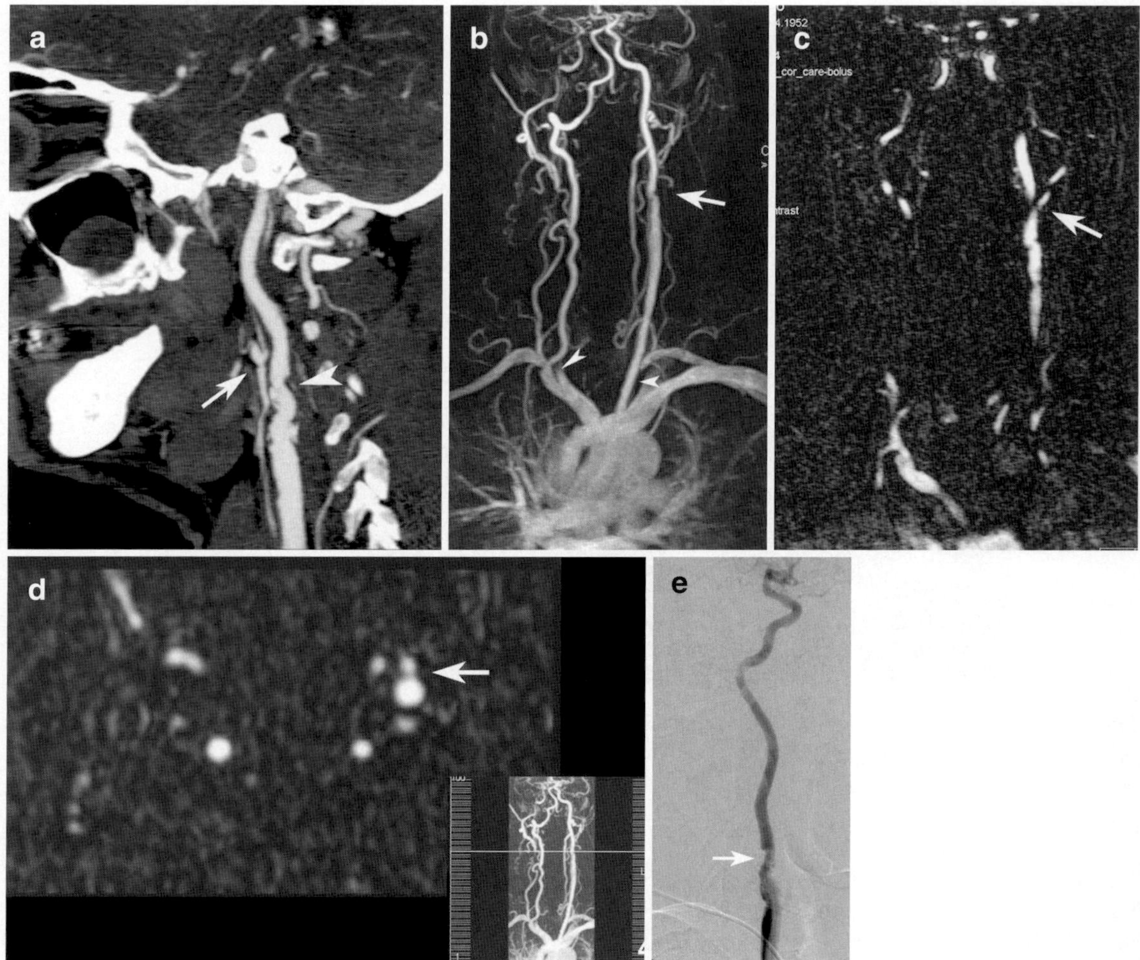

Fig. 5.3. Sagittal CTA image (**a**), demonstrating stenosis of the internal carotid artery (*arrowhead*) and good filling of external carotid artery branches (*arrow*); no communication between common carotid and external artery could be demonstrated. MRA examination (MIP image (**b**), coronal MPR image (**c**), and axial reconstruction (**e**)) revealed the same findings (*arrow* indicating carotid artery bifurcation); note occlusion of the contralateral common and internal carotid artery and left subclavian artery on the MIP image (*arrowheads*); selective angiography during carotid artery stenting procedure confirmed occlusion of the origin of the external carotid artery and stenosis of the internal carotid artery (*arrow*)

an automatic bolus recognition system (bolus triggering) [10–12]. Scanning protocols vary with different systems and manufacturers. With a four-row detector, most examinations are performed with 2.5-mm collimation and a table speed of 15–20 mm per rotation, while using a 16-row detector collimation is reduced to 1.5 mm and table speed can be increased to 36 mm per rotation. Contrast is injected at a flow rate of 3–5 mL s^{-1} with a power injector into an antecubital vein for a total volume of 120 mL. Preferably, injection should take place from the right antecubital vein, to avoid artifacts arising from high-density contrast in the left brachiocephalic vein that may render evaluation of the ostia of the supra-aortic arteries difficult (Fig. 5.5). A CTA image of good quality can be obtained if the patient does not move or swallow for 1 min. Anatomic coverage should include the inner curve of the aortic arch and the circle of Willis.

The radiation dose for CTA is at least 2–3 times lower compared with the dose for angiography [13]. Three-dimensional volume rendering techniques

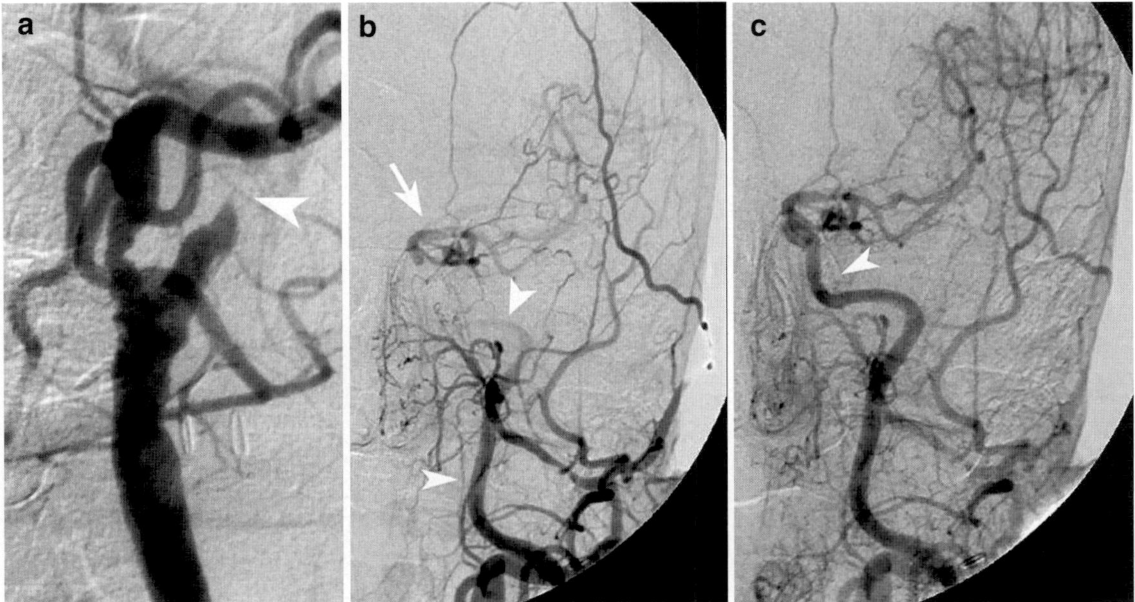

Fig. 5.4. Selective angiographic image of the left carotid artery at the level of the carotid bifurcation (**a**) showing a high-grade stenosis of the internal carotid artery (*arrowhead*). Intracranial angiography (**b**) and (**c**) demonstrates filling of the carotid siphon (*arrow*) through external carotid artery branches, before filling of the distal part of the cervical carotid artery (*arrowheads*) occurs

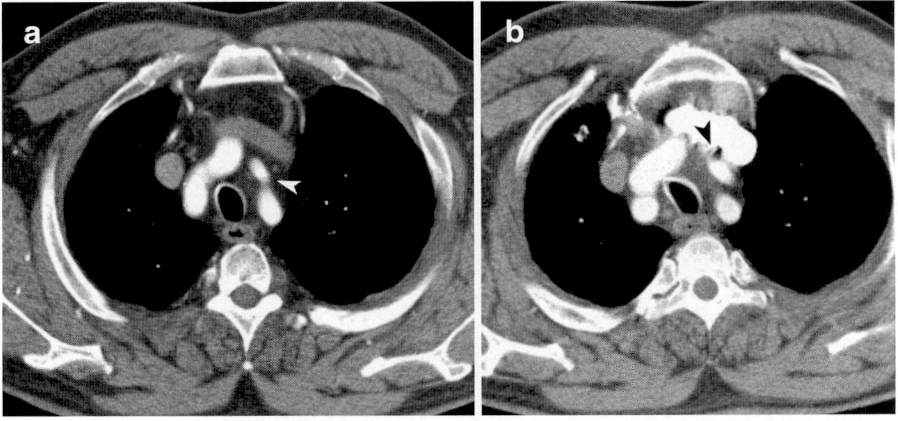

Fig. 5.5. Axial CTA images of one patient with injection of contrast from the right antecubital vein (**a**) and from the left antecubital vein (**b**) performed during control follow-up for thoracic malignancy; good visualization of the supra-aortic arteries is seen (*white arrowhead*); with left-sided injection, strong opacification of the left brachiocephalic vein causes streak artifacts (*black arrowhead*), hampering visualization of the origin of the aortic branches

(VRTs) permit real-time interactive evaluation in any plane and projection. This enhances understanding of degree of stenosis, vessel tortuosity, and plaque characteristics. After obtaining the volumetric data set, a number of postprocessing image reconstruction options are available [13]:

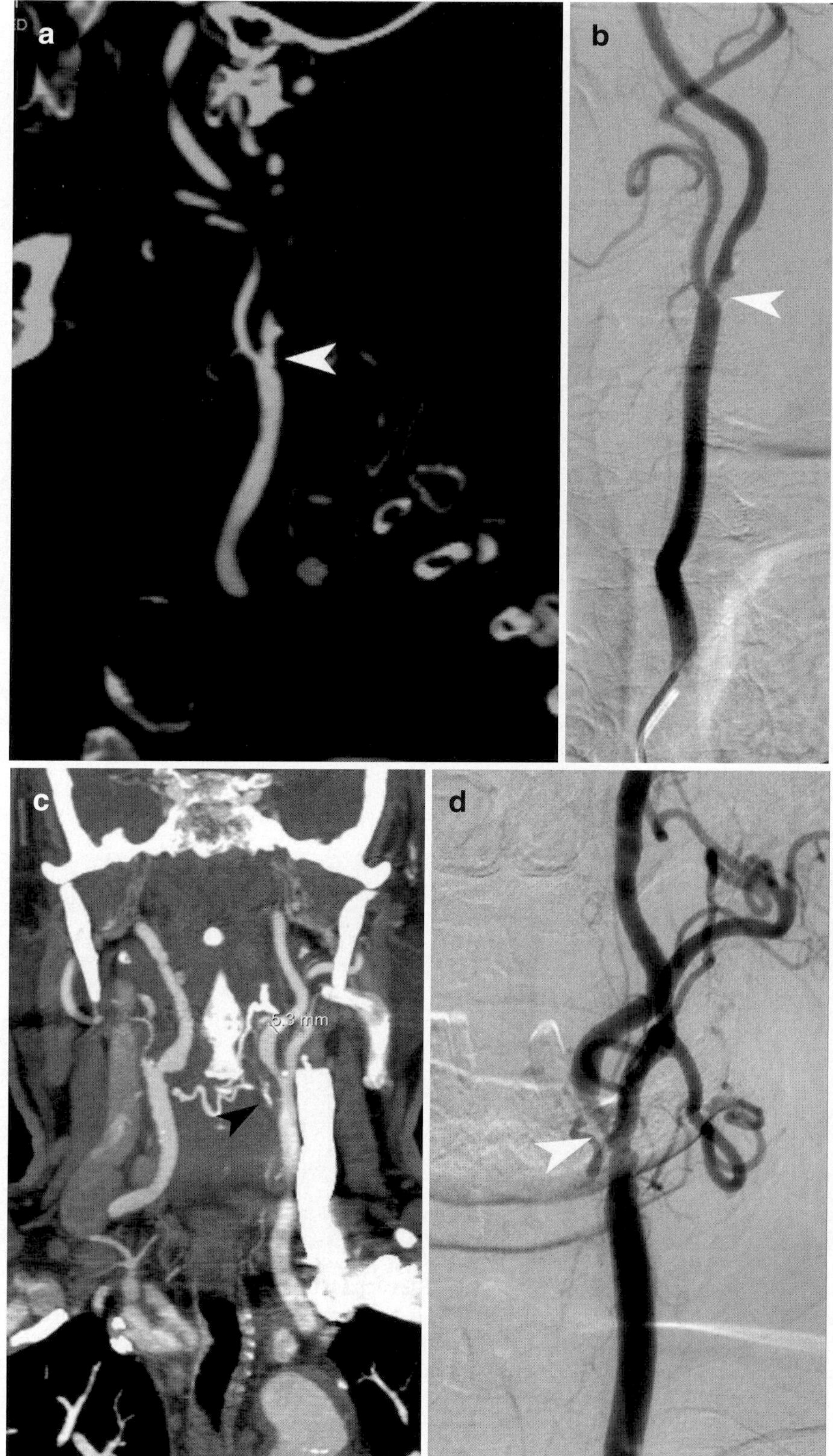

FIG. 5.6. Sagittal CTA image (**a**) of a patient with symptomatic left internal carotid artery stenosis (*arrowhead*); image matches findings at selective angiography (**b**). Coronal CTA image (**c**) of another patient with symptomatic left carotid artery disease, demonstrating stenosis with heterogeneity of plaque (*arrowhead*); excellent correlation with angiographic image (**d**)

- MPR: two-dimensional sections with a thickness of 1 voxel (fast, easily performed at the CT scanner). MPR is typically performed in the coronal and sagittal plane (Fig. 5.6) but curved reformatting is also possible (Fig. 5.7).
- Variable-thickness displays consisting of an assimilation of various sections.
- Maximum intensity projection (MIP) in which images are derived by projecting the highest attenuation voxel in a ray through the scan volume onto an image plane; vessels running in close proximity of osseous structures or calcifications can be easily obscured. Therefore, its use in carotid imaging is relatively limited.
- Shaded surface display: this method uses a single threshold to choose relevant (high-density) voxels; because of the threshold, this method is susceptible to artifacts and may fail to demonstrate vascular calcifications; this method is useful in determining the anatomical relationship between site of stenosis and bony structures and internal jugular vein [14].
- 3D VRTs (require separate workstation): each voxel is adjusted to opacity, color, and brightness according to each CT value, according to preset color and opacity maps; the advantage of this technique is that no threshold levels are being selected, thus avoiding the possibility of altering apparent diameters of vessels [15].
- Reversing window-level transfer function, virtual angioscopic images can be produced [16, 17].

The precision of CTA is more dependent on measurement technique than on acquisition parameters. The ideal scanning plane to obtain magnified transverse oblique images to be used for stenosis measurement is perpendicular to the carotid artery [4]. Especially in cases of a tortuous course of the vessel or a very short stenosis (curved), MPR reformatting can be very helpful (Figs. 5.7 and 5.8). Using CTA, the true cross-sectional area of the normal vessel lumen and the true area of the residual lumen can be definitively visualized and measured [18]. Plaque morphology and characteristics can be evaluated by using pixel density to differentiate fat, fibrosis, calcium, and contrast that permits visualization of plaque composition, intimal hyperplasia, intraplaque hemorrhage, thrombus, and dissection (Fig. 5.8) [18].

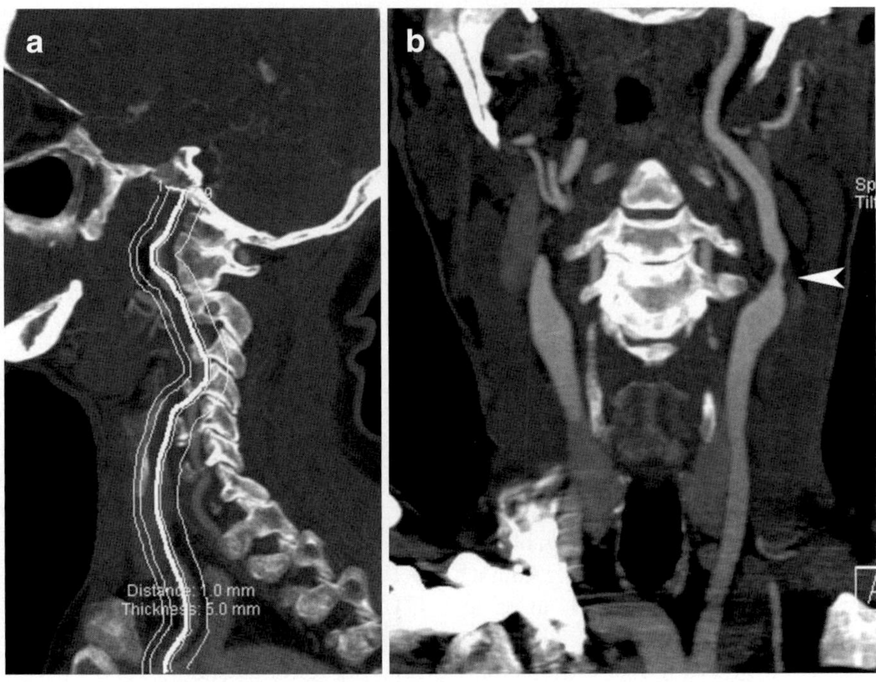

Fig. 5.7. Scanogram (**a**) and curved MPR image (**b**) demonstrating the complete course of the left carotid artery, with stenosis of the internal carotid artery (*arrowhead*)

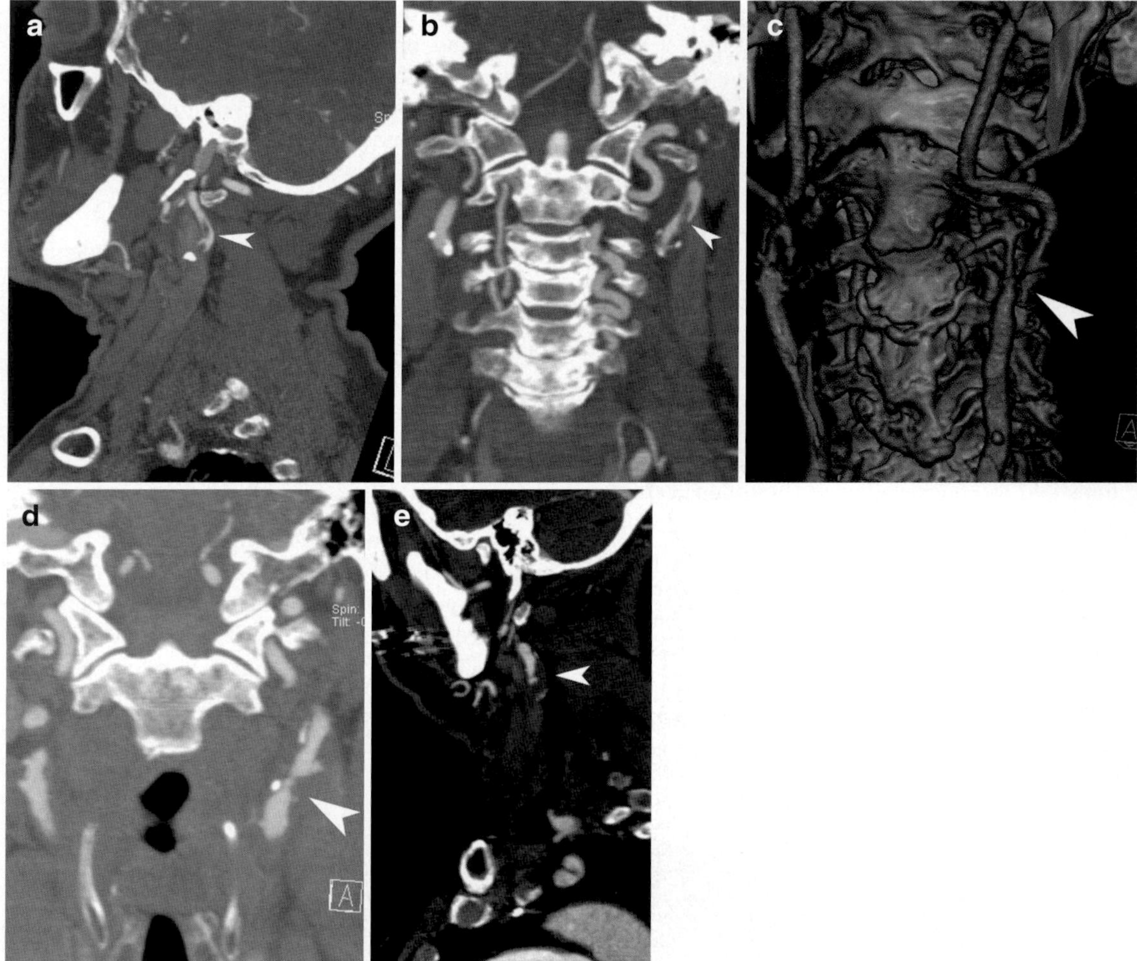

FIG. 5.8. Sagittal (**a**) and coronal (**b**) CTA image of a patient with atrial fibrillation and thrombotic embolus in the internal carotid artery (*arrowhead*). VRT image (**c**) and sagittal (**d**) and coronal (**e**) MPR images of another patient with left carotid artery stenosis (*arrowhead*); the VRT images do not allow for plaque characterization; the MPR images reveal presence of soft plaque and minor calcification

Calcification of plaque should not be considered a limitation of CTA. Heavily calcified eccentric plaque precludes MIP evaluation of CTA, for the reasons indicated above. Overestimation of stenosis in CTA can occur because of "blooming artifacts." By using a so-called "bone window" setting, blooming artifacts can be reduced (Fig. 5.9). Another technique to avoid measurement error is using an incremental reduction of the volume of a multiplanar volume reconstruction [4]. Ring-like calcifications in the arterial wall can mask the patent lumen in MPR images, and here evaluation using axial reconstructions is of use (Fig. 5.10) [12].

A disadvantage of CTA is the inability to detect flow dynamics, and direction of collateral intracranial flow. Swallowing frequently creates motion artifacts, which appear as waviness in the walls of the vessel on reconstructed images, resulting in an image of pseudostenosis (Fig. 5.11). A potential source of error (not specific for CTA, and also occurring with MRA) is collapse of the vessel distally from a severe stenosis. Imaging criteria used in DSA, such as slow filling of the distal segment and evidence of collateral circulation, are not equally applicable in CTA [12].

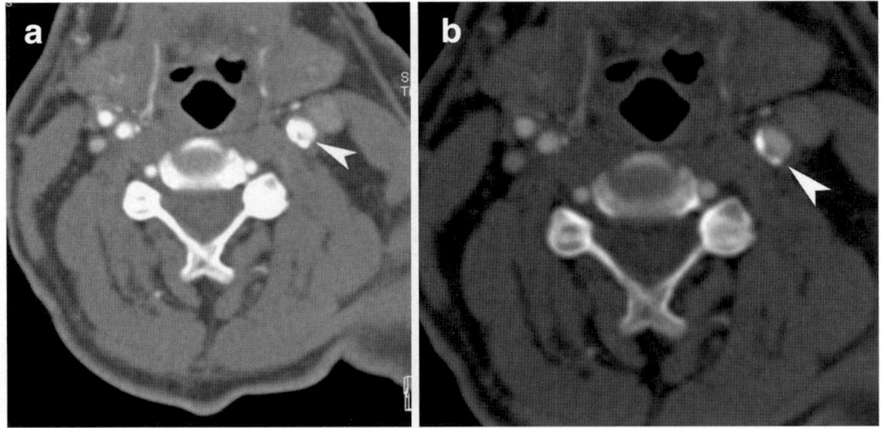

FIG. 5.9. Axial CTA image viewed with standard soft tissue window settings (**a**); differentiation between calcification and intraluminal contrast is difficult, calcifications causing blooming artifacts. Same image viewed with a bone window setting (**b**) reveals true dimensions of lumen and calcification

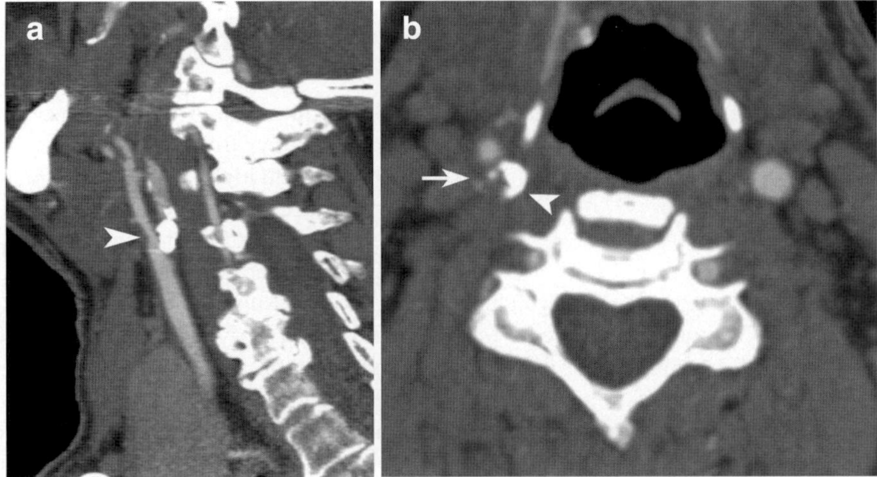

FIG. 5.10. Sagittal MPR image (**a**) of the right carotid artery reveals highly calcified plaque at the level of the carotid bifurcation (*arrowhead*), rendering grading of the stenosis impossible. Axial CTA image (**b**) demonstrates the semicircular configuration of the plaque (*arrowhead*) and allows good visualization of the residual arterial lumen (*arrow*)

A potential problem is that the ascending pharyngeal branch of the external carotid artery can be mistaken as a hairline (trickle) open internal carotid artery. This pitfall can be avoided by following the proximal internal carotid artery into the petrous canal at the skull base. As opposed to MRA, CTA is not contraindicated for patients with pacemakers, or implanted devices and claustrophobic patients. On the other hand, care should be taken in performing CTA in patients with renal insufficiency because of the risk of contrast nephropathy.

In summary, the advantages of MDCT include shorter imaging time, greater axial coverage, motion artifact suppression, improved *z*-axis resolution,

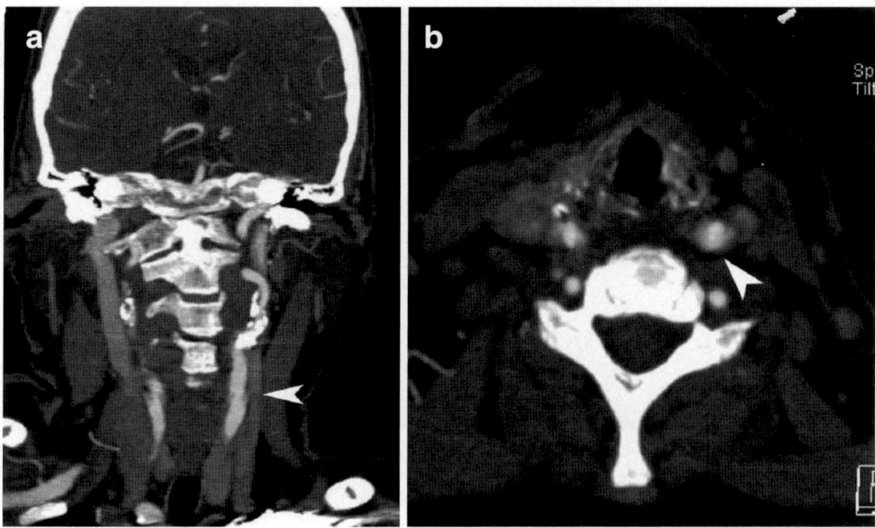

Fig. 5.11. Sagittal MPR image (**a**) demonstrating a step in the left common carotid artery (*arrowhead*), caused by swallowing during image acquisition. Axial CTA image (**b**) at the level of the motion artifact demonstrates blurring of the boundaries of the common carotid artery (*arrowhead*)

higher axial spatial resolution, decreased total dose of iodinated contrast, and real-time interactive 3D display facilities on workstations.

MR Angiography

Traditionally, MRI imaging, using T1-weighted spin-echo (black blood) imaging and cine-MR imaging, is well suited for evaluation of the gross anatomy. Flow-based methods of imaging (using time of flight (TOF) or phase contrast (PC)) properties yield bright blood images using gradient-echo techniques [19]. Limitations of the latter techniques, however, is that they rely on the physical properties of flowing blood (velocity, direction, etc.), making the technique susceptible to artifacts, that may result in overestimation of stenoses or even a false diagnosis of occlusion of a vessel. Furthermore, the spatial resolution and signal-to-noise ratio provided by these two-dimensional techniques do not allow evaluation of small vessel lesions or small side branches [20]. Since portions of the carotid arterial system are orientated relatively perpendicular to the axially directed flow detected with 2D TOF techniques (e.g., carotid siphon), weak flow signals can occur. Similarly for near-occlusion faint cervical and intracranial internal carotid artery flow signals resulting from low velocity, "trickle" flow associated with high-grade stenosis may lack detail to define accurately the length of the lesion and may necessitate additional imaging (Fig. 5.12) [1].

The technique currently most often used in the evaluation of supra-aortic vessels and the internal carotid artery is dynamic subtraction MRA, using gadolinium (0.2 mmol kg^{-1}, flow rate of antecubital injection 2 mL s^{-1}) as an intravenous contrast agent [19, 21–25]. Gadolinium shortens the T1 of blood, allows a larger flip angle to be used, generates a stronger signal with better background suppression, and yields less signal saturation. This results in shorter imaging times. Thus, less flow-related and motion-related artifacts occur, and the technique can demonstrate subtle carotid lesions and allows for imaging from the aortic arch to the circle of Willis (Fig. 5.13a). After a plain MRI, intravenous contrast is administered. Using bolus timing (by using either a test bolus or real-time "fluoroscopic" triggering), the arrival of the contrast can be timed and the contrast-enhanced sequence is performed [19, 26]. This is followed by subtraction of the two series. One limitation of the test bolus technique is the potential for diminished

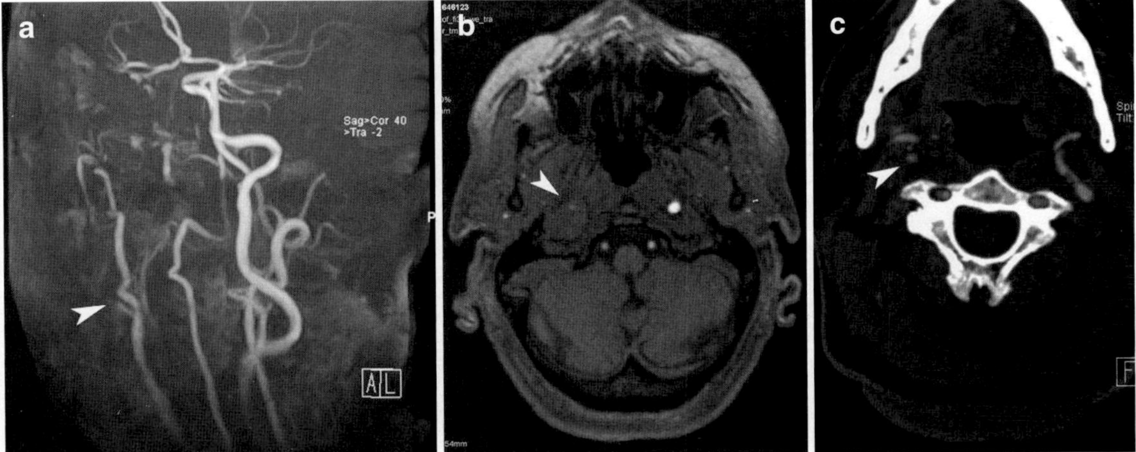

FIG. 5.12. MIP reconstruction (**a**) and axial source images (**b**) of MRA-TOF examination, demonstrating high-grade stenosis of the proximal segment of the right internal carotid artery (*arrowhead*); distal flow is not discernible. Axial CTA image (**c**) of the same patient performed the same day revealed patency of the right internal carotid artery (*arrowhead*) until the carotid siphon; patency was confirmed at surgery

artery-to-vein contrast, associated additional cost of test bolus contrast, and the potential difficulty to observe the test bolus in distal vessels or in cases with slow flow [26]. Considering the arteriovenous transit time of 5–15 s in the normal cerebrovascular system, and maximal selective intraluminal contrast enhancement of the carotid arteries of 10–25 s after intravenous administration of a bolus of contrast material, the problem of venous return into the internal jugular vein can be limited when scanning is performed within 10 s after the start of arterial enhancement. A delay in the arteriovenous transit time due to the presence of an arterial stenosis may actually improve the increase in intraluminal signal intensity during the first pass of the contrast-enhanced blood in the supra-aortic arteries [27].

Obtained images can be either viewed on a slice-to-slice basis or reconstructed on a computer workstation into an MIP image (Fig. 5.13b). It is of importance to evaluate both source images and reconstructed images on a workstation to optimize diagnostic yield (e.g., an occlusion of the origin of the external carotid artery can be easily overlooked evaluating MIP images alone; Fig. 5.3) and increase specificity [28, 29].

False-positive findings are caused by signal voids that result from signal intensity loss due to an increase in velocity at the level of a high-grade stenosis. The use of a contrast agent reduces this effect, but the combination of intravoxel dephasing and limited spatial resolution still leads to signal voids at very small residual vessel lumina [2]. Arterial collapse distally from a high-grade stenosis also contributes to this phenomenon (Fig. 5.14). If the minimal diameter is not perpendicular to the imaging plane, subtle vascular signals may not be distinguished from background signals with the MIP algorithm [30].

Contrast-enhanced MRA demonstrates a low interobserver variability (comparable to that of catheter-based angiography), which implies a high level of reliability in routine clinical practice [31]. Scanning parameters may vary depending on type and manufacturer of the MRI system, and an example is listed in Table 5.2. The discussion of plaque characterization by using MRI is beyond the scope of this chapter but is currently an area for active research.

Three-Dimensional Rotational Angiography

Conventional rotational angiography is obtained by performing a motorized movement at constant

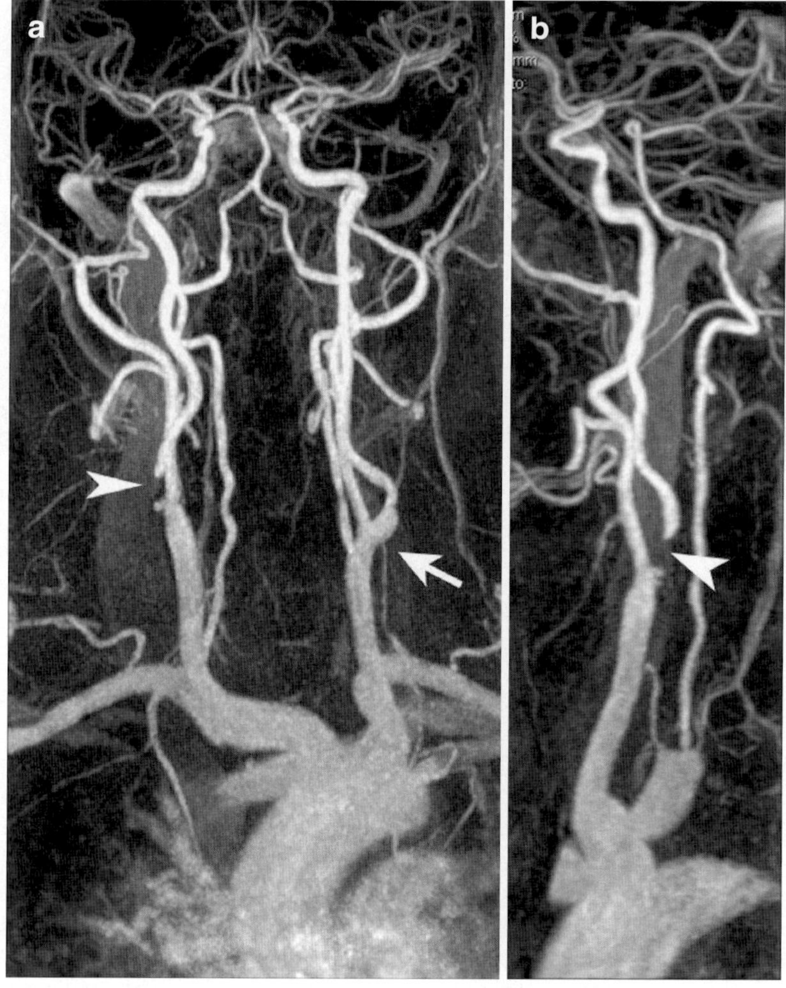

FIG. 5.13. MIP reconstruction of contrast-enhanced MRA, demonstrating vasculature from the aortic arch until circle of Willis. The anteroposterior projection (**a**) reveals a normal left carotid bifurcation (*arrow*), while the right bifurcation (*arrow*) cannot be evaluated. A coned-down lateral view of the right carotid artery (**b**) demonstrates a high-grade stenosis of the right internal carotid artery (*arrowhead*)

speed of the *C*-arc around the patient during continuous contrast injection. To obtain three-dimensional images from a conventional rotational angiographic run, two methods exist. One consists of an examination in two phases, where at first the *C*-arm makes a sweep acquiring images that act as a mask for the subsequent data acquisition. Subsequently, a return sweep is performed while contrast is injected throughout the entire period of data acquisition [32, 33]. The other technique of obtaining 3D-RA is directly based on conventional rotational angiographic images without the use of subtraction [34–36]. With both techniques, images are transferred to a workstation where they are converted into pseudo-computed tomography slices (the image intensifier being considered a multiline detector). Using specific algorithms that correct for image intensifier and contrast distortion, the data set is reconstructed into a volume-rendered image. During this reconstruction process, two different types of image correction are performed to limit visual distortion to a minimum: pincushion distortion correction that is used for diminishing of the environmental influences caused by the earth mag-

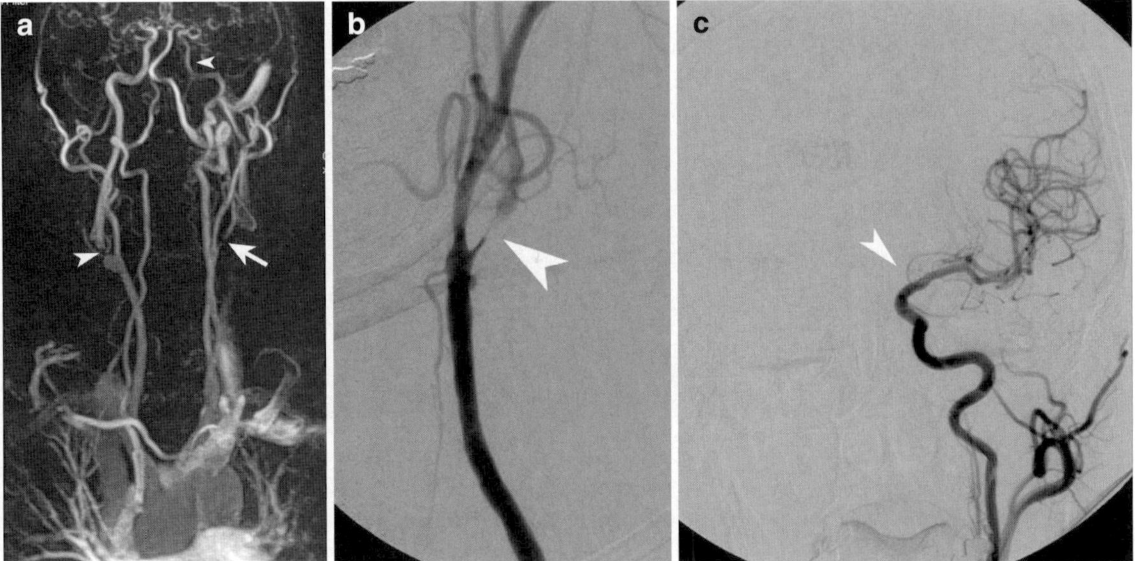

Fig. 5.14. MIP reconstruction of contrast-enhanced MRA (**a**) demonstrating stenosis of right (*large arrowhead*) and left internal carotid artery (*arrow*) with significant reduction of caliber of the distal part of the left internal carotid artery (*small arrowhead*). Selective left carotid arteriography (**b**) confirms the presence of a high-grade stenosis (*arrowhead*) with slow flow into the artery distally from the stenosis. Intracranial angiographic images (**c**) show absence of filling of the anterior cerebral artery (*arrowhead*), indicating anatomical variant

Table 5.2. Scan parameters for MRA examination of carotid arteries.

	CE-MRA	3D-TOF
TE (ms)	1.1	4.24
TR (ms)	3.4	34
rFOV (mm)	320	220/240
Slice thickness (mm)	1.1	0.7
Flip angle (°)	25	30
Voxel size (mm)	1.3 × 0.6 × 1.1	1.0 × 0.8 × 1.0
Matrix	512	512
Scan time	0:19	3:12

netic field and the isocenter correction that corrects all the movement imperfections introduced by the rotating *C*-arc [37]. The 3D volume obtained in this way can be rotated and viewed in any direction, and optimal tube positioning (angulation and skew) can be chosen (Fig. 5.15). Determination of vessel geometrical properties (length, diameter) can be done manually or using automated vessel analysis (AVA) software, yielding shaded surface display images, or volume rendering and MIP images (Fig. 5.16). The measurement error has been established to be acceptably low [34]. The AVA software can also provide an endoscopic view (virtual angioscopy), used for evaluation of the vessel interior. Recent developments in software, using an unenhanced and a contrast-enhanced run, also allow visualization of calcifications. The same method can provide an improved depiction of stent location and its relation to the calcified plaque and vessel wall. Important information on flow dynamics can be gathered from the cine-fluoroscopic angiographic images.

A disadvantage of the first-generation 3D-RA technique is nonvisualization of thrombus. The same is true for conventional angiography. Calcification, however, can be demonstrated using 3D-RA (using either the source images showing some indirect signs of the presence of thrombus – discrepancy between angiographic lumen and location of calcification – or the calcified plaque software). New developments allow for acquisition of CT-like images (XperCT, InnovaCT, DynaCT), which overcome the limitations of the initially available techniques, being able to demonstrate soft plaque (Figs. 5.17 and 5.18).

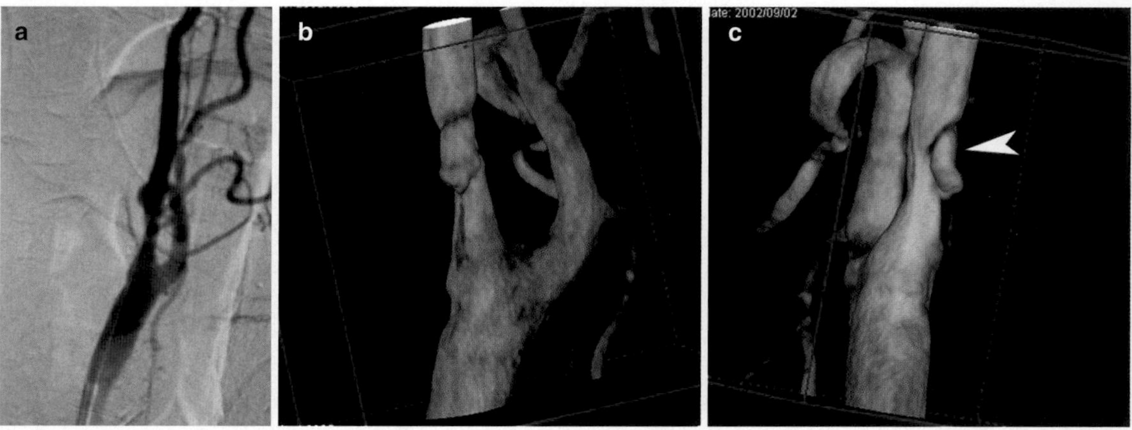

FIG. 5.15. Digital subtraction angiography (**a**) showing carotid bifurcation with slight narrowing of the proximal internal carotid artery. Volume-rendered image obtained with 3D rotational angiography (**b**) with similar projection as (**a**), demonstrating narrowing and irregularities at proximal internal carotid artery. In a different projection (**c**), the stenosis and ulcerative characteristics of the internal carotid artery lesion (*arrowhead*) are demonstrated to advantage

A major use of 3D-RA is in a therapeutic setting in the interventional suite rather than as a diagnostic modality in cases with complex anatomy. The major role in diagnosis has been overtaken mainly by CTA and MRA. However, it has been demonstrated that 3D-RA using nonselective aortic arch injection yields a good correlation with the degree of stenosis when compared with selective angiography using DSA techniques, with the additional advantage of an almost complete exclusion of the risk of neurological complications due to the manipulation of catheters needed for selective angiography [38].

The major advantage of 3D-RA is that due to the short reconstruction times, the interventionalist can optimize projection and make adjustments during the interventional procedure, to ensure optimal outcome, without a significant increase in procedure time, with a significant reduction of radiation exposure of the patient as compared with conventional angiographic imaging, and a decrease in the overall contrast load that can be achieved by eliminating multiple standard angiographic projections [39]. Further reduction in radiation dose can be achieved with the use of flat panel detectors of the direct conversion type [40]. More specifically, for carotid endovascular interventions, 3D-RA allows for determination of length and diameter of stent, and optimal diameter of the protection device.

Comparison of Methods

Review articles comparing duplex ultrasound and MRA and CTA with DSA have demonstrated that all noninvasive tests are highly accurate modalities in detecting severe carotid artery disease [41, 42]. For the distinction between <70% vs. 70–99% stenosis, MRA has a significantly better discriminatory power than duplex ultrasound (Table 5.3). It should be kept in mind in evaluating these studies that both MRA and CTA techniques have made significant advancements ever since the publication of these papers (e.g., high-resolution contrast-enhanced MRA and MDCT). A good correlation exists between MRA (TOF) and CTA regarding measurement of the degree of stenosis of carotid arteries as measured according to the NASCET method and using transverse raw data analysis (Fig. 5.19) [30, 43]. CTA may slightly overestimate the degree of stenosis [44] but reports of underestimation have also been published [12].

Noncontrast-enhanced MRA (using TOF technique) compares favorably with angiography, ultrasound, and excised plaques. A major limitation is its small field of view that does not allow for simultaneous visualization of carotid artery bifurcation, aortic arch anatomy, and the circle of Willis. Contrast-enhanced MRA has emerged and almost completely replaced TOF-MRA because of its

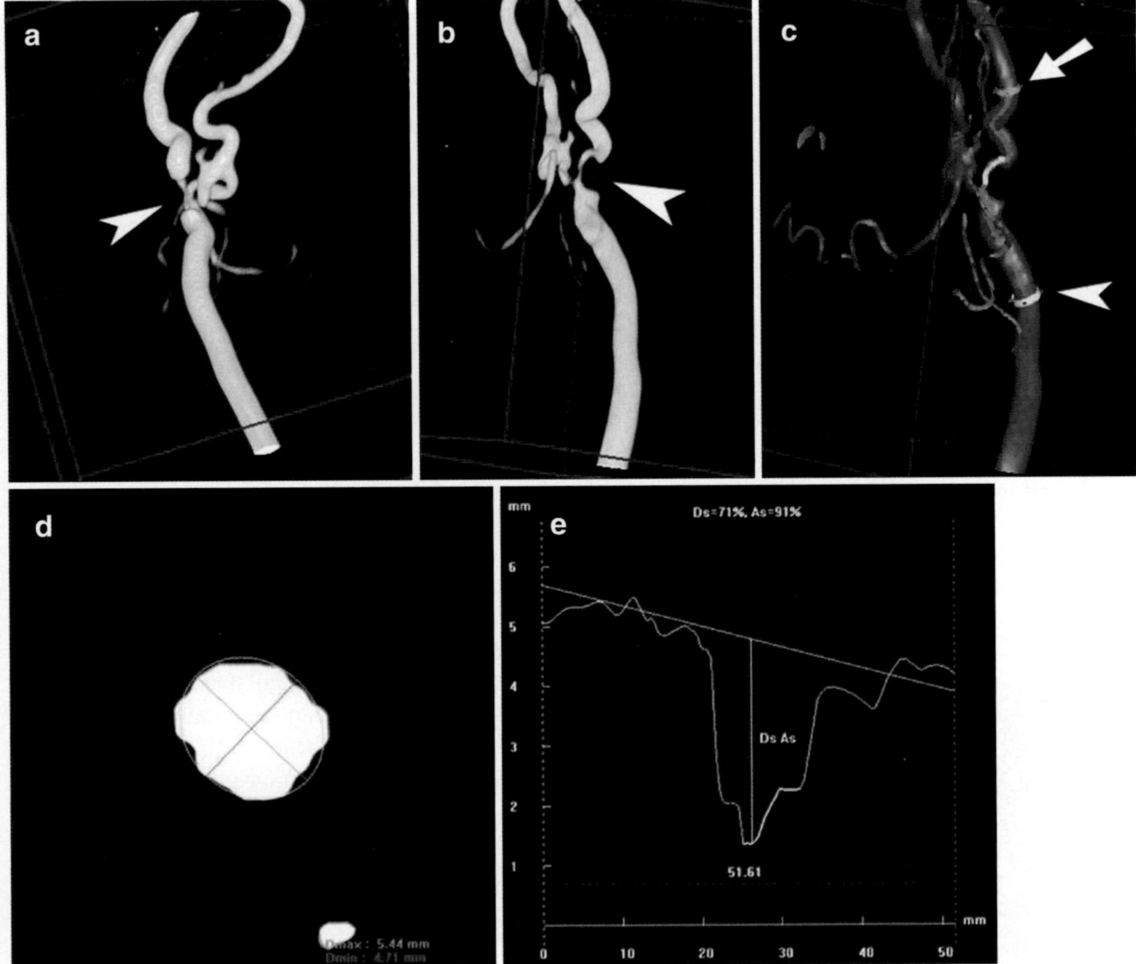

Fig. 5.16. Volume-rendered image in AP projection obtained with 3D rotational angiography (**a**) of carotid artery bifurcation with high-grade stenosis of the internal carotid artery (*arrowhead*). In an oblique projection (**b**), the carotid bifurcation and internal carotid artery stenosis (*arrowhead*) are demonstrated to advantage. Shaded surface display image after application of automated vessel analysis (**c**), demonstrating trajectory from distal common carotid artery (*yellow ring/arrowhead*) to proximal internal carotid artery (*green ring/arrow*). Transverse section (**d**) perpendicular to trajectory as demonstrated in (**c**) at the level of the internal carotid artery showing automated diameter measurements. (**e**) Graphical demonstration of diameters along the course of the trajectory shown in (**c**) with automated calculation of diameter and area stenosis; the AVA features facilitate choice of diameter of protection device and stent dimensions

shorter examination time and improved signal-to-noise ratio. Although several studies indicate a superiority of TOF-MRA as compared with CE-MRA, care should be taken in interpreting these findings since comparison of multiple projections using MRA was made with two- or three-directional DSA, as is described below [45–48]. When using high-resolution contrast-enhanced MRA with integrated parallel acquisition techniques (yielding a resolution of 0.9 × 0.7 × 0.9 mm), most of the problems of overestimation of high-grade stenosis can be reduced but still occur [28, 49]. A combination of three-dimensional TOF and contrast-enhanced MRA therefore seems to be advantageous [45].

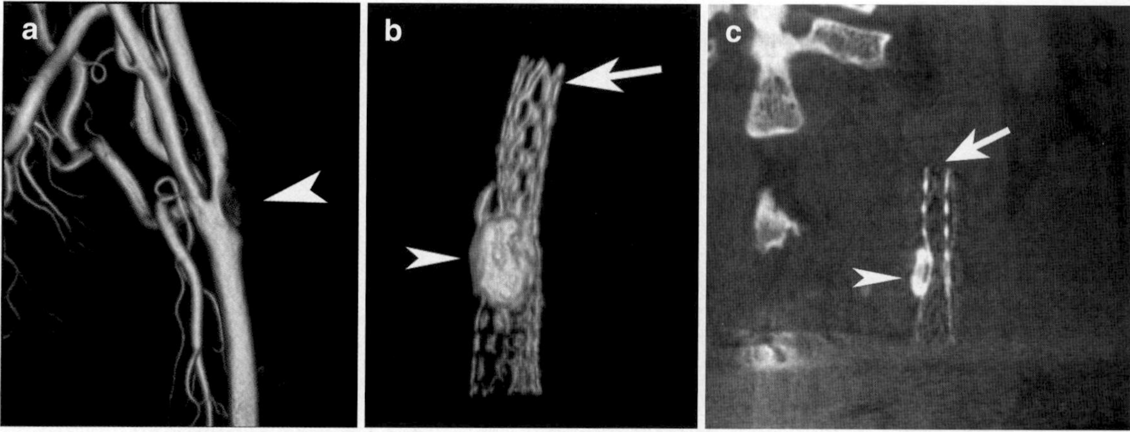

FIG. 5.17. Shaded surface display image of left carotid artery bifurcation (**a**), demonstrating severe stenosis caused by calcified plaque; 3D reconstruction of after stent placement (**b**) and CT-like MPR image (**c**) obtained from rotational run without contrast administration, clearly demonstrating stent struts (*arrow*) and calcified plaque (*arrowhead*). Courtesy of S. Bracard, R. Anxionnat, and L. Picard, Nancy, France

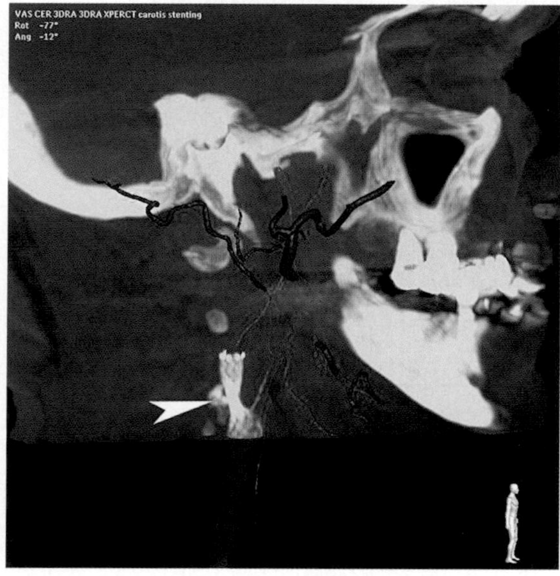

FIG. 5.18. Merged image of shaded surface display and MPR image obtained from rotational angiography run with intra-arterial contrast injection after carotid stent placement

Using state-of-the-art technique contrast-enhanced MRA can yield a sensitivity of 100%, a specificity of 99.3%, a positive predictive value of 93.6%, and a negative predictive value of 100% by using a 70–99% threshold of arterial diameter stenosis. For detection of occlusion, all these values are 100% [28]. Similar results can be obtained when using state-of-the-art CTA [30].

In vitro comparison of conventional angiography using two or three projections and 20-projection rotational angiography demonstrated that conventional angiography significantly underestimates the maximum stenosis [50]. In several studies comparing MRA (both TOF technique and contrast enhanced), conventional DSA, and rotational angiography, underestimation of internal carotid artery stenosis was seen when using DSA while contrast-enhanced MRA correlated best with rotational angiography [51, 52]. These findings can be explained by the inherent limitation of conventional DSA to the depiction of the carotid bifurcation and carotid arteries in only two or three projections. More specifically, for arteries in which the residual stenotic lumen has an asymmetric shape, this limitation can result in an underestimation of the narrowed portion of the noncircular residual lumen on conventional DSA (and explains the findings reporting overestimation of internal carotid artery stenosis on MRA studies as described above). Thus, conventional angiography, despite its higher resolution as compared with MR imaging, does not seem to be the reference standard for carotid artery imaging anymore, and this finding emphasizes the importance of the availability of multiple projections.

TABLE 5.3. Pooled weighted sensitivity and specificity of various imaging modalities as compared with digital subtraction angiography.

	Pooled sensitivity (%)			Pooled specificity (%)		
Stenosis grade	MRA	DUS	CTA	MRA	DUS	CTA
70–99% vs. <70%	95 (92–97)	86 (84–89)	85 (79–90)	90 (86–93)	87 (84–90)	94 (90–96)
<100% vs. 100%	98 (94–100)	96 (94–98)	97 (93–99)	100 (99–100)	100 (99–100)	99 (98–100)

DUS duplex ultrasound. Confidence interval between parentheses.

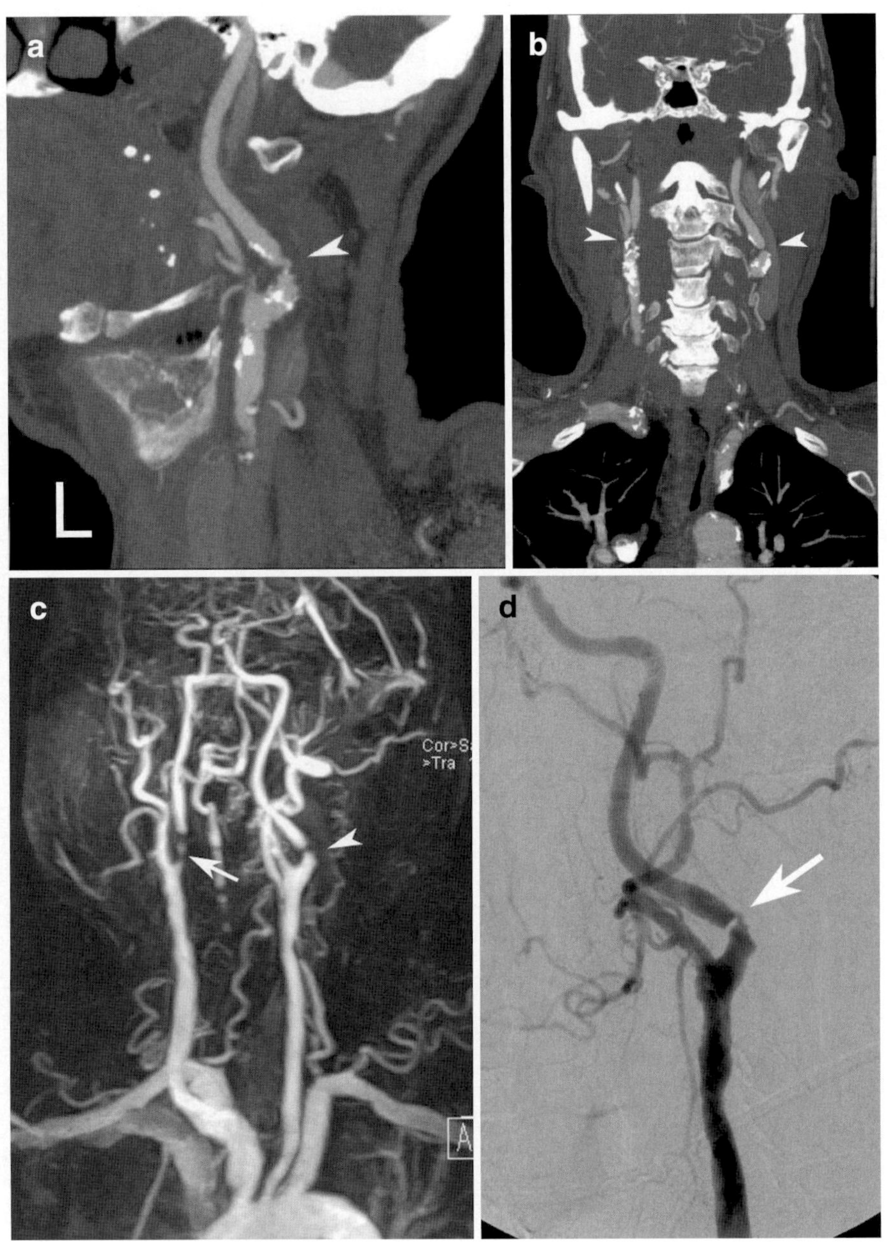

FIG. 5.19. Comparison of CTA, MRA, and DSA; bilateral internal carotid artery stenosis as demonstrated on parasagittal (**a**) and coronal (**b**) CTA MPR images, and MIP reconstruction of contrast-enhanced MRA (**c**) and the corresponding selective carotid arteriography (**d**); note the lack of visualization of calcified plaque and the overestimation of the grade of stenosis on contrast-enhanced MRA

Use of noninvasive imaging techniques further has the inherent advantage of the absence of procedural risk of minor and major stroke, TIAs, and asymptomatic lesions as observed with diffusion-weighted cerebral MRI [53]. When combining duplex ultrasound and another noninvasive diagnostic test, the number of intra-arterial angiographies can be reduced by 80% [2]. If MRA and duplex ultrasound really leave any questions unanswered, CTA using multidetector technology is the next diagnostic step [54]. The role of DSA will be limited to unclear cases [27]. Increasing concern about the costs and risks of angiography and improvements in noninvasive imaging implies that it is increasingly difficult to justify the risk of conventional DSA if the benefit in accuracy is marginal.

The advantages and disadvantages of the various imaging techniques used in the evaluation of carotid artery disease are listed in Table 5.4.

Future Developments

The use of digital subtraction techniques in combination with CTA has been demonstrated feasible. The technique consists of acquisition of a precontrast and postcontrast scan. A three-dimensional model of the bony structures and calcifications is reconstructed from the first nonenhanced data set. The bone model is then combined with the postcontrast data set, and subtraction of both data sets follows (Fig. 5.20) [55]. Crucial factors in obtaining

TABLE 5.4. Overview of advantages and disadvantages of imaging modalities.

	DUS	DSA	CTA	MRA	3D-RA
Gold standard	±	±	±	+	+
Invasiveness	−	+	−	−	+
Ionizing radiation	−	+	+	−	+
Nephrotoxic contrast	−	+	+	−	+
Venous contamination	−	−	+	+	−
Spatial resolution	−	++	+	±	++
Dynamic information	−	+	−	+	+
Anatomical coverage	±	+	++	++	+
Cost	±	++	+	+	++

DUS Doppler ultrasound

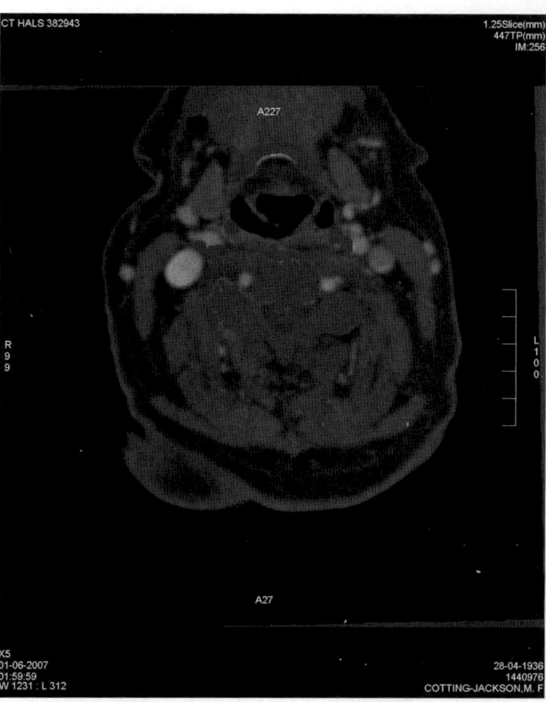

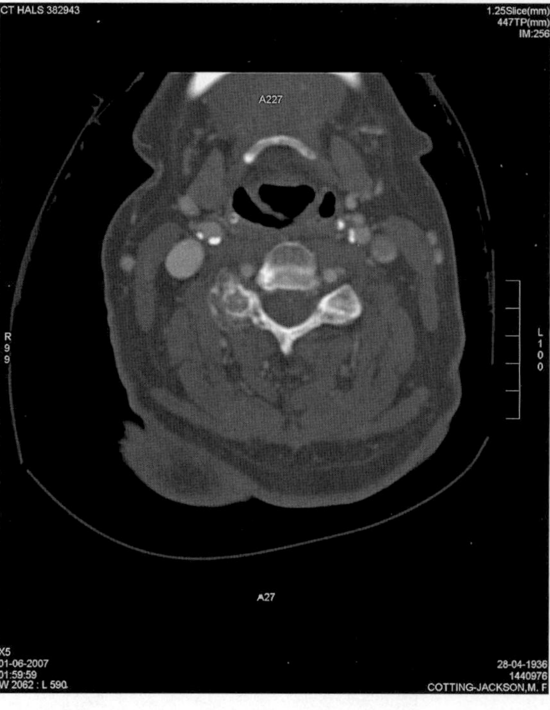

FIG. 5.20. Axial CTA image after intravenous contrast injection (**a**) and axial image (**b**) after subtraction of bony structures and calcified plaque (using an unenhanced image); in this way, artifacts caused by high-density structures can be diminished. Courtesy of R. van den Berg, Amsterdam, The Netherlands

good quality subtraction are avoidance of movement artifacts and accurate registration of both data sets. Digital subtraction CTA offers a potential advantage when separation of the vasculature from bone is important and technically difficult. Automated CTA quantification of internal carotid artery stenosis has been demonstrated feasible, but diagnostic accuracy is not yet sufficient for clinical application [56].

Currently, 3D roadmap functionality that allows for (online) navigation in a three-dimensional fashion during the intervention (even during rotation of the *C*-arm) is available for intracranial interventions (Fig. 5.21), and it is the line of expectation that after clinical validation this option will also become available for peripheral interventions, including carotid interventions. Currently, applications in the peripheral field are still hampered by motion artifacts.

Conclusions

Preprocedure imaging as an addition to duplex ultrasound is useful in selected cases prior to carotid endarterectomy and is of crucial importance and mandatory in the planning of CAS. Both MRA and CTA yield a diagnostic accuracy that is equal or higher to the former "gold standard" DSA, with the additional advantage of a reduction of the adverse events associated with the invasive nature of angiography. Both MRA and CTA can provide the anatomical detail that is necessary to select patients that are suited for an endovascular procedure for stenotic disease of the carotid artery. The role of angiography will continue to decrease and will be limited in the future to procedural guidance.

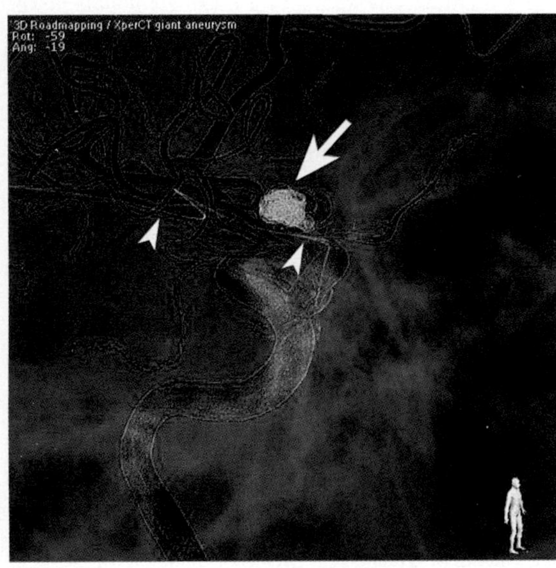

Fig. 5.21. 3D roadmap image based on shaded surface display image after 3D rotational angiography during coiling of intracranial aneurysm (*arrow*); the course of the guidewire of the microcatheter can be clearly seen (*arrowheads*); this feature allows for optimal navigation in tortuous anatomy; the 3D roadmap adjusts automatically with changes in *C*-arm position

Key Points

- "Overview" anatomical imaging is mandatory for evaluation of suitability for CAS.
- Imaging modalities currently used in routine practice are DSA, CTA, MRA, and less frequently 3D-RA.

Catheter Angiography

- Selective catheter angiography in patients with symptomatic cerebrovascular disease may cause disabling stroke and death.
- Arch aortography is associated with much lower neurological complications but access site and contrast-related complications persist.
- 3D rotational angiography is associated with low neurological risk and is useful in a therapeutic setting in the interventional suite rather than as a standalone diagnostic modality.

Computed Tomographic Angiography (CTA)

- Multidetector row CTA has improved spatial resolution, reduced scan time (allowing imaging from the inner curve of the aortic arch to the circle of Willis in one breath-hold), and reduced radiation dose relative to DSA.
- Of a number of postprocessing algorithms, MPR and 3D VRTs are of most use for assessing the extracranial carotid circulation.
- The precision of CTA is more dependent on measurement technique than acquisition parameters. The degree of stenosis is best measured

perpendicular to the carotid artery on magnified transverse oblique images.

- Evaluation of axial reconstructions and use of "bone window" settings can mitigate for ring-like calcification or "blooming artifact" that may cause overestimation of degree of stenosis in heavily calcified vessels.
- CTA is unable to demonstrate flow dynamics and swallowing creates motion artifact that can be misdiagnosed as stenosis.

Magnetic Resonance Angiography

- MRA based on flow-based methods (i.e., time of flight) requires that the blood flow is at 90° to the imaging plane and these techniques are therefore usually limited to the neck.
- Gadolinium-enhanced MRA is not so dependent on vessel orientation but optimization of the diagnostic yield mandates evaluation of both the source and the reconstructed images. Signal voids still occur despite use of gadolinium due to intravoxel dephasing and limited spatial resolution.
- State-of-the-art technique contrast-enhanced MRA can yield a sensitivity of 100%, a specificity of 99.3%, a positive predictive value of 93.6%, and a negative predictive value of 100% by using a 70–99% threshold of arterial diameter stenosis. For detection of occlusion, all these values are 100%.

References

1. Back MR, Rogers GA, Wilson JS, Johnson BL, Shames ML, Bandyk DF. Magnetic resonance angiography minimizes need for arteriography after inadequate carotid duplex ultrasound scanning. J Vasc Surg 2003; 38(3):422–430.
2. Borisch I, Horn M, Butz Bet al., Preoperative evaluation of carotid artery stenosis: Comparison of contrast-enhanced MR angiography and duplex sonography with digital subtraction angiography. Am J Neuroradiol 2003; 24(6):1117–1122.
3. Erdoes LS, Marek JM, Mills JL et al., The relative contributions of carotid duplex scanning, magnetic resonance angiography, and cerebral arteriography to clinical decision making: A prospective study in patients with carotid occlusive disease. J Vasc Surg 1996; 23(5):950–956.
4. Randoux B, Marro B, Koskas F et al., Carotid artery stenosis: Prospective comparison of CT, three-dimensional gadolinium-enhanced MR, and conventional angiography. Radiology 2001; 220(1):179–185.
5. Chong PL, Salhiyyah K, Dodd PD. The role of carotid endarterectomy in the endovascular era. Eur J Vasc Endovasc Surg 2005; 29(6):597–600.
6. Patel SG, Collie DA, Wardlaw JM et al., Outcome, observer reliability, and patient preferences if CTA, MRA, or Doppler ultrasound were used, individually or together, instead of digital subtraction angiography before carotid endarterectomy. J Neurol Neurosurg Psychiatry 2002; 73(1):21–28.
7. Johnston DC, Chapman KM, Goldstein LB. Low rate of complications of cerebral angiography in routine clinical practice. Neurology 2001; 57(11):2012–2014.
8. Berczi V, Randall M, Balamurugan Ret al., . Safety of arch aortography for assessment of carotid arteries. Eur J Vasc Endovasc Surg 2006; 31(1):3–7.
9. Kopp AF, Kuttner A, Trabold T, Heuschmid M, Schroder S, Claussen CD. Contrast-enhanced MDCT of the thorax. Eur Radiol 2003; 13(Suppl 3):N44–N49.
10. Catalano C, Fraioli F, Danti M et al., MDCT of the abdominal aorta: Basics, technical improvements, and clinical applications. Eur Radiol 2003; 13(Suppl 3):N53–N58.
11. Haage P, Schmitz-Rode T, Hubner D, Piroth W, Gunther RW. Reduction of contrast material dose and artifacts by a saline flush using a double power injector in helical CT of the thorax. Am J Roentgenol 2000; 174(4):1049–1053.
12. Silvennoinen HM, Ikonen S, Soinne L, Railo M, Valanne L. CT angiographic analysis of carotid artery stenosis: Comparison of manual assessment, semiautomatic vessel analysis, and digital subtraction angiography. Am J Neuroradiol 2007; 28(1):97–103.
13. Siegel MJ. Multiplanar and three-dimensional multi-detector row CT of thoracic vessels and airways in the pediatric population. Radiology 2003; 229(3):641–650.
14. Sameshima T, Futami S, Morita Yet al., . Clinical usefulness of and problems with three-dimensional CT angiography for the evaluation of arteriosclerotic stenosis of the carotid artery: Comparison with conventional angiography, MRA, and ultrasound sonography.Surg Neurol 1999; 51(3):301–308.
15. Lee EY, Siegel MJ, Hildebolt CF, Gutierrez FR, Bhalla S, Fallah JH. MDCT evaluation of thoracic aortic anomalies in pediatric patients and young adults: Comparison of axial, multiplanar, and 3D images. Am J Roentgenol 2004; 182(3):777–784.
16. Smith PA, Heath DG, Fishman EK. Virtual angioscopy using spiral CT and real-time interactive volume-rendering techniques. J Comput Assist Tomogr 1998; 22(2):212–214.

17. Bartolozzi C, Neri E, Caramella D. CT in vascular pathologies. Eur Radiol 1998; 8(5):679–684.
18. Cinat M, Lane CT, Pham H, Lee A, Wilson SE, Gordon I. Helical CT angiography in the preoperative evaluation of carotid artery stenosis. J Vasc Surg 1998; 28(2):290–300.
19. Ho VB, Corse WR, Hood MN, Rowedder AM. MRA of the thoracic vessels. Semin Ultrasound CT MR 2003; 24(4):192–216.
20. Ho VB, Prince MR. Thoracic MR aortography: Imaging techniques and strategies. Radiographics 1998; 18(2):287–309.
21. Merkle EM, Klein S, Wisianowsky C et al., Magnetic resonance imaging versus multislice computed tomography of thoracic aortic endografts. J Endovasc Ther 2002; 9(Suppl 2):112–113.
22. Leung DA, Debatin JF. Three-dimensional contrast-enhanced magnetic resonance angiography of the thoracic vasculature. Eur Radiol 1997; 7(7):981–989.
23. Holmqvist C, Larsson E-M, Stahlberg F, Laurin S. Contrast-enhanced thoracic 3D-MR angiography in infants and children. Acta Radiol 2001; 42(1):50–58.
24. Willinek WA, Gieseke J, Conrad R et al., Randomly segmented central k-space ordering in high-spatial-resolution contrast-enhanced MR angiography of the supraaortic arteries: Initial experience. Radiology 2002; 225(2):583–588.
25. Wintersperger BJ, Huber A, Preissler Get al., . MR angiography of the supraaortic vessels. Radiologe 2000; 40(9):785–791.
26. Riederer SJ, Bernstein MA, Breen JF et al., . Three-dimensional contrast-enhanced MR angiography with real-time fluoroscopic triggering: Design specifications and technical reliability in 330 patient studies. Radiology 2000; 215(2):584–593.
27. Remonda L, Senn P, Barth A, Arnold M, Lovblad KO, Schroth G. Contrast-enhanced 3D MR angiography of the carotid artery: Comparison with conventional digital subtraction angiography. Am J Neuroradiol 2002; 23(2):213–219.
28. Willinek WA, von Falkenhausen M, Born M et al., Noninvasive detection of steno-occlusive disease of the supra-aortic arteries with three-dimensional contrast-enhanced magnetic resonance angiography: A prospective, intra-individual comparative analysis with digital subtraction angiography. Stroke 2005; 36(1):38–43.
29. Wardlaw JM, Lewis SC, Humphrey P, Young G, Collie D, Warlow CP. How does the degree of carotid stenosis affect the accuracy and interobserver variability of magnetic resonance angiography? J Neurol Neurosurg Psychiatry 2001; 71(2):155–160.
30. Lell M, Fellner C, Baum Uet al., Evaluation of carotid artery stenosis with multisection CT and MR imaging: Influence of imaging modality and post-processing. Am J Neuroradiol 2007; 28(1):104–110.
31. Johnston DC, Eastwood JD, Nguyen T, Goldstein LB. Contrast-enhanced magnetic resonance angiography of carotid arteries: Utility in routine clinical practice. Stroke 2002; 33(12):2834–2838.
32. Klucznik RP. Current technology and clinical applications of three-dimensional angiography. Radiol Clin North Am 2002; 40(4):711–728, v.
33. Unno N, Mitsuoka H, Takei Yet al., . Virtual angioscopy using 3-dimensional rotational digital subtraction angiography for endovascular assessment. J Endovasc Ther 2002; 9(4):529–534.
34. van den Berg JC, Overtoom TT, de Valois JC, Moll FL. Using three-dimensional rotational angiography for sizing of covered stents. Am J Roentgenol 2002; 178(1):149–152.
35. van den Berg JC, Moll FL. Three-dimensional rotational angiography in peripheral endovascular interventions. J Endovasc Ther 2003; 10(3):595–600.
36. van den Berg JC. Three-dimensional rotational angiography. In: Wyatt MG, Watkinson AF (eds). Endovascular Intervention – Current Controversies. Shrewsbury, UK: tfm Publishing, 2004, pp. 247–256.
37. Bridcut RR, Winder RJ, Workman A, Flynn P. Assessment of distortion in a three-dimensional rotational angiography system. Br J Radiol 2002; 75(891):266–270.
38. Pozzi MF, Calgaro A, Bruni S, Bottaro L, Pozzi MR. Three-dimensional rotational angiography of the carotid arteries with high-flow injection from the aortic arch. Preliminary experience. Radiol Med (Torino) 2005; 109(1–2):108–117.
39. Racadio JM, Fricke BL, Jones BV, Donnelly LF. Three-dimensional rotational angiography of neurovascular lesions in pediatric patients. Am J Roentgenol 2006; 186(1):75–84.
40. Hatakeyama Y, Kakeda S, Korogi Y et al., Intracranial 2D and 3D DSA with flat panel detector of the direct conversion type: Initial experience. Eur Radiol 2006; 16(11):2594–2602.
41. Nederkoorn PJ, van der Graaf Y, Hunink MG. Duplex ultrasound and magnetic resonance angiography compared with digital subtraction angiography in carotid artery stenosis: A systematic review.Stroke 2003; 34(5):1324–1332.
42. Koelemay MJ, Nederkoorn PJ, Reitsma JB, Majoie CB. Systematic review of computed tomographic angiography for assessment of carotid artery disease. Stroke 2004; 35(10):2306–2312.
43. Binaghi S, Maeder P, Uske A, Meuwly JY, Devuyst G, Meuli RA. Three-dimensional computed tomography angiography and magnetic resonance angiography

of carotid bifurcation stenosis. Eur Neurol 2001; 46(1):25–34.

44. Hacklander T, Wegner H, Hoppe Set al., . Agreement of multislice CT angiography and MR angiography in assessing the degree of carotid artery stenosis in consideration of different methods of postprocessing. J Comput Assist Tomogr 2006; 30(3):433–442.
45. Fellner C, Lang W, Janka R, Wutke R, Bautz W, Fellner FA. Magnetic resonance angiography of the carotid arteries using three different techniques: Accuracy compared with intraarterial x-ray angiography and endarterectomy specimens. J Magn Reson Imaging 2005; 21(4):424–431.
46. Townsend TC, Saloner D, Pan XM, Rapp JH. Contrast material-enhanced MRA overestimates severity of carotid stenosis, compared with 3D time-of-flight MRA. J Vasc Surg 2003; 38(1):36–40.
47. Nederkoorn PJ, Elgersma OE, Mali WP, Eikelboom BC, Kappelle LJ, van der Graaf Y. Overestimation of carotid artery stenosis with magnetic resonance angiography compared with digital subtraction angiography. J Vasc Surg 2002; 36(4):806–813.
48. Muhs BE, Gagne P, Wagener J et al., Gadolinium-enhanced versus time-of-flight magnetic resonance angiography: What is the benefit of contrast enhancement in evaluating carotid stenosis? Ann Vasc Surg 2005; 19(6):823–828.
49. Clevert DA, Johnson T, Michaely H et al., High-grade stenoses of the internal carotid artery: Comparison of high-resolution contrast enhanced 3D MRA, duplex sonography and power Doppler imaging. Eur J Radiol 2006; 60(3):379–386.
50. Zhang WW, Harris LM, Dryjski ML. Should conventional angiography be the gold standard for carotid stenosis? J Endovasc Ther 2006; 13(6):723–728.
51. Anzalone N, Scomazzoni F, Castellano Ret al., . Carotid artery stenosis: Intraindividual correlations of 3D time-of-flight MR angiography, contrast-enhanced MR angiography, conventional DSA, and rotational angiography for detection and grading. Radiology 2005; 236(1):204–213.
52. Elgersma OE, Wust AF, Buijs PC, van der Graaf Y, Eikelboom BC, Mali WP. Multidirectional depiction of internal carotid arterial stenosis: Three-dimensional time-of-flight MR angiography versus rotational and conventional digital subtraction angiography. Radiology 2000; 216(2):511–516.
53. Bendszus M, Koltzenburg M, Burger R, Warmuth-Metz M, Hofmann E, Solymosi L. Silent embolism in diagnostic cerebral angiography and neurointerventional procedures: A prospective study. Lancet 1999; 354(9190):1594–1597.
54. Forsting M, Wanke I. Funeral for a friend. Stroke 2003; 34(5):1324–1332.
55. Jayakrishnan VK, White PM, Aitken D, Crane P, McMahon AD, Teasdale EM. Subtraction helical CT angiography of intra- and extracranial vessels: Technical considerations and preliminary experience. Am J Neuroradiol 2003; 24(3):451–455.
56. Bucek RA, Puchner S, Kanitsar A, Rand T, Lammer J. Automated CTA quantification of internal carotid artery stenosis: A pilot trial. J Endovasc Ther 2007; 14(1):70–76.

6 Cerebral Arterial Anatomy

Ridwan Lynn and Alex Abou-Chebl

Cerebrovascular Anatomy

Disorders of the cerebrovascular system constitute a major class of diseases affecting the central nervous system. A detailed understanding of the cervical and cranial vascular anatomy and physiology is essential for successful diagnostic and interventional management of cerebrovascular disorders. This chapter will provide a basic overview of angiographic arterial anatomy of the cervicocranial circulation while emphasizing clinical considerations pertinent to interventions of the cervicocranial vasculature.

The Aortic Arch

Diagnostic and interventional studies of the cervicocranial vasculature typically begin in the aortic arch. The complex embryological development of the aortic arch leads to several anatomical variants that must be recognized for safe and efficient performance of interventions (Fig. 6.1) [1]. In the typical aortic arch configuration (65% of cases), the aortic arch gives rise first, proximal to distal, to the brachiocephalic trunk (the innominate artery), followed by the left common carotid artery (LCCA), and finally the left subclavian artery (Fig. 6.2). This is the so-called "left aortic arch" and is also the "friendly arch" configuration as it is the easiest for cannulation of the great vessels. The most common normal variant of the aortic arch (~25% of cases) is one in which the brachiocephalic trunk and the LCCA share a common origin, which can make LCCA cannulation more demanding. In approximately 7% of cases, the LCCA arises from the proximal brachiocephalic artery rather than from the aortic arch, the so-called "bovine" configuration, which makes LCCA cannulation even more difficult (Fig. 6.3).

Much less common variants include a left aortic arch with an aberrant right subclavian artery (˜0.4–2% of cases) that arises from the aortic arch near to or distal to the origin of the left subclavian artery (Fig. 6.4). The arch will therefore have four branches and often there is some tortuosity of the origins of the great vessels. When the left vertebral artery (VA) arises from the aortic arch (~0.5% of cases), typically in between the LCCA and left subclavian artery, the unsuspecting interventionalist may inadvertently cannulate the significantly smaller caliber VA, increasing the risk of causing a dissection and hindbrain stroke. Other rare variants (<<1% of cases) include a left brachiocephalic trunk giving rise to the LCCA and the left subclavian artery, a right aortic arch, a right aortic arch with mirror image branching, or even a double aortic arch.

Acquired abnormalities of the aortic arch can have a significant impact on carotid cannulation, especially in the population of patients at risk for carotid atherosclerosis. A type 1 aortic arch is the normal configuration and is one in which all three great vessels arise from the apex of the aortic arch, so that a horizontal line drawn in the axial plane (i.e., perpendicular to the long axis of the human body) at the apex of the arch will intersect the origin of all three vessels, or the origins will be at most within one carotid width below the apex. With increasing age, atherosclerosis

S. Macdonald and G. Stansby (eds.), *Practical Carotid Artery Stenting*,
DOI: 10.1007/978-1-84800-299-9_6, © Springer-Verlag London Limited 2009

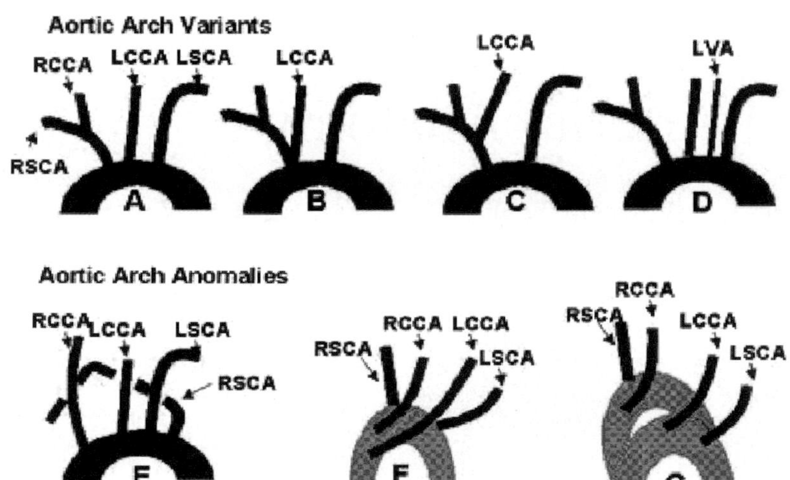

FIG. 6.1. Diagrammatic schema illustrating the most common variations in aortic arch configuration. Normal aortic arch as shown in (**a**) is found in about 65%. In (**b**), the left common carotid artery (LCCA) and brachiocephalic trunk share a common origin (25%). In (**c**), the so-called "bovine arch," the LCCA arises from the proximal brachiocephalic artery (7%). In (**d**), the left vertebral artery (LVA) arises directly from the aortic arch proximal to the origin of the left subclavian artery (LSCA) (0.5%) rather than from the LSCA itself. *RSCA* right subclavian artery, *RCCA* right common carotid artery

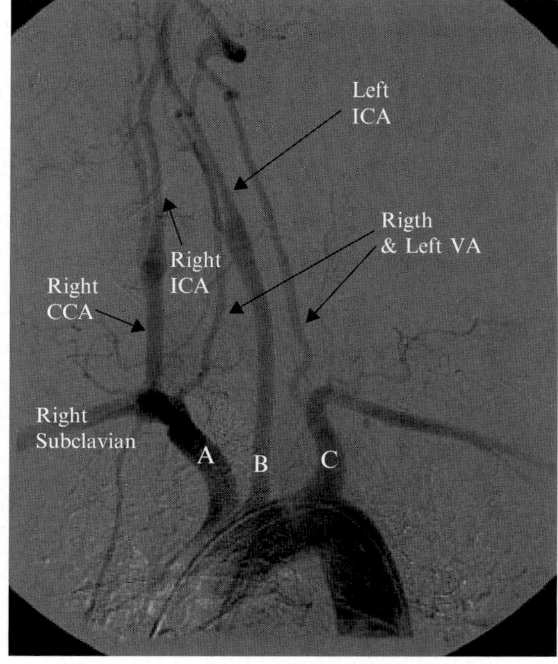

FIG. 6.2. Left anterior oblique aortic arch digital subtraction angiogram revealing a normal configuration of the aortic arch and great vessels. Note that this is a type 1 arch as the origins of the brachiocephalic trunk (**a**), left common carotid artery (**b**), and left subclavian artery (**c**) arise from the apex of the aortic arch. The great vessels have only mild tortuosity and the common carotid arteries (CCA) are relatively straight. Note also that the vertebral arteries (VA) are both large in caliber and are therefore codominant. In this view, the origin of the right VA (arrow head) is usually well visualized but the left is overlapped with the subclavian

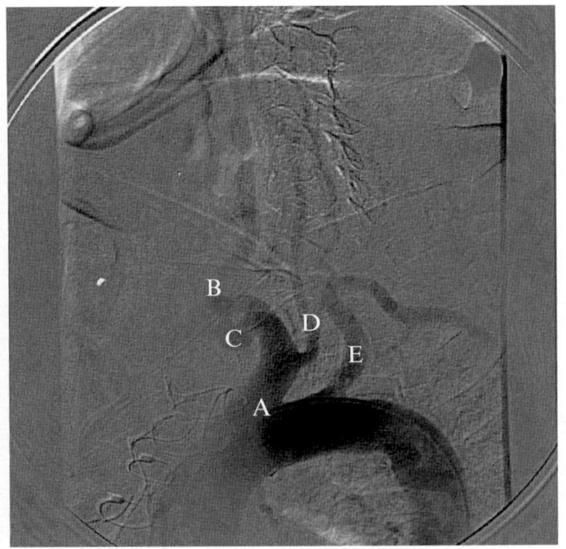

FIG. 6.3. Left anterior oblique aortic arch digital subtraction angiogram revealing a left aortic arch without a brachiocephalic trunk and an aberrant right subclavian artery origin. The right common carotid is the first branch of the arch (**a**). The second branch is the left common carotid (**b**). The right subclavian artery (**c**) arises directly from the aorta and its origin is overlapped with the left subclavian (**d**) and can arise distal to it

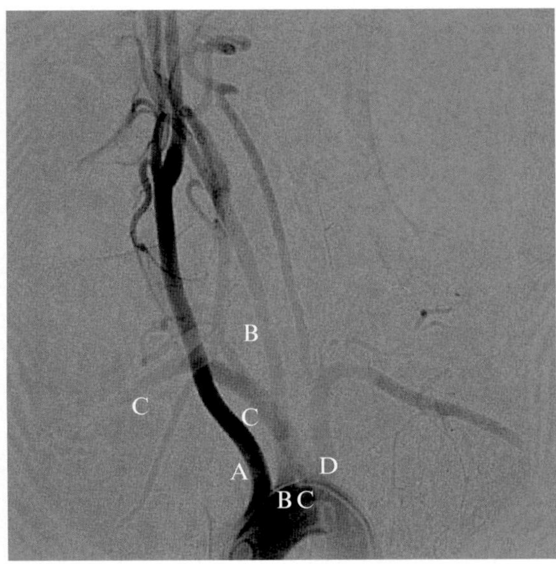

FIG. 6.4. A left anterior oblique aortic arch angiogram showing a type 3 arch configuration. Note that the aortic arch apex is narrow and higher than the origins of the great vessels. The innominate artery has a low origin (greater than two carotid widths below the arch apex) from the arch. Note also the tortuosity of the great vessels in this patient with longstanding severe hypertension

and uncontrolled hypertension can lead to elongation and rostral migration of the distal aortic arch and a change in the relative positions of the great vessels. As the LCCA and the left subclavian artery migrate rostrally along with the distal arch, the arch itself begins to take on a narrowed and peaked appearance rather than a smooth convex shape. As a result, the innominate appears to arise lower than usual, i.e., from the ascending aorta. The LCCA and the left subclavian artery can also arise from this ascending segment. These changes combine to make cannulation of the innominate and LCCA difficult if not impossible particularly with type 3 arches, the most extreme configuration with the innominate artery arising more than two carotid widths below the apex of the arch (Fig. 6.5). A type 2 arch lies somewhere in between types 1 and 2 and the innominate will arise between one and two carotid widths below the apex [2, 3].

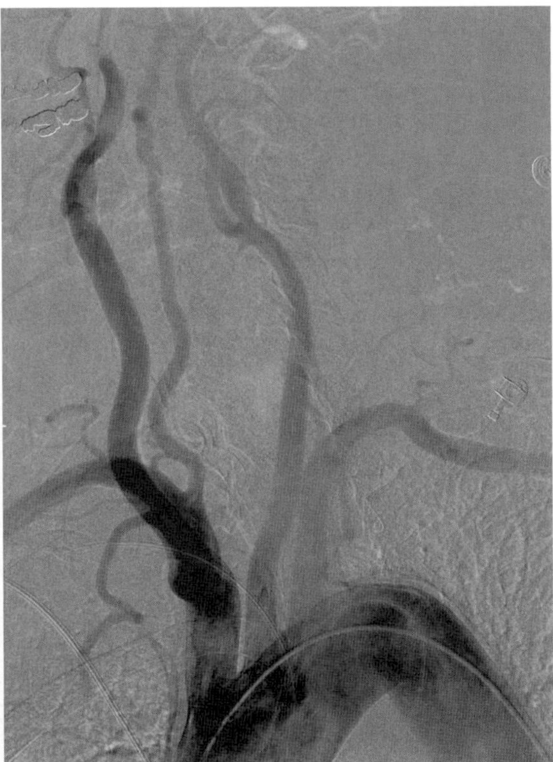

FIG. 6.5. Left anterior oblique arch angiogram showing a "bovine configuration" wherein the left common carotid artery (**d**) arises from the innominate artery (**a**). The remainder of the great vessels have normal origins including the right common carotid (**b**) and right subclavian (**c**) arteries which arise normally from the innominate artery leaving the left subclavian artery (**e**) as the second branch of the aorta

The Cervical Vessels

The vascular supply to the brain is derived from two pairs of cervical vessels: the internal carotid arteries (ICAs) and VAs. The ICAs supply blood to the anterior intracranial circulation while the VAs contribute to the posterior intracranial circulation, also known as the *vertebrobasilar circulation*. The ICA and VA systems are interconnected via anastomoses that can be clinically significant when one or more vessels become(s) occluded. Occlusion of the ICAs or VAs causes unique clinical vascular syndromes. However, due to the presence of intracranial collateral channels, namely the circle of Willis, some pathological conditions may be clinically silent or may affect unexpected regions of the brain (e.g., an occipital stroke from an ICA stenosis) leading to diagnostic uncertainty for the unwary.

The right CCA arises medially and rostrally from the innominate artery, whereas the left CCA arises directly from the aortic arch and runs posterolaterally (Fig. 6.2). CCAs are approximately 7–8 mm in diameter and generally have no branches prior to their bifurcations. They are straight vessels although they can become quite tortuous with age and prolonged hypertension. Loops in the CCA are unusual. The CCA bifurcates into the ICA and the external carotid artery (ECA) (Fig. 6.6). The CCA bifurcation occurs most commonly at the level of the third to fourth cervical vertebrae (C3–C4), which is also at the level of the angle of the jaw, but it can be as low as the first thoracic (T1) and as high as the first cervical vertebra (C1). The relative position of this bifurcation is critical to note on angiography since very high and very low anatomical bifurcations can make surgical exposure very difficult and risky and such patients may be better treated endovascularly.

The ECA is the smaller of the two terminal branches of the CCA and is distinguished from the ICA by its numerous branches in the neck (Fig. 6.6). The ECA branches supply blood to the soft tissues of the face, mouth, pharynx, larynx, and the neck.

They also serve as potential sources of collateral blood flow to the intracranial circulation in the setting of high-grade proximal internal carotid stenosis or occlusion. The ECA has a rich anastomotic network between its branches and the contralateral ECA, so that complete occlusion of one ECA is rarely of clinical consequence. In addition to supplying collaterals to the internal carotid circulation, the ECA supplies collaterals to the VA, most commonly via the occipital artery through the muscular and spinal branches of the VA at the level of the first and second cervical vertebrae. There is significant variability in the configuration of the ECA and its branches. In regards to the cerebral circulation, the most important branches of the ECA are the ascending pharyngeal, occipital artery, middle meningeal artery, and several small branches of the

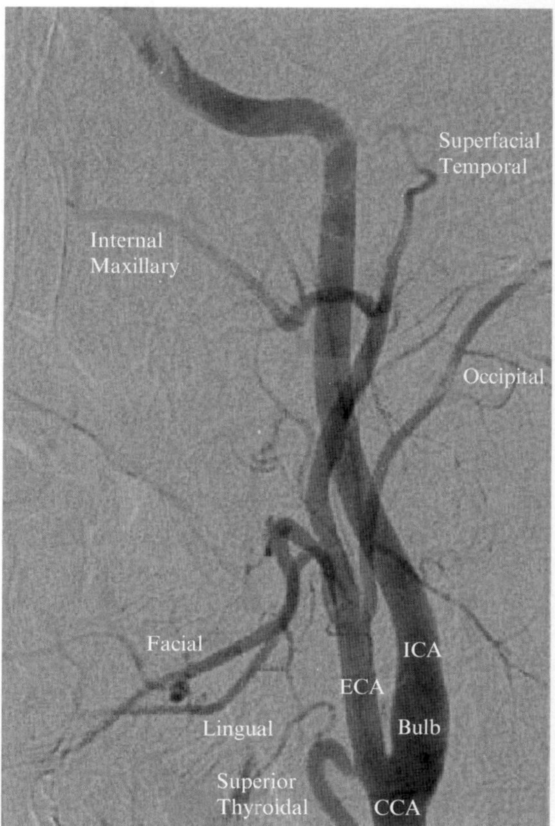

FIG. 6.6. Left anterior oblique view of a left common carotid artery (CCA) angiogram showing a normal carotid bifurcation. Note the dilatation of the internal carotid artery (ICA) known as the *carotid bulb*. The remainder of the cervical ICA is straight and has no branches. The external carotid artery (ECA) originates anteromedially off the CCA; it is smaller than the ICA, does not have a bulb, and has multiple branches, some of which (the superior thyroidal, facial, lingual, occipital, internal maxillary, and superficial temporal arteries) are seen in this figure

internal maxillary artery, all of which anastomose with the intracranial circulation. Intracranial ICA collateral sources include the vidian artery, caroticotympanic artery, artery of the foramen rotundum, the inferiolateral trunk, and the ophthalmic artery, which can fully reconstitute intracranial ICA flow.

The ICA (measuring 4–6 mm) is the larger of the two branches of the CCA and arises posterolaterally from the CCA, while the ECAs arise anteromedially (Fig. 6.6). The two ICAs supply 80% of cerebral blood flow (CBF). They supply the majority of the cerebrum including the frontal, parietal, anterior and lateral temporal lobes, and the deep gray structures except for the thalamus. The ICA contains two important sensory organs involved in the maintenance of brain tissue perfusion and oxygenation. The proximal 1.5 cm of the ICA dilates to 7–9 mm in diameter and is known as the *carotid bulb* (Fig. 6.6). This is a richly innervated structure and is also called the *carotid sinus*, which is involved in arterial blood pressure regulation. Raised arterial pressure and increased wall tension within the bulb trigger reflex bradycardia (mediated via the vagal nerve) and vasodilation (via sympathetic inhibition) and consequently a reduction in arterial pressure. A reduction in tension on the wall of the carotid bulb results in an opposite response. The purpose of the carotid sinus baroreflex therefore is to maintain cerebral perfusion constant. The other organ of the carotid bulb is the carotid body, a sensory organ with chemoreceptors that respond to arterial oxygen tension. Activation of afferents by the chemoreceptors in the carotid body results in an increase in ventilation to increase tissue oxygenation. Surgical and endovascular procedures on the carotid bulb may affect the function of the carotid sinus and result in hemodynamic perturbations (e.g., injury to the carotid sinus from endarterectomy is associated with increased sympathetic outflow and hypertension, whereas stimulation of the carotid sinus during angioplasty can cause bradycardia and hypotension) [4] (see Chap. 14).

The carotid artery distal to the bulb is generally straight and migrates medially before it enters the carotid canal in the petrous bone. The cervical ICA lies within the carotid sheath along with the jugular vein and the vagus nerve. Several other nerves (i.e., the recurrent laryngeal, hypoglossal, and the sympathetic nerves) course either with the ICA or across it and are therefore prone to injury during carotid surgery, trauma, or dissection. The ICA does not have any branches in the neck although rarely the ascending pharyngeal or superior thyroid arteries can arise from the bulb. Also rarely found is the persistence of fetal connections between the cervical ICA and the VA (i.e., the proatlantal intersegmental arteries, types 1 and 2). Hypoplasia or atresia of the ICA are very rare and can be differentiated from acquired occlusion by the small size of the carotid canal on plain skull X-rays.

The paired VAs arise from the subclavian arteries and ascend in the neck within the transverse foramina of the cervical vertebrae before entering the cranium (Fig. 6.2). The VAs are classically divided into four segments (V1–V4). The first (V1) segment extends from the VA origin off the subclavian artery through its posterior–rostral course toward the C6 transverse foramen. The V2 segment of the VA courses rostrally within the transverse foramina of the C6 to C2 vertebral bodies. The V3 segment consists of the VA segment that projects posteriorly over the superior surface of the ring of the atlas (C1) before making a sharp anterior–superior turn to pierce the atlanto-occipital membrane to become the intracranial segment (V4). The cervical VAs give off small cervical branches to supply the cervical muscles, spinal cord and periosteum of the cervical vertebrae, and meningeal branches to supply the dura in the posterior fossa.

Asymmetry in the size of the VAs is common. In 50% of cases, the left VA is larger and dominant, whereas the right VA is larger in 25% and the vessels are codominant in the remainder (Fig. 6.2). Atherosclerotic narrowing of the dominant VA therefore can be symptomatic if the contralateral VA is hypoplastic; however, ECA to VA anastomoses (through the ascending cervical artery, occipital artery, and ascending pharyngeal artery) may also account for variability in the symptomatology.

Intracranial Vessels

The anterior and posterior circulations are interconnected at the base of the brain via a circular anastomosis known as the *circle of Willis*. The ICA circulation is connected to the vertebrobasilar circulation via a pair of posterior communicating arteries (PCom). Anteriorly, a single anterior communicating artery (ACom) unites the paired anterior cerebral arteries (ACAs), thus completing the circular anastomosis (Fig. 6.7a). The circular network provides an important collateral source of blood flow, so that even if three of the four cervical vessels (i.e., ICAs and VAs) are occluded, the entire brain can potentially be supplied from the remaining vessel. In reality, the circle of Willis and all of its components are complete in only about 25% of individuals, so the majority of humans are at some risk of cerebral ischemia if one of the four main cerebral vessels shuts down [5]. Figure 6.7 illustrates the variants in the circle of Willis. The most common variant involves a hypoplastic or absent PCom (unilateral or bilateral). The other common variant is the persistence of a large PCom (fetal posterior cerebral artery – PCA) that feeds the entire PCA, so that the PCA becomes a branch of the ICA rather than the basilar artery (BA) (Fig. 6.8). In such cases, the proximal PCA segment between the basilar artery apex and the PCom (i.e., the P1 segment) is hypoplastic or atretic. The PCom on the side of the fetal PCA is therefore not a source of collateral blood supply to the ICA territory. If a fetal PCA is combined with another common variant, an absent ACom or an absent or atretic A1 segment of the ipsilateral ACA (i.e., the horizontal ACA segment between the ICA terminus and the ACom), the ICA territory on that side is considered to be isolated and has no direct potential collateral sources (Fig. 6.8). In these cases, significant flow-limiting stenoses of the proximal ICA are often symptomatic.

The intracranial ICA can be subdivided into several segments and there are several naming schemata. The easiest nomenclature is to refer to each segment by the name of an adjacent structure or by the name of the structure through which it courses (Fig. 6.9). The ICA enters the skull via the carotid canal within the dense petrous portion of the temporal bone, hence its name is the petrous carotid segment. The petrous segment takes a horizontal and anteromedial course before turning rostrally

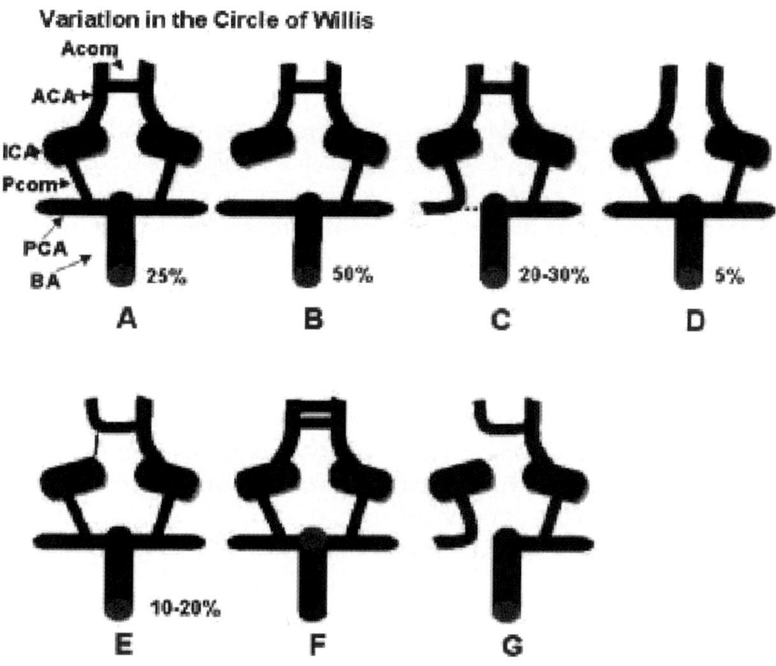

Fig. 6.7. Simplified schema illustrates the variations in the circle of Willis. (**a**) Complete circle of Willis (25%), (**b**) absent PCom (25–50%), (**c**) fetal PCA (20–30%), (**d**) absent ACom (5%), (**e**) hypoplastic or atretic ACom (10–20%), (**f**) duplicated ACom (18%), and (**g**) isolated ICA (coexistence of absent A1 segment of ACA and fetal PCA). *ACom* anterior communicating artery, *ACA* anterior cerebral artery, *ICA* internal carotid artery, *PCom* posterior communicating artery, *PCA* posterior cerebral artery, *BA* basilar artery

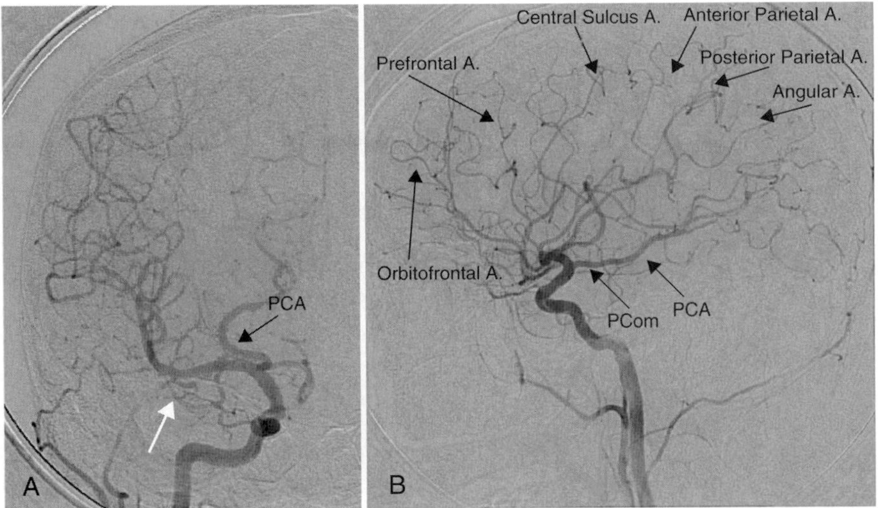

FIG. 6.8. An anteroposterior (**a**) and lateral (**b**) common carotid angiogram highlighting common anatomical variants of the circle of Willis. In the AP view (**a**), the A1 segment of the anterior cerebral artery (ACA) is absent (note the absence of any vessels running in the usual location of the ACA parallel to the black line) and only the frontopolar artery fills (*dashed arrow*). The posterior communicating artery (PCom) is large in caliber (**b**) and is seen filling the posterior cerebral artery (PCA) which is seen with the typical "S" curve appearance lateral to the midline in the AP plane (**a**) and coursing posteriorly on the lateral view (**b**). This is the so-called "fetal PCA" suggesting that the P1 segment of the PCA normally arising from the basilar artery is either absent or atretic. In this angiogram, the lack of the ACA branches makes identification of the middle cerebral artery (MCA) branches simpler, particularly in the lateral view (**b**). The MCA trunk or M1 segment (*white arrow* in (**a**)) divides into a superior (*s* in (**b**)) and an inferior division (*i* in (**b**)). The relevant MCA cortical branches are shown in (**b**)

as it emerges from the carotid canal and enters the cavernous sinus forming the cavernous ICA. In the cavernous sinus, the ICA takes a rostral turn and makes a *C*-loop adjacent to the sphenoid bone before exiting the cavernous sinus and becoming intradural. The anterior clinoid process lies in this region. Therefore, the short segment of ICA, as it exits the cavernous sinus but before it becomes intradural, is the infraclinoidal ICA, which gives off an anteriorly directed ophthalmic artery (the first major and constant intracranial branch of the ICA). The supraclinoidal ICA courses posteriorly and rostrally and gives off the posteriorly directed PCom (Fig. 6.9). The PCom connects with the ipsilateral PCA and is the most constant of the fetal connections between the anterior and posterior circulations. Next, the ICA gives off the very important anterior choroidal artery, which is also directed posteriorly but which is very small and not always seen angiographically. The ICA ends at the carotid terminus (also carotid "T" or siphon) by bifurcating into the middle cerebral artery (MCA) and the ACA (Fig. 6.9).

The MCA is the most important vessel of the anterior circulation and supplies the largest portion of the cerebral hemispheres. It feeds important cortical regions including the primary sensory and motor cortices, Broca's area, Wernicke's area, the angular and superior temporal gyri (primary language areas in the dominant hemisphere), and their counterparts in the nondominant hemisphere (subserving visuospatial functions). Due to its larger size (compared with the ACA) and the typical configuration of the carotid terminus being one in which the ICA essentially becomes the MCA giving off the ACA at an extreme angle, the MCA is the recipient artery for the majority of cerebral emboli, whether emanating from ICA stenoses or from more proximal sources [6].

The MCA has several named branches and segments (Figs. 6.8 and 6.9). The most proximal segment is the M1 segment or the MCA trunk.

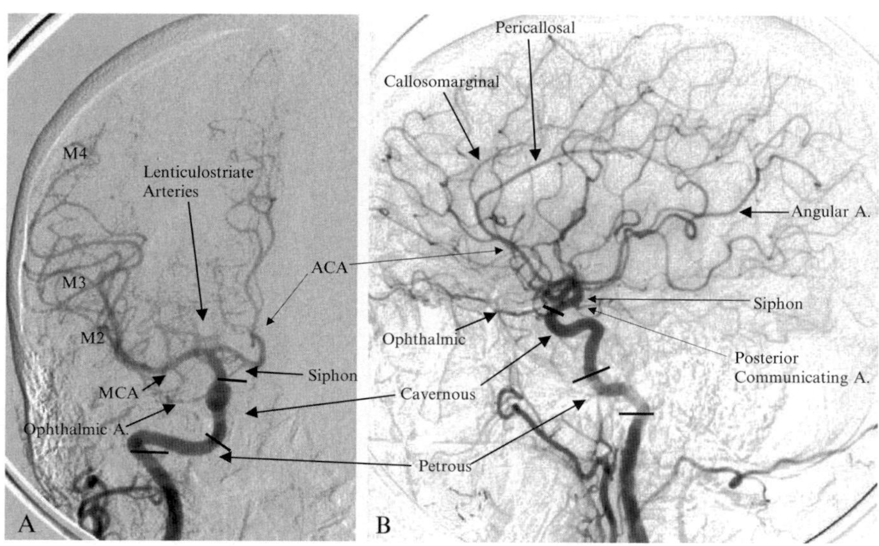

FIG. 6.9. Anteroposterior (**a**) and lateral (**b**) common carotid injection digital subtraction angiographic images showing normal intracranial carotid territory vascular anatomy. The three major segments of the intracranial internal carotid artery (petrous, cavernous, and siphon – also known as *terminus or carotid T*) are labeled. The ophthalmic artery is well visualized in both views whereas the posterior communicating artery is typically best seen arising from the carotid siphon in the lateral view (**b**). The middle cerebral artery (MCA) trunk is best seen in the AP plane as it is foreshortened and overlapped with its own branches on the lateral view. The MCA segments are named as a group by their general location and orientation relative to the Sylvian fissure (M2–M4). The M1 segment is by definition the horizontal segment of the MCA, which most often is the MCA trunk. The *angular artery* is labeled in the lateral view (**b**) as the posterior-most branch of the MCA as it exits from the Sylvian fissure. The lenticulostriate arteries arising from the MCA trunk are seen faintly as a collection of small vessels on the AP view (**a**). The anterior cerebral artery (ACA) segments (A1–A2) are shown in the AP projection and the two major branches of the ACA are best seen on the lateral view

This segment projects laterally toward the Sylvian fissure and also supplies multiple small perforating vessels (the lenticulostriate arteries) to the basal ganglia. Within the Sylvian fissure, the MCA trunk bifurcates (or trifurcates) into vertically oriented M2 segments, also known as the superior and inferior divisions, or the anterior and posterior divisions, respectively. The M3 segments are the next horizontal segments as the MCA branches take a turn laterally toward the surface of the Sylvian fissure. After exiting through the Sylvian fissure, the M4 segments travel over the lateral convexity of the cerebral hemisphere. Each M4 branch is named for the cortical gyrus it supplies. Similarly, the horizontal (and first) segment of the ACA is called the *A1 segment*. The A1 segment ends where the ACom connects the pair of ACAs and it continues rostrally in between the cerebral hemispheres and over the corpus callosum as the A2 segment. There are two major named branches of the ACAs: the pericallosal and callosomarginal arteries (Fig. 6.9).

The intracranial posterior circulation consists of the paired intracranial VAs (V4 segments), the BA, and its terminal branches, the PCAs (Fig. 6.10). The V4 segments of the VAs converge anterior to the caudal pons to form a single BA. Each VA gives off the posterior inferior cerebellar artery (PICA) in its mid-V4 segment before supplying a small but critical artery to the spinal cord, the anterior spinal artery, as well as small feeders to the medulla oblongata. In some cases, a non-dominant VA can terminate in PICA and not supply any flow to the BA which becomes effectively a continuation of the dominant contralateral VA. Also, the PICA can sometimes arise extracranially from the V3 segment and enter the intracranial cavity via the foramen magnum. The BA supplies critical structures within the brainstem that regulate motor function, eye movements, respiration, and wakefulness. The BA gives off small median and paramedian perforating arteries (to the pons primarily), the paired anterior inferior cerebellar arteries (AICA), and the paired superior cerebellar arteries (SCA) (Fig. 6.10). It terminates at the pontomesencephalic junction into the paired PCAs. The PCAs themselves supply perforators to the midbrain and thalamus before supplying the bulk of the blood flow to the occipital lobes and medial temporal lobes.

In addition to variations of the circle of Willis, there is also variability in the size, configuration, and branching patterns of the MCAs, VAs, and BA. Normal variants that may be of clinical consequence are persistent anterior-to-posterior circulation anastomoses other than the normal anastomosis, the PCom [7]. Early in fetal development, the carotid arteries develop first and supply flow to the vestigial vertebral arteries via multiple channels. At this stage, the VAs are not fully formed and consist of a rete mirabile or network of numerous small channels, which will fuse and eventually form the VAs and BA. The feeding channels from the ICAs will eventually regress as the VAs are formed leaving only the PComs as the sole anterior–posterior circulation connection. When these vestigial connections fail to regress, persistent anterior–posterior connections other than the PCom will be seen angiographically. The most commonly found connection, and the most rostral, is the primitive trigeminal artery which is found in approximately 0.5% of individuals. This vessel originates from the dorsal aspect of the proximal cavernous ICA and connects with the middle to proximal BA. If it is large in caliber, the trigeminal artery will supply the bulk of flow to the BA and the PCAs, therefore the VAs will be small or atretic. Saccular aneurysms are seen commonly (~25%) with this anomaly. Recognition of this vessel is also important because it may be a complicating factor in patients with ICA stenosis. Not only can these patients have VB ischemia from carotid stenosis, but also if during intervention ICA blood flow is sufficiently reduced the brainstem may become ischemic and the patient can become comatose. The other persistent fetal connections from rostral

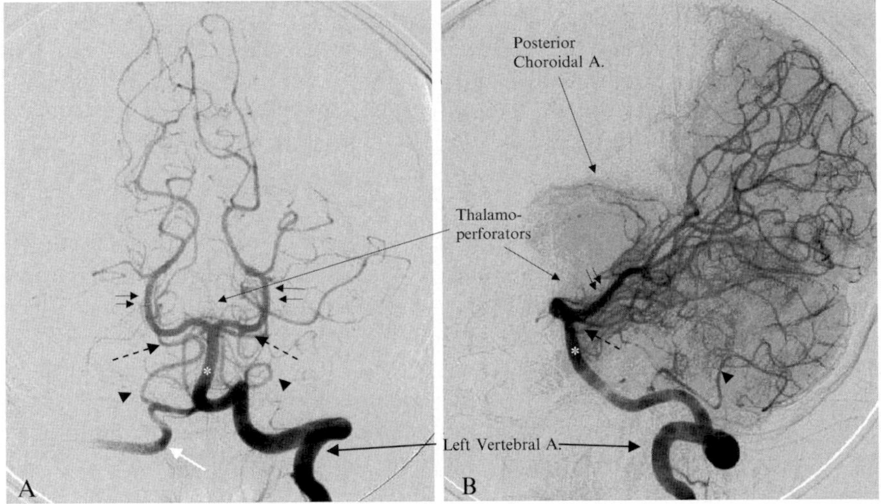

Fig. 6.10. Anteroposterior and lateral digital subtraction angiograms of a selective left vertebral artery (VA) angiogram with reflux into the right VA (*white arrow* in (**a**)). The first intracranial branch of each VA is the posterior inferior cerebellar artery (*arrowheads* in (**a**) and (**b**)). The two VAs then merge to form the basilar artery (*asterisk* in (**a**) and (**b**)). The basilar artery supplies perforators to the pons and midbrain (not seen) as well as two anterior inferior cerebellar arteries (also not well seen in these images) proximally and the two superior cerebellar arteries (*dashed arrows* in (**a**) and (**b**)). The basilar artery terminates by dividing into the two posterior cerebral arteries (*double arrows* in (**a**) and (**b**)). The posterior cerebrals and the basilar artery apex give rise to thalamoperforators and the posterior choroidal artery, among others, to supply critical feeders to the diencephalon

to caudal are very rare and include the otic artery originating from the petrous carotid, a hypoglossal artery originating from the distal cervical ICA to BA through the hypoglossal canal, and the proatlantal intersegmental arteries types 1 and 2 which connect the cervical ICA to the BA or VA through the foramen magnum.

Cerebral Circulation: Unique Features

The cerebral arteries are histologically different from comparably sized peripheral arteries. The walls of the cervical ICAs and VAs are, like other muscular arteries, composed of an intimal layer, internal and external elastic laminae, a thick and muscular tunica media, and an adventitial layer [8]. Within millimeters after the ICAs enter the petrous bone and the VAs penetrate the dura at the foramen magnum, the vessels lose their adventitia and external elastic lamina, making these arteries much more fragile than their coronary or peripheral counterparts. Another important feature is that the intracranial vessels (ICA, MCA, ACA, PCA, VA, and BA) are situated within the subarachnoid space. The ICAs enter the subarachnoid space as they exit the cavernous sinus becoming intradural, and the VAs become intradural at the foramen magnum. Therefore, perforation or rupture of these vessels may result in subarachnoid hemorrhage (SAH), which can be rapidly fatal. This quality should lead to extreme caution during endovascular interventions. Another feature of the intracranial circulation is that there are surface or pial (after the pia matter of the brain) collaterals between the ACA, MCA, and PCA. These anastomoses between terminal arterioles are not as robust as the collaterals from the circle of Willis but in certain conditions, particularly slowly progressive pathological states, they can supply significant amounts of collateral flow to the underperfused region.

The cerebral circulation is rigidly regulated to maintain CBF constant since low CBF can cause ischemia and excessive CBF can cause intracerebral hemorrhage (ICH). The physiological mechanism by which this is achieved is called *cerebral autoregulation*. Throughout a broad range of arterial blood pressures, mean arterial pressures of ~50–175, CBF is maintained constant around a value of 50–60 ml/100 g min^{-1}. Beyond these limits, there is a critical decrease or increase in CBF leading to ischemia or ICH, respectively. This mechanism is effective under normal conditions but in pathological conditions causing cerebral ischemia there is a loss of autoregulation. This occurs because of maximal arteriolar vasodilation to maintain CBF. As a consequence, CBF becomes linearly dependent on mean arterial pressure. Therefore, since the brain cannot decrease its energy demands, any reduction in blood pressure will necessarily reduce CBF and can worsen cerebral ischemia. This is in contrast with coronary ischemic conditions where reduction in systolic blood pressure can actually reduce myocardial oxygen demand and attenuate ischemic injury. The converse situation, excessive CBF due to hypertension, even if the hypertension is relative to previous values such as in a patient who has had a recent carotid revascularization, can result in ICH due to endothelial and vascular injury [9].

Finally, the brain is extremely sensitive to embolization. In the peripheral tissues, except for massive embolization in a patient with poor collaterals, embolization is not often of clinical consequence. Even minute emboli to a small caliber cerebral vessel can cause major clinical syndromes if an eloquent area of brain is affected, particularly if it is an end artery without collaterals. For example, the anterior choroidal artery (300–500 μm) supplies among other structures, the posterior limb of the internal capsule, which contains the corticospinal tract. Infarction of this region often causes a complete, dense hemiplegia. Large emboli of course can be quite devastating if they occlude specific portions of the cerebral vasculature. Carotid terminus (i.e., siphon) occlusion carries a particularly poor prognosis with 40–60% mortality and has a poor recanalization rate with intravenous and even intra-arterial thrombolysis. This is because occlusion in that location often prevents collateral flow from the contralateral ICA, via the ACom, from reconstituting the MCA [10]. In addition, if there is poor collateral flow to the ipsilateral ACA, patients can develop both MCA and ACA territory infarcts, which frequently, and rapidly, lead to brain swelling and herniation.

Conclusions

The cerebral arterial tree is complex and differs significantly from the peripheral and coronary vasculature due to both anatomical and physiological qualities. Combined with the complex anatomy and physiology of the brain, these factors necessitate that a systematic approach to the patient with cerebrovascular disease be founded on a solid understanding of cerebrovascular anatomy and physiology.

Key Points

Clinical/Pathological

- Due to variability in the circle of Willis (which is complete in only 25% of individuals), some conditions may be clinically silent or affect unexpected regions of the brain (e.g., an occipital stroke from an ICA stenosis) leading to diagnostic uncertainty for the unwary.
- There is a loss of cerebral autoregulation in pathological conditions causing cerebral ischemia.
- The brain cannot decrease its energy demands; therefore, any reduction in blood pressure will reduce CBF which can worsen cerebral ischemia.
- This is in contrast with coronary ischemic conditions where reduction in systolic blood pressure can actually reduce myocardial oxygen demand and attenuate ischemic injury.

Anatomical/Technical

- The complex embryological development of the aortic arch leads to several anatomical variants that must be recognized for safe carotid intervention.
- Increasing age, atherosclerosis, and uncontrolled hypertension can lead to elongation and rostral migration of the distal aortic arch and a change in the relative positions of the great vessels, increasing the technical complexity of carotid stenting (see Chaps. 7 and 11).
- There is variation in the position of the carotid bifurcation. Very high (C1) or low bifurcations (T1) can make surgical exposure difficult; such patients may be better treated endovascularly.
- Intracranial ICA collateral sources include the vidian artery, caroticotympanic artery, artery of the foramen rotundum, the inferiolateral trunk, and the ophthalmic artery, which can fully reconstitute intracranial ICA flow.
- If a fetal PCA is combined with another common variant, an absent ACom or an absent or atretic A1 segment of the ipsilateral ACA, the ICA territory on that side is considered to be isolated and has no direct potential collateral sources, which can lead to intraprocedural problems if the blood pressure falls precipitously.
- The MCA is the recipient artery for the majority of cerebral emboli, whether emanating from ICA stenoses or from more proximal sources.
- Identification of the primitive trigeminal artery (0.5% of individuals) is important during carotid stenting as these individuals may suffer brainstem ischemia and coma if ICA blood flow is sufficiently reduced intraprocedurally.
- In their intracranial portions, vessels lose their adventitia and external elastic lamina, making them much more fragile than their coronary or peripheral counterparts. As the intracranial vessels are situated within the subarachnoid space, perforation/rupture may result in SAH, which can be rapidly fatal.
- Even minute emboli to a small caliber cerebral vessel can cause major clinical syndromes if an eloquent area of brain is affected. For example, the anterior choroidal artery (300–500 μm) supplies the posterior limb of the internal capsule, which contains the corticospinal tract. Infarction of this region often causes a complete, dense hemiplegia.
- Carotid terminus (i.e., siphon) occlusion carries a particularly poor prognosis with 40–60% mortality and has a poor recanalization rate with intravenous and even intra-arterial thrombolysis. If there is poor collateral flow to the ipsilateral ACA, patients can develop both MCA and ACA territory infarcts, which frequently, and rapidly, lead to brain swelling and herniation.

References

1. Osborn A. The aortic arch and great vessels. *In* Diagnostic Cerebral Angiography, 2nd edn. 1999. Lippincott Williams & Wilkins, Philadelphia.
2. Lin SC, Trocciola SM, Rhee J, Dayal R, Chaer R, Morrissey NJ, et-al. Analysis of anatomic factors and age in patients undergoing carotid angioplasty and stenting. *Ann Vasc Surg* 2005; 19(6): 798–804.
3. Lam RC, Lin SC, Derubertis B, Hynecek R, Kent DC, Faries PL. The impact of increasing age on

anatomic factors affecting carotid angioplasty and stenting. *J Vasc Surg* 2007; 45: 875–880.

4. Gupta R, Abou-Chebl A, Bajzer CT, Schumacher HC, Yadav JS. Rate, predictors, and consequences of hemodynamic depression after carotid artery stenting. *J Am Coll Cardiol* 2006; 47(8): 1538–1543.
5. Krabbe-Hartkamp MJ, van der Grond J, de Leeuw FE, de Groot JC, Algra A, Hillen B, Breteler MM, Wali WP. Circle of Willis: Morphologic variation on three-dimensional time-of-flight MR angiograms. *Radiology* 1998; 207: 103–111.
6. Hegedus K, Fekete I, Tury F, Molnar L. Experimental focal cerebral ischemia in rabbits. *J Neurol* 1985; 232(4): 223–230.
7. Caldemeyer KS, Carrico JB, Mathews VB. The radiology and embryology of anomalous arteries of the head and neck. *Am J Roentgenol* 1998; 270: 297–304.
8. Lee RM. Morphology of cerebral arteries. *Pharmacol Therapeut* 1995; 66(1): 149–173.
9. Abou-Chebl A, Yadav J, Reginelli J, Bajzer C, Bhatt D, Krieger D. Intracranial hemorrhage and hyperperfusion syndrome following carotid artery stenting: Risk factors, prevention, and treatment. *J Am Coll Cardiol* 2004; 43(9): 1596–1601.
10. Harrison MJ, Marshall J. The variable clinical and CT findings after carotid occlusion: The role of collateral blood supply. *J Neurol Neurosurg Psychiatry* 1988; 51(2): 269–272.

7 Patient Selection: Anatomical

Robin Williams and Sumaira Macdonald

Careful case selection is an absolute prerequisite for safe carotid artery stenting (CAS) practice. All patients being considered for CAS require "overview" anatomic imaging, i.e., from the arch origins of the great vessels to the circle of Willis. This may be achieved by arch aortography, or if there is local enthusiasm and expertise (and bearing in mind that noninvasive imaging modalities have not been validated for assessment of the arch origins), by contrast-enhanced magnetic resonance angiography (CEMRA) or computed tomographic angiography (CTA) (see Chap. 5).

Absolute contraindications to carotid stenting are an occluded ICA or visible thrombus. A difficult origin of the brachiocephalic artery from the ascending aorta or of the left CCA from the brachiocephalic artery may make selective catheterization difficult or impossible. Because of problems with access, any severe tortuosity of the brachiocephalic artery or CCA is a relative contraindication to endovascular treatment. Tortuosity of the ICA above the stenosis may prevent use of a cerebral protection system other than reverse flow. This same tortuosity may be turned into a kink or occlusion by a stent. In all these situations, consideration should be given to carotid endarterectomy (CEA).

The concept of anatomic suitability for endovascular repair of abdominal aortic aneurysm (EVAR) has been accepted for some time. Those with unfavorable infrarenal necks and severe iliac tortuosity, e.g., may be less suited to an endovascular solution. The procedural risks of EVAR are not necessarily increased but the durability of an endovascular treatment may be inferior to open repair in this patient population. What has evidently been less clear until recently is that there may be certain anatomic features that render a patent less suitable for an endovascular treatment option for carotid stenosis. For CAS, it is less an argument of poor durability than one of increased procedural risk. The ultimate goal of any carotid intervention is, of course, survival free of ipsilateral stroke. As procedural risk is offset against longer-term stroke-free survival, measures to reduce procedural stroke are vitally important.

Level of operator experience for CAS is an important consideration in the attendant procedural hazards of that intervention, but the influence of anatomic suitability should not be overlooked. Indeed, operator experience and anatomic suitability are closely linked. Experienced interventionists are able to safely treat a wider range of challenging anatomies than novice.

This chapter seeks to explore and define some of the anatomic factors that may increase procedural risks of CAS.

Learning Curve Is More Than the Acquisition of Technical Ability

Dr. Mark Wholey, an experienced carotid interventionist who has performed more than 1,000 carotid stenting procedures, was recently quoted as saying "When the surgical high-risk carotid stent trials

S. Macdonald and G. Stansby (eds.), *Practical Carotid Artery Stenting,*
DOI: 10.1007/978-1-84800-299-9_7, © Springer-Verlag London Limited 2009

were initiated, we presumed we could stent all patients who met the entry criteria" [1]. He subsequently concluded, in an article for Endovascular Today, "We know that with CAS, there are two critical ways to avoid stroke: patient selection and operator experience" [2].

The carotid interventionists at Lenox Hill Heart and Vascular Institute of New York, comprising interventional cardiologists and an interventional neuroradiologist, were instrumental in the development of CAS and its FDA approval. They are experienced interventionists working in a high-throughput center, having performed more than 2,000 CAS procedures. They evaluated their outcomes for CAS early in their experience, i.e., between 1994 and 1998 [3]. At that time, their treated population amounted to 390 patients. Dedicated carotid stents were only just becoming available toward the end of this 4-year period, as were rapid-exchange systems and the importance of the dual antiplatelet regime during CAS was only just being realized. This period in time predates commercially available cerebral protection devices. What was clearly demonstrated was a year-on-year decrease in procedural stroke and death.

Some may argue that this reduction in adverse event rate simply represents the interventionists' learning curve for the technicalities of the procedure. Indeed, there was a clear linear correlation between number of patients treated and adverse event rate within the CAVATAS trial – both the outcomes for carotid endarterectomy and carotid angioplasty (the percutaneous carotid intervention was fairly rudimentary in this early randomized trial) improved with increasing patient throughput [4].

However, the authors of the early Lenox Hill experience came to a different conclusion: "At the start, only pedunculated thrombus was considered a contraindication" [3]. Later a number of relative contraindications became apparent. These factors – that included stenoses >90%, length and multiplicity of stenoses, concentric calcification and kinks, and tortuosity and angulated takeoff of the internal carotid artery – were associated with a poorer outcome during CAS, i.e., they incurred a higher procedural risk.

Interval	Stroke and death rate (%)
1994–1995	6.8
1995–1996	5.8
1996–1997	5.3
1997–1998	4.1

"Knowledge rests not upon truth alone, but upon error also" (Carl Gustav Jung 1875–1961)

The learning curve is arguably more than the acquisition of technical ability; it also encompasses an understanding of appropriate patient selection.

Subsequent work from the Lenox Hill group has further refined the anatomic features that were associated with increased risk [5]. The authors considered that some lesion characteristics (e.g., degree of stenosis and length) were associated with increasing technical difficulty, but that the two most important anatomic features predicting increased procedural risk were heavy concentric calcification (≥3 mm in width and deemed by at least two orthogonal views to be circumferentially situated around the lesion) and excessive tortuosity (defined as ≥2 flexion points that exceed 90°, within 5 cm of the lesion, including the takeoff of the internal carotid artery from the common carotid artery). In the authors' experience of 1,500 CAS cases at that time, whilst it was accepted that complex anatomy could be dealt with by special techniques, it was clear that the presence of two or more risk factors significantly increased procedural risk.

The association between aortic arch anomalies and procedural risk was explored in a recent study [6]. Two hundred nineteen consecutive patients undergoing CAS were evaluated. One hundred eighty-nine (88.3%) were categorized as having "normal anatomy," defined by the authors as types I–III arches, and the remaining 25 (11.7%) were considered to have abnormal anatomy, i.e., bovine-type arch, direct arch origin of great vessel, or agenesis of the CCA. Technical failure occurred overall in 26 cases (12%) and neurological complication in 14 cases (6.5%). Technical failure was higher in the arch anomaly group; however, the difference did not reach statistical significance (89.6 vs. 76.4%, $p = 0.1$). Neurological complications occurred more frequently in the arch anomaly group (20 vs. 5.3%, $p = 0.039$). Type of arch was the only variable independently associated with neurological complications (OR = 2.01, $p = 0.026$). The authors concluded that aortic arch anomalies were not infrequent and were associated with increased risk of neurological complications. Complex arterial anatomy is more common in the elderly and, although the safety of CAS in octogenarians is the subject of ongoing debate, this might explain, in part, why the event rate reported in the lead-in phase of the CREST trial increased with age and why the effect was not seen to be mediated by potential clinical confounding factors [7].

The relationship between patient age, certain anatomic features, and outcome following CAS was recently explored [8]. Anatomic characteristics that were considered to have the potential to impact on the outcome of CAS were evaluated in 135 procedures performed in 133 patients. Anatomic factors were judged to be either favorable or unfavorable and these included aortic arch elongation, arch calcification, arch vessel origin stenosis, common and internal carotid artery tortuosity, degree of stenosis, lesion calcification, and length. Thirty-seven patients (28%) were ≥80 years of age. Those patients who were ≥80 years old had an increased incidence of unfavorable arch elongation ($p = 0.008$), arch calcification ($p = 0.003$), common carotid or innominate artery origin stenosis ($p = 0.006$), common carotid artery tortuosity ($p = 0.0009$), internal carotid artery tortuosity ($p = 0.019$), and an increased degree of treated lesion stenosis ($p = 0.007$). No significant difference was found for treated lesion calcification or length. The combined stroke, myocardial infarction, and death rate for the entire population was 3.7%. The rate was significantly increased in patients aged ≥80 years old (10.8%) compared with those aged <80 years old (1%, $p = 0.012$). The authors concluded that elderly patients, defined as those aged ≥80 years, had a higher incidence of anatomic features that increased the technical difficulty of CAS. This increase in unfavorable anatomy seemed to be associated with an increased complication rate during CAS. Although the small number of perioperative events did not allow for determination of a direct relationship with specific anatomic characteristics, it was argued that the presence of unfavorable anatomy warranted serious consideration during evaluation of patient suitability for CAS, especially in elderly patients.

It would seem that certain anatomic factors influence outcome for CAS. But the world literature is limited and there have been no attempts at a systematic evaluation of these anatomic factors. One way of evaluating those anatomic factors that may impact on outcome for CAS is to use consensus methodology.

There are a number of formal consensus methods and these include consensus development conferences, nominal group techniques (NGT), and the Delphi consensus method (named after the oracle at Delphi). The former is not infrequently used in medicine, the latter two are less commonly used in medicine – they both require specialist statistical analysis – but are gaining favor. For the consensus development conference, the interaction is not structured, the data aggregation method is implicit – there is no statistical analysis applied – and there is face-to-face interaction amongst panelists, thereby allowing more charismatic (or aggressive!) members of the group to dominate opinions and the outcome. The NGT and Delphi methods involve complex statistical analysis in which judgments are combined according to strict mathematical rules and, in both, interaction is structured. However, the Delphi method has the advantage of no face-to-face contact; panelists' decisions are made in isolation and subsequently reviewed by an experienced statistician.

Because of its advantages as a consensus methodology, the Delphi method was proposed as a means of deriving a simple scoring system of anatomic suitability based on a panel of experts' responses to an electronic questionnaire. The specific aim was to guide novice interventionists (i.e., those who had performed <50 CAS cases) in their selection of patients for CAS. To make the results and the scoring system relevant to the wide range of practitioners who perform CAS and to reduce "group think," the panelists, chosen primarily because of their CAS expertise, included representation from interventional cardiology, interventional radiology, and vascular surgery and were geographically diverse. For Delphi methodology, six panelists are the minimal requirement. For between 6 and 11 panelists, there is a linear relationship between increasing number and increasing yield but no additional advantage is demonstrated after the inclusion of 11 experts.

The panelists:
- **Interventional Cardiology**: Alberto Cremonesi and Robert Fathi
- **Interventional Radiology**: Peter Gaines, Sumaira Macdonald, Claudio Schönholz, and Jos van den Berg
- **Vascular Surgery**: Jean-Pierre Becquemin, Marc Bosiers, Michel Makaroun, Jon Matsumura, and Peter Schneider

The exercise was divided into four sections. In "Round 1," panelists were asked to propose individual anatomic criteria that were thought to be important considerations during CAS, and these were duly subdivided according to anatomical level, i.e., "access," "arch," and "target vessel."

There was consensus on the inclusion of the following anatomic criteria:

- Access:
  - Low bifurcation/short CCA
  - Tortuous CCA
  - Diseased CCA
  - Diseased/occluded ECA
- Arch:
  - Severe arch atheroma
  - Severe arch origin disease
  - Type III arch
  - Bovine arch
- Target vessel:
  - Pinhole stenosis (flow beyond)
  - Angulated ICA origin
  - Angulated distal ICA
  - Circumferential calcification of ICA

In "Round 2," each anatomic criterion was judged individually in terms of the level of difficulty it imparted. The panelists scored the isolated factors on a scale of 1 "easy" to 9 "difficult" using a simple visual analog scale (Fig. 7.1). The panelists were instructed to imagine that they were advising novices who were going to perform a filter-protected CAS case themselves on each anatomy. The panelists' responses were analyzed by the statistician. Mathematical agreement was defined as those scores lying within three points of each other on a scale of 1–9. Figure 7.2a demonstrates an example of good agreement and Fig. 7.2b represents an example of poor agreement.

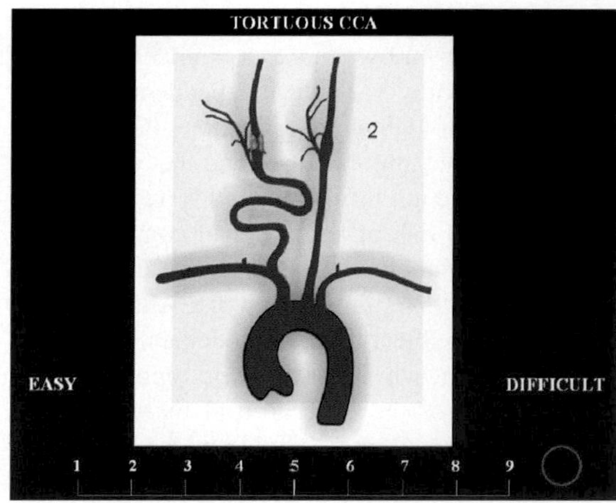

Fig. 7.1. An example of an individual anatomic parameter and the scoring scale in "Round 2"

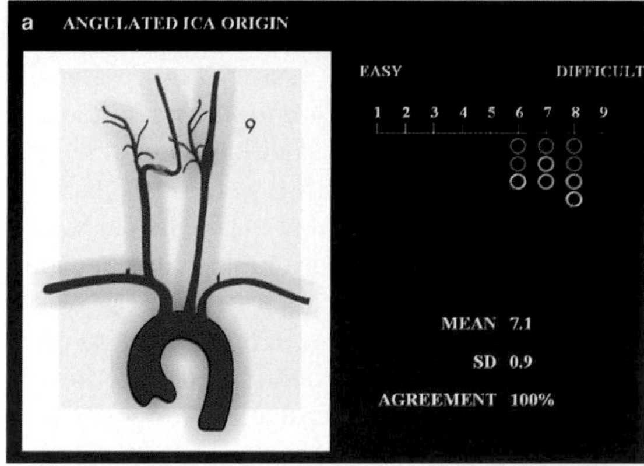

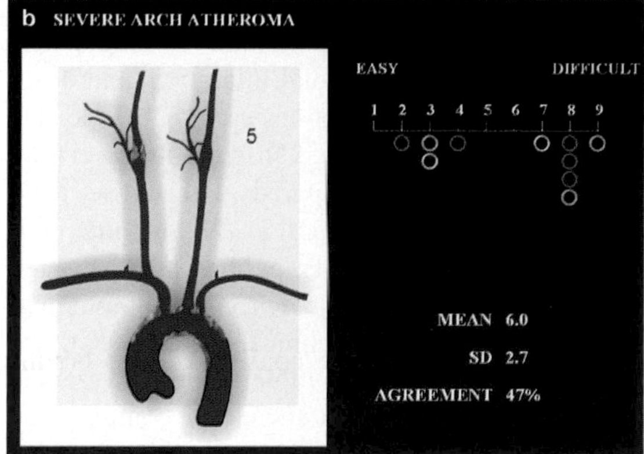

Fig. 7.2. (**a**) "Round 2": an example of good agreement between the panelists on the level of difficulty of an individual anatomic parameter. (**b**) "Round 2": an example of a poor level of agreement between panelists on the level of difficulty of an individual anatomic parameter

TABLE 7.1. Difficulty rating and interobserver agreement for individual anatomic criteria.

Round 2	Difficulty median ± SD	Agreement (%)
Low bifurcation	2.0 (0.9)	93
Occluded/severely diseased ECA	3.1 (1.3)	84
Bovine arch	4.5 (1.5)	76
99% stenosis (pinhole) but flow beyond	5.4 (1.9)	60
Diseased CCA (>50%)	5.6 (0.8)	100
Angulated distal ICA	5.6 (1.6)	73
Severe arch atheroma	6.0 (2.7)	47
Type III arch	6.4 (2.2)	64
Circumferential calcification of ICA	7.0 (1.6)	78
Angulated ICA origin	7.1 (0.9)	100
Severe arch origin disease	7.6 (1.3)	80
Tortuous CCA	8.4 (1.0)	87

SD standard deviation

In Table 7.1, the anatomic factors assessed individually are listed in terms of increasing difficulty, alongside their judged median level of difficulty, and level of agreement between panelists for that parameter.

It is notable that tortuosity of the common carotid artery scores as "very difficult" for novice interventionists, with a mean score of 8.4. Excessive tortuosity increases the difficulty of lesion access and even if access is gained in this type of anatomy, it may not be maintained, with the potential of losing access when one least wants to, part way through the procedure. Angulated distal ICA scored 5.6, i.e., it was judged as a less difficult anatomic entity but tortuosity here may make device delivery difficult, and can prevent positioning of a distal embolic protection device (but can be managed using flow reversal as a means of cerebral protection). These two sites of tortuosity may expose the patient to the risks of atheroembolism from the arch, to air embolism, excessive contrast administration, bifurcation plaque disruption, and ICA dissection. Of the two main arch variants to be considered, the bovine arch was considered to be less of a challenge than the type III arch and of two "lesion" characteristics, circumferential calcification scored as more technically challenging than a "pinhole" stenosis (with flow beyond).

In "Round 3," panelists were asked to propose which of the anatomic criteria from "Round 1" could be lost without loss of discrimination, to reduce the final number of combinations. "Round 4," the final round, or "derivation phase" represents a full factorial design, incorporating 96 combination anatomies and this round is ongoing. Once the "derivation" phase is completed, the aim is to validate the scoring system proposed. This will be done by evaluating patient anatomy on "overview" anatomic imaging obtained within completed randomized trials such as EVA3S [9], thereby comparing patient anatomies that score as "difficult" for CAS as judged objectively by the expert panel with the procedural outcomes in these patients. It must be borne in mind that 85% of those performing CAS within EVA3S had performed ≤50 cases, thereby qualifying as "novices" in the Delphi consensus.

Summary

There is evidence to support the fact that certain anatomic features increase the technical difficulty and thus the procedural risks of CAS and that these features may be more frequently encountered in the elderly. A formal mathematical consensus method is ongoing, with the aim of developing a scoring system to quantify technical difficulty and thus guide inexperienced practitioners to safer patient selection for CAS.

References

1. Wholey, MH. Commentary. Best suited for stenting versus endarterectomy. The controversial issue. J Endovasc Ther 2007;14:687–688.
2. Wholey, MH. Improving trial design. Endovasc Today February;2007;29–35.
3. Vitek, JJ, Roubin, GS, Al-Mubarek, N, et al. Carotid artery stenting: Technical considerations. Am J Neuroradiol 2000;21:1736–1743.
4. Endovascular versus surgical treatment in patients with carotid stenosis in the Carotid and Vertebral Artery Transluminal Angioplasty Study (CAVATAS): A randomised trial. Lancet 2001;357(9270):1729–1737.
5. Roubin, G, Iyer, S, Halkin, A, et al. Realizing the potential of carotid artery stenting. Proposed paradigms for patient selection and procedural technique. Circulation 2006;113:2021–2030.
6. Faggioloi, GL, Ferri, M, Freyrie, A, Gargiulo, M, Fratesi, F, Rossi, C, et al. Aortic arch anomalies are associated with increased risk of neurological events

in carotid stent procedures. Eur J Vasc Endovasc Surg 2007;33:436–441.

7. Hobson, RW, II, Howard, VJ, Roubin, GS, Brott, TG, Ferguson, RD, Popma, JJ, et al. Carotid artery stenting is associated with increased complications in octogenarians: 30-day stroke and death rates in the CREST lead-in phase. J Vasc Surg 2004;40:1106–1111.
8. Lam, RC, Lin, SC, DeRubertsi, B, et al. The impact of increasing age on anatomic factors affecting carotid angioplasty and stenting. J Vasc Surg 2007;45:875–880.
9. Mas, JL, Chatellier, G, Beyssen, B, et al. Endarterectomy versus stenting in patients with symptomatic severe carotid stenosis. N Engl J Med 2006;355:1660–1671.

8
Plaque Stability and Carotid Stenting

M. Bosiers, K. Deloose and P. Peeters

Introduction

Carotid angioplasty and stenting (CAS) is increasingly being performed for the treatment of severely stenotic carotid disease [1–5]. Despite, this growing acceptance, the recently published data of the Eva-3S trial [6], performed in France, and the SPACE trial [7] in Germany failed to prove superiority of CAS over CEA. Nevertheless, earlier publications show that with growing experience and the development of dedicated CAS equipment and devices, CAS can be performed safely and efficiently [2, 8].

The term "vulnerable" or "unstable plaque" refers to a plaque at increased risk of causing thrombosis and lesion progression. Therefore, plaque stability is an important predictor for both primary stroke [9] and the outcome of CAS [10]. Patients presenting with unstable or vulnerable plaque are at increased risk for stroke due to the emboligenic nature of the plaque. The plaques that can be defined as most vulnerable are these with a thin fibrous cap which are inflamed, noncalcified and lipid-filled [11–13].

This chapter reviews available diagnostic methods for identifying unstable plaque and provides important guidelines for stenting patients presenting with the highly emboligenic unstable plaque.

Diagnostic Tools

Different possible diagnostic tools are available to identify unstable plaque. The value of ultrasound imaging in the evaluation of plaque stability has been well documented. Biasi et al. [14] and el-Barghouty et al. [15] simultaneously developed a computerized methodology to evaluate carotid plaque morphology based on color flow duplex examination. A digitized B-mode image at the level of the highest stenosis as determined by the peak flow velocity measurement is transferred to the computer and analyzed for the gray-scale median (GSM) of the carotid plaque (Fig. 8.1). The GSM represents the median of the frequency distribution of gray tones of the pixels included in the region of interest (median echo level, GSM of the region) in a scale of 256 gray tones (0–5 darkest tone; 255–5 brightest tone) and describes the overall brightness of the region of interest. Dark regions are associated with a GSM close to 0, whereas the GSM of bright regions can approach 255.

For the GSM analysis, first a blood region and an adventitia region are outlined on the selected image. The normalized gray scale for the blood is defined as 0 and 195 for the adventitia. Based on the GSM of these two echo-anatomic reference points, the total carotid plaque is normalized by automatic linear scaling. The imaging processing for GSM calculation can be performed by means of the commercially available and user-friendly Adobe Photoshop software®, as follows [16–18]:

1. The color information in the image is omitted so that all the processing and analysis is performed on images in gray mode.
2. An area in the blood (free of noise) is selected. The GSM is obtained by using the histogram

S. Macdonald and G. Stansby (eds.), *Practical Carotid Artery Stenting*,
DOI: 10.1007/978-1-84800-299-9_8, © Springer-Verlag London Limited 2009

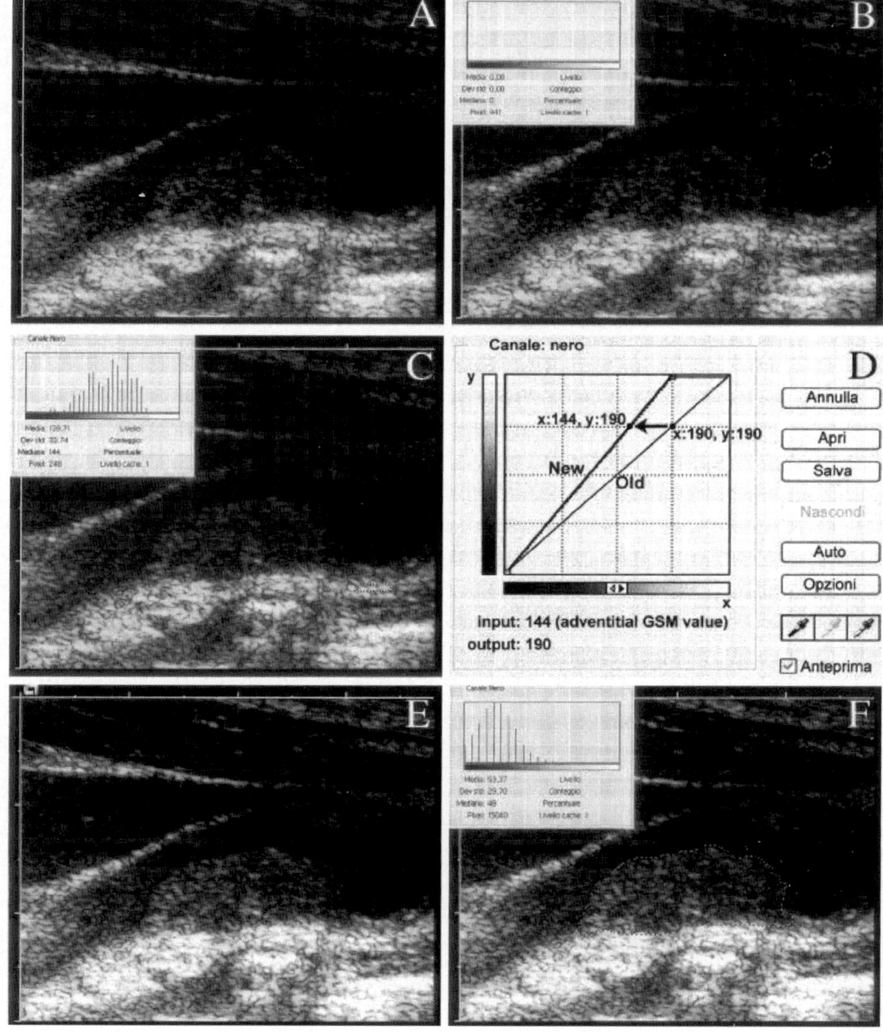

FIG. 8.1. GSM calculation. (**a**) B-mode image of plaque. (**b**) Measurement of GSM in blood. (**c**) Measurement of GSM in adventitia. (**d**) Normalization (standardization) based on algebraic linear scaling of image using "curve" function of software. Gray-scale values of all pixels in image are adjusted according to input and output values of two reference points (blood: input value is measured GSM before linear scaling and output value is 0–5; adventitia: input value is measured GSM before linear scaling and output value is 185–195). In the resultant image, GSM of blood equals 0–5 and that of the adventitia equals 185–195. (**e**) Normalized image. (**f**) Calculation of GSM in normalized plaque (GSM = 48) [10]

facility in the program and the median value of the gray levels of all the pixels.

3. Similarly, part of the adventitia is selected. The measurement of the GSM has to be made at the brightest part of the adventitia on the same arterial wall as the plaque.
4. Image standardization. Algebraic scaling of the whole image is performed using the "curves" facility of the software. This is linear and based on the two reference points: blood and adventitia. The scale is adjusted so that the gray value of the blood is in the region of 0–5 and that of

the adventitia in the region of 185–195. Thus, the gray values of all pixels will change as defined by this new linear scale.

5. Measurement of echodensity (gray levels of the pixels) of the plaque. In standardized images, the plaque is outlined by the mouse of a personal computer and the GSM, defined as the median of overall gray shades of the pixels in the plaque, can be obtained from the histogram of the gray shades of plaque pixels.

It has been shown that the GSM gives a good measure of overall plaque echogenicity and can be used as a predictor for the stroke risk in CAS. Biasi et al. [10] performed the ICAROS trial (Imaging in Carotid Angioplasty and Risk of Stroke) and concluded that carotid plaques with GSM $\leq$ 25 are defined as echogenic and that in these patients the risk of stroke in CAS is significantly increased. The ICAROS investigators included 418 CAS patients that received a preprocedural echographic evaluation of carotid plaque with GSM measurement. The onset of neurological deficits during the procedure and the postprocedural period was recorded. It was shown that patients with a GSM $\leq$ 25 had a significantly increased ($p = 0.005$) stroke rate (7.1%) if compared with patients with GSM > 25 (1.5%) [10].

Carotid intimal medial thickness (IMT) can also be considered as a marker for plaque vulnerability. According to the recommendations of the American Society of Echocardiography and the Society of Vascular Medicine and Biology, carotid plaques with an IMT of >1 mm are strong predictors of carotid disease progression [19] and stroke [20].

Another new approach to identify plaque instability by means of duplex is the pixel distribution analysis (PDA) described by Lal et al. [21]. With this PDA technique, which is based on the fact that different tissues reflect US differently, it is possible to localize and quantify the amount of intraplaque hemorrhage, lipid, fibromuscular tissue, and calcium in the plaque. Furthermore, this technique allows comparison of the architectural features (lipid core size and core location) of different plaques. Using the PDA technique, the authors did find significant differences between plaques in symptomatic and asymptomatic patients. Plaques from symptomatic patients demonstrated with significantly larger quantities of intraplaque hemorrhage and the lipid cores were larger and were located closer to the flow lumen as these in asymptomatic plaques. Asymptomatic plaques were characterized by smaller amounts of calcium. For fibromuscular tissue, no difference was observed between the two groups [22].

To date, the use of MRI, CT scanning, or PET scanning has limited value in the diagnosis of vulnerable plaque. Mohler [23] has pointed out that MRI usually confirms presence of vulnerable plaque as diagnosed on duplex. In the future, high-resolution MRI may be helpful for characterizing plaque, but to date those programs are not readily available. Also, CT scanning may have a role in the future to diagnose unstable plaque. With a CT scan with or without X-ray contrast dye, the lipid content of plaque can be identified, but the fact the calcium in the plaque can create shadowing on CT makes it difficult to determine the degree of stenosis and the component of the plaque [23].

Carotid Stenting

Unlike carotid endarterectomy (CEA), where the plaque is completely removed from the body, the plaque remains in the artery after CAS. As this source of potentially hazardous debris stays in the artery, there is a requirement for protection against embolization potentially leading to devastating neurological complications. As shown in different publications, embolic protection devices (EPDs) offer good brain protection during the intervention, resulting in optimal procedural success rates with low neurological complication rates in all patients [1, 3, 4]. All EPD systems currently on the market can be classified under three main groups, each with its own working principle (1) distal occlusion devices, (2) distal filters, and (3) proximal occlusion devices. Specifically for vulnerable lesions, proximal occlusion devices seem attractive as they do not require potentially hazardous lesion passage before complete cerebral protection is established [24]. Nevertheless to data, there is insufficient evidence to prove the case.

It has been shown by Cremonesi et al. [25] that in centers with good experience in CAS, since the introduction of dedicated CAS equipment and devices, there has been a clear shift from intraprocedural to postprocedural complications. They

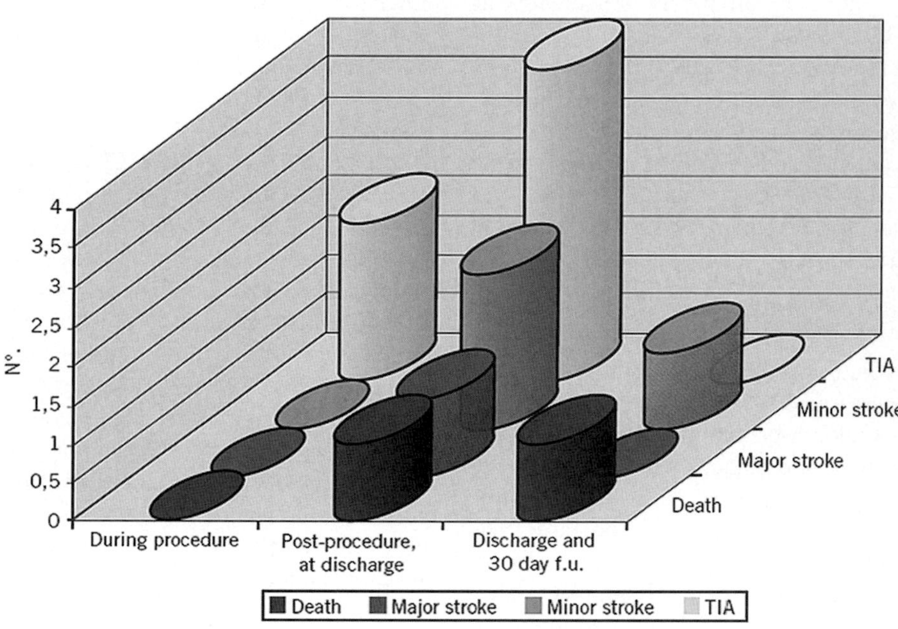

FIG. 8.2. Temporal distribution of embolic events [25]

observed, as presented in Fig. 8.2, that approximately two third of all events occur after the procedure, which are probably caused by late emboli through the struts of the stent.

Vulnerable Plaque and Stent Scaffolding

After the procedure, as soon as the EPD is removed, the only protection against brain embolization remains the selected carotid stent. Therefore, the stent scaffolding capacities of the stent are potentially of major importance to obtain a stroke-free CAS outcome. It is the mesh design of the stent that has to guarantee that no debris is dislodged through the stent interstices. Logically, stents with a smaller free cell area and hence a greater percentage of wall coverage may better contain the fractured and dilated plaque after CAS resulting in a lower number of postprocedural events.

With this in mind, we recommend that the stent manufactures improve the stent scaffolding capacities of their stents by downsizing the free cell areas of there stents, but according to Wholey and Finol [26] this is unfortunately easier said than done. They stated that, in their quest for the ideal carotid stent, the stent designers have to ideally balance long-term stent performance characteristics such as axial and circumferential stiffness and strength, scaffolding properties, conformability, and side branch preservation with acute considerations relating to deliverability and deployment, such as constrained profile and flexibility. The design team has to consider numerous interrelated parameters, such as strut length and width, wire diameter and pitch, bridge configuration, material selection, and processing conditions to achieve optimal performance [26]. So, changing one stent design feature, such as free cell area to improve the scaffolding potential of the stent, has an immediate and direct impact on overall stent behavior.

An often used classification for stent design is the binary "open" and "closed" cell design one, in which the differentiation is made by the number and arrangement of bridge connectors. In closed-cell stents, the adjacent ring segments are connected at every possible junction with flexible

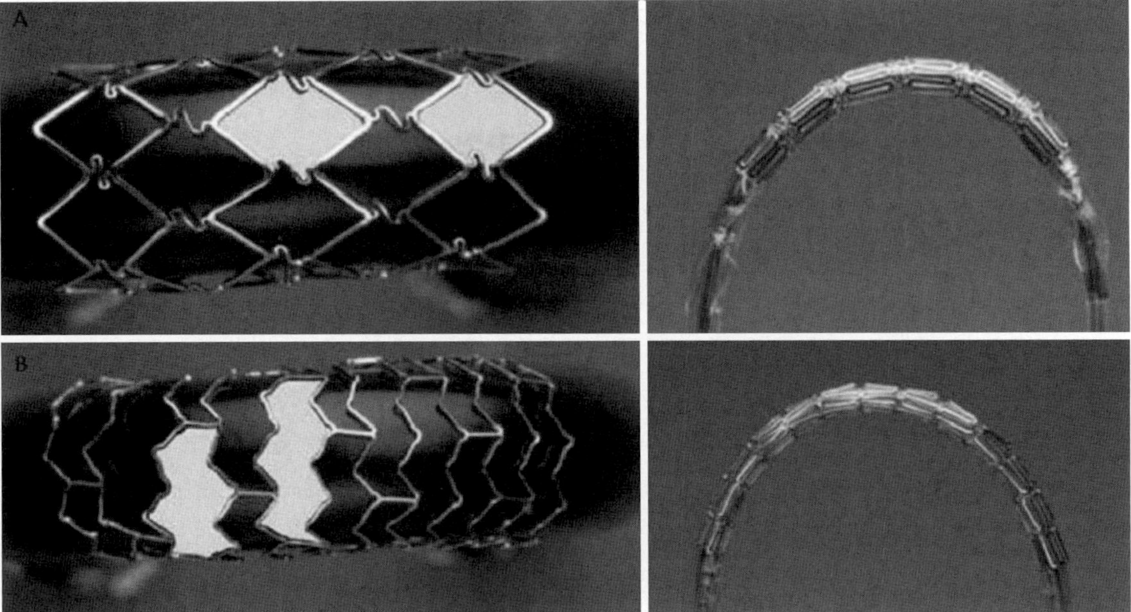

FIG. 8.3. (**a**) Fully supported closed-cell design demonstrating comparable flexibility to the (**b**) unsupported open-cell design [26]

bridge connectors, allowing some limited degree of flexion between adjacent rings (Fig. 8.3). In the open-cell stents, not all junction points are interconnected, which allows more between adjacent ring segments. The flexion benefits of an open-cell design have a cost in scaffolding uniformity, just as the scaffolding benefits of a closed-cell design have a cost in flexion and conformability [26].

In our first publication on the effects of stent design on CAS outcome, the binary "open" and "closed" cell design classification was used. We retrospectively reviewed 701 CAS patients and found a total 30-day stroke, death, and TIA event rate of 11.1% in the patients treated with open-cell designed stents vs. 3% for the group treated with closed-cell stents [27]. Wholey and Finol [26] stated that this classification may be too general for comparison and concluded that cell size and surface area coverage appears to be more important. They gave the example that a closed-cell stent with a diameter of 1,000 μm is more likely to be responsible for plaque prolapse and embolization than an open cell of 500 μm.

In our later publication on the correlation between carotid stent design and clinical event rates using the data of the Belgian–Italian Carotid (BIC) registry [28], it was decided to categorize the stent according to their free cell area. Stents were classified into four subgroups according to the free cell area of the stents (Fig. 8.4):

1. <2.5 mm^2: Wallstent (1.08 mm^2) and X-Act (2.74 mm^2)
2. 2.5–5 mm^2: NexStent (4.07 mm^2)
3. 5–7.5 mm^2: Precise (5.89 mm^2) and Exponent (6.51 mm^2)
4. >7.5 mm^2: Protégé (10.71 mm^2) and Acculink (11.48 mm^2)

The BIC registry was performed in four highly experienced CAS centers in Belgium and Italy (Department of Vascular Surgery of the AZ St-Blasius in Dendermonde, Belgium; Department of Cardiovascular and Thoracic Surgery of the Imelda Hospital in Bonheiden, Belgium; Department of Vascular and Endovascular Surgery, University of Siena, Italy; and Interventional Cardio-Angiology Unit, Villa Maria Cecilia Hospital, Cotignola, Italy) the importance of stent selection. A total population of 3,179 CAS patients was available for analysis, of which

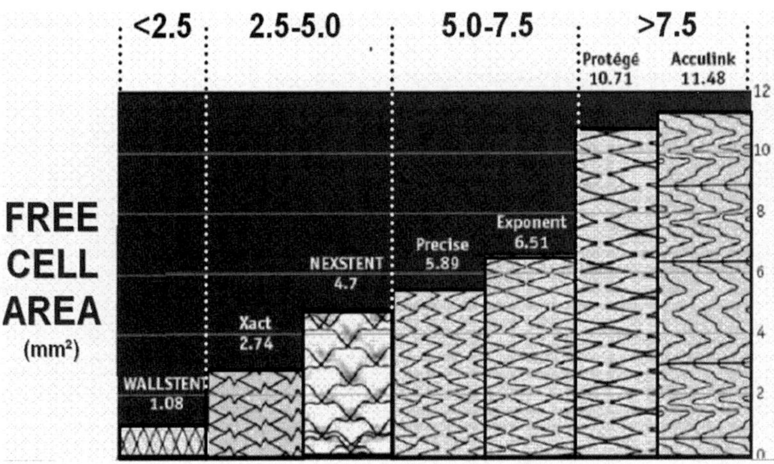

FIG. 8.4. Overview of the investigated stents and their free cell areas (based on Houdart CIRSE 2005)

41.4% presented as baseline as symptomatic and 58.6% as asymptomatic. Protected CAS was performed in 3,049 patients (95.9%): distal filters were used in 92.9%, proximal occlusion devices in 6.4%, and distal occlusion systems in only 0.8% of the cases. Stenting was performed in all patients; 66.3% received stents with a free cell area <2.5 mm^2, 4.2% between 2.5 and 5 mm^2, 10.3% between 5 and 7.5 mm^2, and 19.2% of the patients received a stent larger than 7.5 mm^2. Table 8.1 overviews the distribution of the used EPDs and carotid stents used in the BIC registry.

Both for the total population and for the symptomatic and asymptomatic subgroups, events were subdivided into procedural (until removal of all endovascular material) and postprocedural (until 30 days) events. The neurological complications were defined as death, major stroke (i.e., clinically persisting >24 h), minor stroke (i.e., persisting <24 h), and TIA.

Table 8.2 reports the overview of event rates related to the free cell area groups for the total population, symptomatic and asymptomatic subgroup in absolute numbers and percentage.

For the total population, we revealed significant differences in event rates according to free cell area. The differences were most clear for the events that occurred in the postprocedural phase, in which, as mentioned earlier, it is only the selected carotid stent that protects against embolization. Postprocedural event rates equal 1.2, 2.2, 3.4, and 3.4% for free cell areas lower than 2.5 mm^2, between 2.5 and 5 mm^2, between 5 and 7.5 mm^2, and higher than 7.5 mm^2, respectively. The differences in complication rates were substantially more pronounced among symptomatic patients. However, there was no evidence of differences according to free cell area in the asymptomatic population. In detail, testing showed that important significant differences were observed in the symptomatic population between stents with free cell areas lower than 2.5 mm^2 on the one hand and larger than 5 mm^2 on the other hand and this for both event types (all events and postprocedural events). Specifically, (all) event rates equal 2.3, 6.5, and 7.5% for free cell areas lower than 2.5 mm^2, between 5 and 7.5 mm^2, and higher than 7.5 mm^2, respectively, in the symptomatic patient population. Postprocedural event rates equal 1.2, 5.2, and 7.0%, respectively, in that population.

Also in a second publication of the BIC registry in which we aimed in finding differences between the EPDs used [29], we had to conclude that all of the observed differences in event rates between the

TABLE 8.1. Distribution of selected embolic protection devices and carotid stents.

EPD		
Design	Brand: manufacturer	*N* (%)
Distal filtration	FilterWire: Boston Scientific, Natick, MA, USA	1,640 (51.6)
	Angioguard: Cordis, Miami Lakes, FL, USA	514 (16.2)
	Accunet: Abbott Vascular Devices, Redwood City, CA, USA	204 (6.4)
	Emboshield: Abbott Vascular Devices, Redwood City, CA, USA	177 (5.6)
	Rubicon Filter: Boston Scientific, Natick, MA, USA	6 (0.2)
	Spider: ev3, Plymouth, MN, USA	191 (6.0)
	Trap: ev3, Plymouth, MN, USA	82 (2.5)
	Interceptor: Medtronic Vascular, Santa Rosa, CA, USA	13 (0.4)
Proximal occlusion	Mo.Ma: Invatec, Roncadelle, Italy	150 (4.7)
	NPS: W. L. Gore & Associates, Flagstaff, AZ, USA	42 (1.3)
Distal occlusion	Percusurge: Medtronic Vascular, Santa Rosa, CA, USA	26 (0.8)
Unprotected		130 (4.1)
	Stent	
Free cell area (mm2)	Brand: manufacturer	*N* (%)
<2.5	Carotid Wallstent: Boston Scientific Corp., Natick, MA, USA	2,107 (66.3)
2.5–5	X-Act: Abbott Vascular Devices, Redwood City, CA, USA	105 (3.3)
	NexStent: Endotex, Cupertino, CA, USA	30 (0.9)
	Precise: Cordis, Miami Lakes, FL, USA	293 (9.2)
5–7.5	Exponent: Medtronic Vascular, Santa Rosa, CA, USA	34 (1.1)
>7.5	Protégé: ev3, Plymouth, MN, USA	201 (6.3)
	Acculink: Abbott Vascular Devices, Redwood City, CA, USA	409 (12.9)

TABLE 8.2. Event rates related to free cell area.

Free cell area (mm2)	Total population			Symptomatic population			Asymptomatic population		
	Patients	All events (%)	Postprocedural events (%)	Patients	All events (%)	Postprocedural events (%)	Patients	All events (%)	Postprocedural events (%)
<2.5	2,107	2.3	1.2	882	2.3	1.2	1,225	2.3	1.2
2.5–5	135	2.2	2.2	52	1.9	1.9	83	2.4	2.4
5–7.5	327	4.9	3.4	155	6.5	5.2	172	3.5	1.7
>7.5	610	3.8	3.4	228	7.5	7.0	382	1.6	1.3
Total	3,179	2.83	1.9	1,317	3.6	2.73	1,862	2.25	1.3

different EPDs and EPD types were explained by the stent-type selected. We crosschecked the 3,030 CAS procedures in the registry which were performed with commercially available EPDs, to see whether any relation could be found between events and the selected EPD. Eccentric filters (FilterWire, Spider) were used in 1,831 (60.4%), concentric filters (Emboshield, Angioguard, Trap, Accunet) in 981 (32.4%), proximal occlusion (NPS, Mo.Ma) in 192 (6.3%), and distal occlusion (Percusurge) in 26 (0.9%) of the 3,030 cases in the analysis. There was no significant difference in procedural adverse neurological events observed for any of the EPDs or types of EPDs. The observed differences in 30-day events for different EPDS selected are largely attributable to the difference in stent-type used in conjunction with the EPD. A statistically significant difference was found in favor of eccentric filters compared with concentric filters at 30 days only ($p = 0.04$), but after adjustment for risk factors and stent design this difference was no longer apparent ($p = 0.51$). Taking the 30-day event rate after CAS using the FilterWire (2.2%) as control reference value, a statistically significant increased 30-day event rate was only found for the Accunet (5.9%) concentric filter. Stents with a free cell area larger than 5.0 mm^2 were used over 65% of the Accunet cases, the predominant one being the Acculink stent which has the highest free cell area of the stents used in this study.

The findings of the BIC registry are supported by a subanalysis of the SPACE trial [7], which was performed by Prof. Jansen. He found a 30-day event rate of 11.0% in patients treated with stents with an open-cell design, while it was "only" 6.0% for the patients treated with a closed-cell stent.

Vulnerable Plaque and Tortuous Anatomy

Regarding the necessity of optimal scaffolding to treat vulnerable carotid plaque, the presence of vulnerable carotid plaque in a tortuous vessel poses difficulties. Stents with high scaffolding characteristics, small free cell area or closed-cell design, currently have a limited flexibility. If placed in a tortuous carotid, they tend to alter the vessels original curve. If not placed accurately, the insertion of a stent with good scaffolding capacities, but more rigid design, can result in kinking of the carotid vessel just distal of the implanted stent (Fig. 8.5).

In these tortuous bends, the flexibility of the open-cell design may be required comprising the potential scaffolding. This increases the risk of plaque prolapse especially in the vulnerable lesions (Fig. 8.6).

Furthermore, with the placement of open-cell stents, the cells open on the concave surface of the bend, which can cause prolapse and fish scaling on the open surface. Fish scaling can lead to intimal disruption with contrast extending to the adventitia (Fig. 8.7).

These factors mean that CAS of vulnerable plaques in tortuous lesions may require a compromise approach. On the one hand, the vulnerable plaque requires excellent scaffolding to prevent embolization and on the other hand, the stent needs to be flexible enough to accommodate to the vessel's tortuosity. In our practice, plaque scaffolding, especially in the vulnerable lesion, is our prime determinator for selecting a stent with a small free cell area, if we believe it is feasible to implant the stent without significantly altering the vessel's anatomy. Alternatively, we will go for CEA in this specific patient population.

Opimization Vulnerable plaque Before CAS

Statins inhibit the enzyme 3-hydroxy-3-methylglutaryl coenzyme A reductase (HMG-CoA reductase) which results in the inhibition of the body's synthesis of cholesterol and an increase in the number of low-density lipoprotein (LDL) receptors expressed on both hepatic and extrahepatic tissues. Both actions lead to a decrease in plasma cholesterol levels. Beside the LDL lowering effect, statins also reduce inflammation, inhibit macrophage function, reverse endothelial dysfunction, and decrease thrombogenicity [30, 31]. The combined effect of statins "stabilizes" the vulnerable carotid plaque against disruption. It has been demonstrated that in individuals with carotid artery disease with moderately elevated LDL cholesterol levels, aggressive LDL cholesterol lowering with statins can reduce cardiovascular events and overall mortality [32, 33].

Crisby et al. [34] investigated the use of pravastatin as an adjunct to CEA, treating patients with pravastatin to stabilize plaque preoperatively and then investigating the composition of these plaques after they were surgically removed. Patients with symptomatic carotid artery stenosis received 40 mg day^{-1} pravastatin or no lipid-lowering therapy for 3 months prior to scheduled CEA. They found that pravastatin administration resulted in a decrease in lipids, lipid oxidation, inflammation, matrix metalloproteinase 2, and cell death and an increase in tissue inhibitors of metalloproteinase 1 and collagen content in the investigated plaques, which are all consistent with a proposed plaque-stabilizing effect.

Gröschel et al. [35] investigated a group of 180 CAS patients of which 53 (29.4%) received statin therapy for at least a week prior to CAS (atorvastatin: $n = 40$, 10–40 mg day^{-1}; simvastatin: $n = 6$, 40 mg day^{-1}; pravastatin: $n = 5$, 10–40 mg day^{-1}; cervistatin: $n = 1$, 0.3 mg day^{-1}; and lovastatin: $n = 1$, 40 mg day^{-1}). They found that preoperative

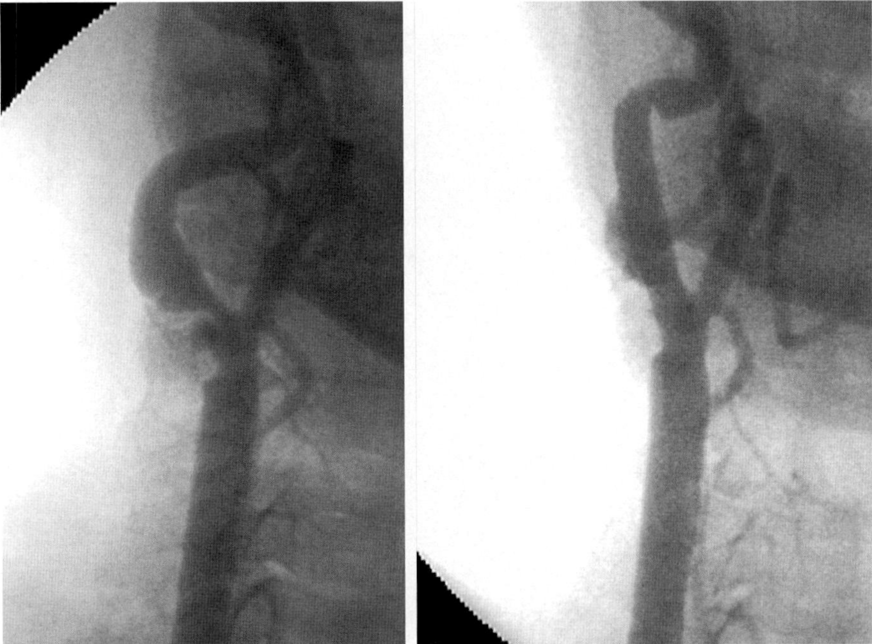

Fig. 8.5. Stent selection for tortuous carotid lesions: (**a**) pre- and (**b**) postprocedural angiography of carotid artery stenting (CAS), a closed-cell cobalt chromium alloy stent (Carotid Wallstent) causing kinking of the artery distal of the lesion

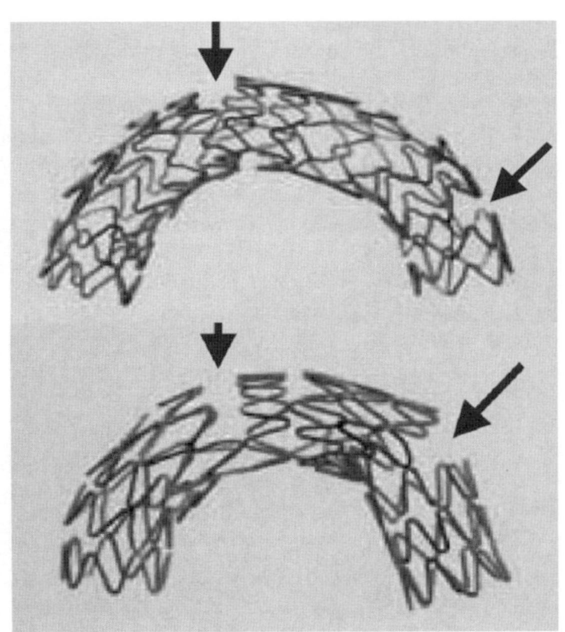

Fig. 8.6. Larger open-cell designed stents insufficiently scaffold vulnerable lesions in tortuous anatomy [26]

statin prescription effectively reduced ($p < 0.05$) the 30-day incidence of stroke, myocardial infarction, and death after CAS in symptomatic patients.

Key Points

- Different diagnostic methods are available to check plaque stability. To date, the most commonly used method is the GSM analysis. Carotid plaques with GSM ≤ 25 are defined as echogenic and have a significantly increased risk of stroke after CAS.
- Protected CAS can be safely performed in patients with vulnerable lesions. Theoretically, the use of proximal occlusion devices has the advantage that the vulnerable lesion does not need to be passed to install the EPD. To date, there is no evidence available confirming this theory.
- While during CEA the debris completely removed from the body, the plaque remains in the artery after CAS. As after the intervention the stent is the only protector against potential embolization,

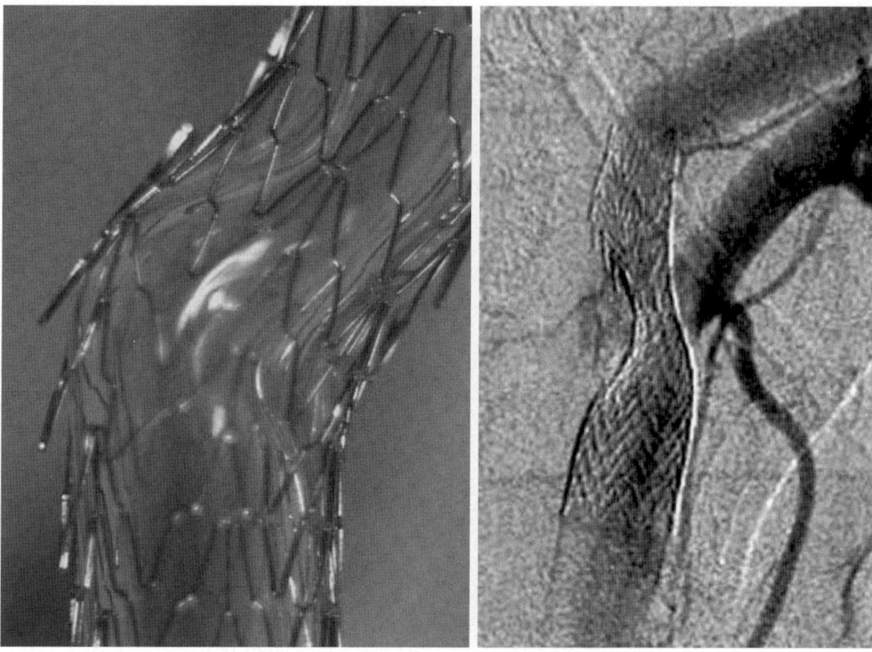

FIG. 8.7. (**a**) Fish scaling of open-cell design at the concave surface of the stent. (**b**) Open-cell struts extending beyond the intima with focal contrast extravasation after CAS [26]

the most important feature of the stent is scaffolding and its late embolization prevention.

- To provide the mandatory scaffolding of the vulnerable lesion, we advocate the use of stents with a small free cell area to perform CAS in especially symptomatic patients.
- In patients with combined vulnerable plaque and tortuous lesions, we either perform CAS with the small free cell area stents if we believe it can be implanted without significant alteration of the vessel's original anatomy, or prefer to transfer the patient to CEA.
- Statin administration prior to CAS lowers the complication rate after CAS. Especially in vulnerable lesions, it is recommended to prescribe statins in order to "stabilize" the plaque before performing CAS.

Acknowledgments. The authors take great pleasure in thanking the staff of Flanders Medical Research Program (http://www.fmrp.be), with special regards to Koen De Meester for performing the systematic review of the literature and providing substantial support to the writing of the chapter.

References

1. Wholey MH, Al-Mubarek N, Wholey MH. Updated review of the global carotid artery stent registry. *Catheter Cardiovasc Interv* 2003; 60:259–266.
2. Bosiers M, Peeters P, Deloose K, Verbist J, Sievert H, Sugita J, et al. Does carotid artery stenting work on the long run: 5-year results in high-volume centers (ELOCAS Registry). *J Cardiovasc Surg (Torino)* 2005; 46:241–247.
3. Kastrup A, Groschel K, Krapf H, Brehm BR, Dichgans J, Schulz JB. Early outcome of carotid angioplasty and stenting with and without cerebral protection devices: A systematic review of the literature. *Stroke* 2003; 34:813–819.
4. Cremonesi A, Manetti R, Setacci F, Setacci C, Castriota F. Protected carotid stenting: Clinical advantages and complications of embolic protection devices in 442 consecutive patients. *Stroke* 2003; 34:1936–1941.
5. Kastrup A, Schulz JB, Raygrotki B, Gröschel K, Ernemann U. Comparison of angioplasty and stenting with cerebral protection versus endarterectomy for treatment of internal carotid artery stenosis in elderly patients. *J Vasc Surg* 2004; 40:945–951.
6. Mas JL, Chatellier G, Beyssen B, Branchereau A, Moulin T, Becquemin JP, et al. Endarterectomy versus

stenting in patients with symptomatic severe carotid stenosis. *N Engl J Med* 2006; 355:1660–1671.

7. SPACE Collaborative Group, Ringleb PA, Allenberg J, Bruckmann H, Eckstein HH, Fraedrich G, et al. 30 day results from the SPACE trial of stent-protected angioplasty versus carotid endarterectomy in symptomatic patients: A randomised non-inferiority trial. Lancet 2006; 368:1239–1247.
8. Verzini F, Cao P, De Rango P, Parlani G, Maselli A, Romano L, et al. Appropriateness of learning curve for carotid artery stenting: An analysis of periprocedural complications. *J Vasc Surg* 2006; 44:1205–1211.
9. Gronholdt ML, Nordestgaard BG, Schroeder TV, Vorstrup S, Sillesen H. Ultrasonic echolucent carotid plaques predict future strokes. *Circulation* 2001; 104:68–73.
10. Biasi GM, Froio A, Diethrich EB, Deleo G, Galimberti S, Mingazzini P, et al. Carotid plaque echolucency increases the risk of stroke in carotid stenting: The Imaging in Carotid Angioplasty and Risk of Stroke (ICAROS) study. *Circulation* 2004; 110:756–762.
11. Kolodgie FD, Burke AP, Farb A, Gold HK, Yuan J, Narula J, et al. The thin-cap fibroatheroma: A type of vulnerable plaque: The major precursor lesion to acute coronary syndromes. *Curr Opin Cardiol* 2001; 16:285–292.
12. Virmani R, Burke AP, Kolodgie FD, Farb A. Pathology of the thin-cap fibroatheroma: A type of vulnerable plaque. *J Interv Cardiol* 2003; 16(3):267–272.
13. Hunt JL, Fairman R, Mitchell ME, Carpenter JP, Golden M, Khalapyan T, et al. Bone formation in carotid plaques: A clinicopathological study. *Stroke* 2002; 33:1214–1219.
14. Biasi GM, Mingazzini PM, Sampaolo A. Echographic characterization of carotid plaque and risk for cerebral ischemia. In: Progress in Angiology and Vascular Surgery, Castellani LD (ed.). Torino, Italy: Minerva Medica, 1995, pp 59–65.
15. el-Barghouty N, Geroulakos G, Nicolaides A, Androulakis A, Bahal V. Computer-assisted carotid plaque characterisation. *Eur J Vasc Endovasc Surg* 1995; 9:389–393.
16. Elatrozy T, Nicolaides A, Tegos T, Zarka AZ, Griffin M, Sabetai M. The effect of B-mode ultrasonic image standardisation on the echodensity of symptomatic and asymptomatic carotid bifurcation plaques. *Int Angiol* 1998; 17:179–186.
17. Sabetai M, Tegos T, Nicolaides A, Dhanjil S, Pare GJ, Stevens JM. Reproducibility of computer-quantified carotid plaque echogenicity: Can we overcome the subjectivity? *Stroke* 2000; 31:2189–2196.
18. Biasi GM, Froio A, Deleo G, Piazzoni C, Camesasca V. What have we learned from the Imaging in Carotid Angioplasty and Risk of Stroke (ICAROS) study? *Vascular* 2004; 12:62–68.
19. Roman MJ, Naqvi TZ, Gardin JM, Gerhard-Herman M, Jaff M, Mohler E, et-al.. Clinical application of noninvasive vascular ultrasound in cardiovascular risk stratification: A report from the American Society of Echocardiography and the Society of Vascular Medicine and Biology. *J Am Soc Echocardiogr* 2006; 19:943–954.
20. Lorenz MW, Markus HS, Bots ML, Rosvall M, Sitzer M. Prediction of clinical cardiovascular events with carotid intima-media thickness: A systematic review and meta-analysis. *Circulation* 2007; 115:459–467.
21. Lal BK, Hobson RW, Pappas PJ, Kubicka R, Hameed M, Chakhtoura EY, et al. Pixel distribution analysis of B-mode ultrasound scan images predicts histologic features of atherosclerotic carotid plaques. *J Vasc Surg* 2002; 35:1210–1217.
22. Lal BK, Hobson RW. Pixel distribution analysis to identify unstable carotid plaques. *Endovasc Today* 2006; 5:88–92.
23. Mohler ER. Overview of vulnerable plaque. *Endovasc Today* 2006; 5:79–82.
24. Bosiers M, Deloose K, Verbist J, Peeters P. Embolic protection devices. *J Vasc Endovasc Surg* 2006; 13:125–130.
25. Cremonesi A, Setacci C, Manetti R, de Donato G, Francesco S, Balestra G, et al. Carotid angioplasty and stenting: Lesion related treatment strategies. *EuroIntervention* 2005; 1:289–295.
26. Wholey MH, Finol EA. Designing the ideal stent. *Endovasc Today* 2007; 6:25–34.
27. Hart J, Peeters P, Verbist J, Deloose K, Bosiers M. Do device characteristics impact outcome in carotid artery stenting? *J Vasc Surg* 2006; 44:725–730; discussion 730–731.
28. Bosiers M, de Donato G, Deloose K, Verbist J, Peeters P, Castriota F, et al. Does free cell area influence the outcome in carotid artery stenting? *Eur J Vasc Endovasc Surg* 2007; 33:135–141.
29. Iyer M, de Donato G, Deloose K, Verbist J, Peeters P, Castriota F, et al. The type of embolic protection does not influence the outcome in carotid artery stenting. *J Vasc Surg* 2007; 46(2):251–256.
30. Nighoghossian N, Derex L, Douek P. The vulnerable carotid artery plaque: Current imaging methods and new perspectives. *Stroke* 2005; 36:2764–2772.
31. Smilde TJ, van den Berkmortel FW, Wollersheim H. The effect of cholesterol lowering on carotid and femoral artery wall stiffness and thickness in patients with familial hypercholesterolaemia. *Eur J Clin Invest* 2000; 30:473–480.
32. Furberg CD, Adams HP, Jr., Applegate WB, Byington RP, Espeland MA, Hartwell T, et al. Effect of lovastatin on early carotid atherosclerosis and cardiovascular

events. Asymptomatic Carotid Artery Progression Study (ACAPS) Research Group. *Circulation* 1994; 90:1679–1687.

33. Byington RP, Furberg CD, Crouse JR III, Espeland MA, Bond MG. Pravastatin, lipids, and atherosclerosis in the carotid arteries (PLAC-II). *Am J Cardiol* 1995; 76:54C–59C.
34. Crisby M, Nordin-Fredriksson G, Shah PK, Yano J, Zhu J, Nilsson J. Pravastatin treatment increases collagen content and decreases lipid content, inflammation, metalloproteinases, and cell death in human carotid plaques: Implications for plaque stabilization. *Circulation* 2001; 103:926–933.
35. Gröschel K, Ernemann U, Schulz JB, Nägele T, Terborg C, Kastrup A. Statin therapy at carotid angioplasty and stent placement: Effect on procedure-related stroke, myocardial infarction, and death. *Radiology* 2006; 240:145–151.

9 Pharmacological Support

D.R. Turner and S.M. Thomas

Pharmacotherapy in Patients Undergoing Carotid Artery Stenting

Introduction

Stroke is a major cause of morbidity and mortality worldwide, and its occurrence has major implications for the individual, family, and healthcare system alike. Cerebral infarction accounts for approximately 70% of stroke, and atheroembolism from carotid artery disease is implicated in 15–30% of cases [1].

Survivors of ischemic cerebrovascular events are not only at high risk of recurrent stroke, but also of other adverse vascular outcomes, such as myocardial infarction (MI) and vascular-related death, by as much as 4–11% per annum [2, 3].

Some 15–23% of patients who present with stroke will have experienced a prior transient ischemic attack (TIA) [4, 5], nearly half of these within the preceding 7 days [4]. Various clinical and investigational tools have been proposed to identify those patients at high risk of early recurrence [6–9].

Although carotid stenosis accounts for a relatively small proportion of cases of cerebrovascular ischemic events, its diagnosis is important, as it is two to three times more likely to cause early recurrent stroke than other subtypes [1, 9–11].

The risk of future stroke in those recently symptomatic patients is considerable, particularly if the stenosis is severe and associated with exhausted cerebrovascular reactivity [12]. In patients presenting with hemispheric transient cerebral ischemia, 8–12% of patients will suffer a stroke within a week, and 11–15% within a month of presentation [13], presumably reflecting the ongoing unstable nature of the atherosclerotic lesion. Thus, early intervention is warranted to minimize the chance of recurrent cerebrovascular events, as well as address the risk of adverse vascular events in other territories. It is known that carotid endarterectomy is beneficial in reducing stroke rates in patients with recently symptomatic high-grade carotid stenosis [14, 15] and a smaller benefit is seen in treated moderate stenoses [16]. Current evidence suggests that early intervention is necessary to maximize benefit [17].

Carotid artery stenting (CAS) is an evolving therapeutic technique to treat carotid artery stenosis. Debate still exists regarding its place in the management of carotid stenosis, but in experienced hands it is probably as efficacious as surgery and has become a widely performed intervention. The role of modern pharmacotherapy as an adjunct to CAS cannot be overstated. Drug treatment in patients undergoing CAS following recent TIA or ischemic stroke can be divided into "best medical therapy," i.e., those interventions which are deemed to reduce the risk of subsequent stroke and other vascular-related events, independent of the carotid artery intervention, and CAS-specific pharmacological agents which are used during the stenting procedure itself. Best medical therapy also encompasses those aspects of lifestyle modification which

S. Macdonald and G. Stansby (eds.), *Practical Carotid Artery Stenting*,
DOI: 10.1007/978-1-84800-299-9_9, © Springer-Verlag London Limited 2009

may improve outcome in the recently symptomatic patient with carotid artery disease. These are discussed along with the evidence supporting their use.

This evidence is sometimes very difficult to tease from the literature, as there is a great deal of heterogeneity in study design, timing and measured outcome. For example, some studies reporting on secondary prevention of ischemic stroke have recruited patients up to 5 years following their most recent event [18, 19]. The pathogenesis of carotid atherosclerotic stroke dictates that risk of a recurrent event is greatest early and diminishes with time. Thus, any pharmacological intervention instituted late is unlikely to have a significant effect on reducing recurrent stroke, although it may have a beneficial effect on other vascular-related outcomes. Studies focusing on early intervention following acute carotid atheroembolism are sparse, and more data are required to advise optimal management. Despite this, guidelines for best medical management following acute stroke, and in pursuit of secondary prevention exist [20, 21]. A cumulative early approach seems to offer the best chance of significant and sustained reduction in recurrent stroke risk [22–24].

Best Medical Therapy

It should not be forgotten that atherosclerosis is a generalized process. Patients presenting with transient cerebral or retinal ischemia or stroke, as well as having a high risk of recurrent stroke, have a considerable risk of noncarotid territory vascular events, including myocardial infarction. Addressing this increased risk in those patients with recently symptomatic cerebrovascular disease, by pharmacological intervention, is a cornerstone of effective management and should be considered as first-line therapy in all patients. Aggressive treatment of underlying contributory conditions such as diabetes and hypertension are mandatory, and pharmacological intervention should be augmented, where necessary, by lifestyle modification.

Lifestyle Modifications

The evidence to support lifestyle modification in order to decrease the risk of recurrent stroke is largely based on epidemiological studies (particularly with reference to primary stroke prevention) and common sense. Measures such as smoking cessation, weight reduction, regular exercise, moderation or cessation of alcohol intake, and a healthy balanced diet should all be actively encouraged [21].

Treatment of Background Medical Conditions

A number of comorbid states increase the risk of atherosclerosis and stroke, and therapy should be optimized to control or reverse these.

Diabetes Mellitus

Diabetes is strongly associated with an increased risk of primary ischemic stroke, particularly the microvascular subtype. The presence of diabetes doubles the risk of stroke recurrence, and poor glycemic control in acute stroke leads to worse outcomes [25]. Hyperglycemia in acute stroke is also found in patients not known to be diabetic. Its management is controversial. Intensive insulin therapy following acute myocardial infarction is known to improve outcome [26], but the evidence of benefit in acute stroke is lacking and work is ongoing to define the role of aggressive glycemic control in this setting [27–30]. However, current guidelines, based on level II category C evidence, recommend treating prolonged hyperglycemia occurring within the first 24 h of acute ischemic stroke with insulin in the form of a glucose–potassium–insulin infusion (GKI) [20].

Data on secondary stroke prevention in patients with diabetes are relatively sparse, as most of the evidence relates to primary stroke prevention. This paucity of data is especially true when considering macrovascular ischemic stroke, although there is a trend toward a reduction in macrovascular complications with improved glycemic control. There is good evidence that improved glycemic control reduces the risk of future microvascular complications. Thus, current guidelines suggest normalization of blood glucose levels following ischemic stroke. Furthermore, the benefit derived from the best medical therapeutic measures described in this chapter is even greater in diabetic patients, and these are also advocated [21, 25].

Hypertension

There is a strong link between elevated blood pressure and all types of primary stroke. Although some controversies exist regarding the exact relationship in ischemic stroke [31], most reports point to a linear association and a reduction of blood pressure may reduce primary stroke risk by about 30–40% [31, 32]. The choice of agent seems of secondary importance [31].

Acute stroke is frequently associated with elevated BP. This may reflect a heightened level of stress following the neurovascular insult, and frequently improves spontaneously. Very high or indeed very low blood pressures following stroke are indicative of a poor outcome. This may purely be a reflection of the severity of neurological damage. Conversely, hypertension could theoretically increase the risk of cerebral edema or secondary hemorrhage, whilst hypotension may increase the chance of cerebral thrombosis or of underperfusion and extended ischemia by jeopardizing the ischemic penumbra. The management of hypertension in acute stroke remains controversial, with little convincing data to suggest that lowering blood pressure improves outcome [33]. Current guidelines suggest that consideration of hypotensive agents may be given to facilitate thrombolysis in hyperacute stroke [20]. The role of blood pressure reduction outside of this setting is the subject of ongoing study [34].

The evidence for blood pressure reduction to prevent ischemic recurrent stroke is gathering. Interpretation of the literature is hampered by the diverse nature of the data, with a variety of differing agents commenced at hugely variable time periods following the primary event, which often is not categorized by subtype. Primary stroke caused by severe carotid artery disease was thought to be particularly susceptible to hypoperfusion-induced secondary stroke with blood pressure reduction. However, this only appears to be true in the presence of bilateral high-grade stenoses [35].

Results of the UK TIA trial suggested that lowering blood pressure following TIA reduces the risk of future recurrence [36]. Subsequent trials have provided further evidence. The Post-stroke Antihypertensive Treatment Study (PATS) demonstrated a 29% decrease in recurrent stroke in patients treated with indapamide, a thiazide diuretic, despite only a modest average BP reduction (5/2 mmHg). Seventy-one percent of the 5,665 recruited patients had had an ischemic primary event [37].

Supporting these findings, the results of the Perindopril pROtection aGainst REcurrent Stroke Study (PROGRESS) [18], which compared combination therapy with indapamide and the ACE inhibitor perindopril, perindopril alone or placebo, showed a highly significant reduction in recurrent stroke (RRR 43%) in the combination group, with a mean BP decrease of 12/5 mmHg. However, the perindopril-alone group, despite a similar average BP decrease to that seen in PATS (5/3 mmHg), showed only a nonsignificant reduction (RRR 5%) in secondary stroke risk. A potential source of bias in PROGRESS, which was not randomized, was reflected in the tendency toward allocation of dual therapy in patients with higher background risk.

Conversely, a subgroup analysis of the Heart Outcomes Prevention Evaluation (HOPE) trial, which focused on patients with high vascular risk and history of previous stroke, showed that patients with a history of ischemic stroke treated with the ACE inhibitor ramipril had a significant reduction in the composite endpoint of fatal and nonfatal stroke and transient ischemic attack, with a similar small magnitude of BP reduction (4/3 mmHg). This improvement, despite apparent minimal BP lowering, has invoked the theory that such improvement may be due to other mechanisms of action of ACE inhibitors, such as a direct effect on atherosclerosis progression [38, 39]. However, these small reductions in office blood pressure measurement may not tell the whole truth, as ambulatory or night-time measurements may be altered to a greater degree [40].

Further evidence from these trials suggests that clinically stable patients with normal baseline blood pressures suffering stroke may also benefit from blood pressure reduction to prevent recurrence.

Recent interest has centered on the angiotensin receptor blockers (ARBs), with experimental evidence suggesting that these drugs may have neuroprotective characteristics above and beyond their effect on blood pressure. This beneficial effect is probably mediated by angiotensin II Type 2 receptors in the brain, which are not affected by the ARBs that have a predilection for the angiotensin II type 1 receptor. The MOSES study compared eprosartan with nitredipine, a calcium channel blocker, and found the former more effective in preventing recurrent stroke. A much larger trial, Prevention Regimen For Effectively avoiding Secondary Strokes (PROFESS), is currently further evaluating the role of ARBs in secondary stroke prevention.

At present, the literature supports blood pressure reduction following large vessel ischemic stroke, and a combination therapy of complimentary agents is likely to provide the best level of protection. The threshold for treatment and optimal regime is unknown, but based on class 1, level A evidence, hypertension following ischemic stroke or TIA should be treated in all clinically stable patients beyond the hyperacute period, and treatment should be considered in all patients, irrespective of whether hypertensive or not (IIa, B) [21].

Soberingly, the impact of healthcare measures on hypertension following stroke may be disappointingly low, as significant numbers of patients remain hypertensive in the longer term [41].

Hyperlipidemia

The association between hypercholesterolemia and primary or secondary stroke is much less clear than for coronary heart disease (CHD). Observational studies have failed to show an association between dyslipidemia and stroke, although there may a weak association with ischemic subtypes, counterbalanced by an inverse association with intracerebral hemorrhage [42, 43].

Numerous studies of 3-hydroxy-3-methylglutaryl coenzyme A reductase inhibitor (statin) therapy in patients with CHD have shown considerable improvement in cardiac outcomes [44]. The Cholesterol Treatment Trialists' meta-analysis of 14 randomized studies of statin therapy, involving over 90,000 patients, mostly asymptomatic or with CHD, showed that a 1 mmol L^{-1} decrease in LDL cholesterol concentration over a mean of 5 years is associated with a significant relative risk reduction of ischemic stroke of about 20%, with a trend toward increasing benefit with larger LDL concentration reductions. Furthermore, ongoing benefit was demonstrated with longer-term treatment [45]. However, the specific question of statin therapy in secondary stroke prevention was not considered. A subgroup analysis of the Heart Protection Study (HPS), one of the 14 trials studied above, which featured 3,280 people who had a history of nondisabling ischemic stroke, transient ischemic attack, or carotid artery procedure prior to randomization failed to demonstrate any significant reduction in the stroke rate, although a nonsignificant trend toward fewer ischemic strokes was identified. This was despite a 1 mmol L^{-1} decrease in LDL cholesterol level and a 20% decrease in any vascular events [19]. The lack of response in this setting, given the clear reduction in risk in other high-risk participants, merited further study. Consequently, the Stroke Prevention by Aggressive Reduction in Cholesterol Levels (SPARCL) trial [46] was published, specifically investigating the effect of high-dose atorvastatin on secondary stroke prevention in those patients without clinically manifest coronary heart disease or hypercholesterolaemia, who had been recently symptomatic with a TIA/minor stroke in the preceding 1–6 months. A significant decrease in recurrent stroke was found in the active treatment group (HR 0.84, absolute risk reduction 2.2%). High-dose atorvastatin was also associated with significantly reduced coronary and other vascular adverse events. Notably, 25% of patients allocated to placebo in SPARCL received a commercially available statin outside of the trial, possibly masking an even greater benefit of active therapy. Furthermore, post-hoc analysis suggests that greater reductions in cholesterol levels may further reduce recurrent stroke risk [47].

The contradictory results of the HPS stroke subgroup and SPARCL may be explained in a number of ways, not least because the confidence intervals of the two results overlap, and thus the difference may represent a random error. Furthermore, recruitment in HPS specifically excluded those patients who had experienced a cerebrovascular event in the preceding 6 months (time of highest risk), and the average time from symptoms to enrolment was 4.7 years. Other methodological differences mean that the results may not be directly comparable [19, 46, 48].

Some evidence exists to suggest that the beneficial effect of statins may in part be due to known pleiotropic effects rather than their cholesterol lowering properties. Statin therapy is known to lead to plaque stabilization and possible regression, as well as improving endothelial function and reducing inflammation [49, 50]. The Study to Evaluate Carotid Ultrasound with Ramipril and vitamin E (SECURE) showed a dose-dependent reduction in carotid intimomedial thickness with ramipril therapy. Whilst these effects could theoretically improve outcome in secondary stroke prevention, there are little data to suggest they play a major role, and the chance of improved outcome seems to correlate with greater degrees of LDL cholesterol concentration reduction. The results of SPARCL have led some to advocate immediate commencement of atorvastatin following TIA or minor stroke [51]. Current recommendations suggest that high vascular risk patients with dyslipidemia and recent ischemic stroke or TIA should engage in measures to reduce cholesterol, including lifestyle modification and statin therapy (I, A). In recently symptomatic patients with presumed atherosclerotic origin but no other features of dyslipidemia, statin therapy may be considered to reduce risk of future vascular events (IIa, B) [21]. Further studies are required to gain a greater insight into the relative merits of statins following acute large vessel ischemic stroke.

Anticoagulants

Antithrombotics

Anticoagulants have a defined role in the management of cardioembolic stroke secondary to atrial fibrillation, but numerous studies comparing anticoagulation with warfarin at high and low intensity with antiplatelets have failed to show significant benefit, whilst possibly increasing risk of hemorrhage [52, 53]. Anticoagulant therapy is thus not recommended in the secondary prevention of ischemic stroke, other than in the context of AF [21].

Antiplatelets

There is compelling evidence that all patients who suffer cerebral ischemia should be placed on antiplatelet agents, due to a 28 and 16% reduction in nonfatal and fatal strokes, respectively [54], and that therapy should commence as early as possible following diagnosis to prevent early recurrent ischemic stroke [55, 56]. Hypothetically, the benefits of early antiplatelet therapy are likely to be greater in large artery-induced ischemic stroke, where platelet-rich microemboli associated with the unstable carotid plaque may be reduced by aggressive antiplatelet therapy, than with lacunar infarction, where platelet-mediated mechanisms are less likely to play a role.

Aspirin

Aspirin has been the most widely studied antiplatelet drug and has been shown to reduce the risk of further ischemic stroke and other vascular events by 15–25% [53, 54, 57]. A dose of 75–150 mg is at least as effective as higher doses, and higher doses are likely to lead to greater complications [54, 57–59]. A very favorable cost-benefit profile means that it is generally considered the agent of choice in secondary prevention of ischemic stroke.

Thienopyridines

Thienopyridines act by blocking the ADP-mediated activation of platelets. Ticlopidine, the first to be developed, has been shown to be efficacious in the prevention of adverse vascular events, with a nonsignificant relative odds reduction of 10% compared with aspirin [60]. However, it is uncommonly associated with significant gastrointestinal and hematological side effects. Subsequently, clopidogrel has been introduced into clinical practice and has become more widely utilized due to its better safety profile. It is a prodrug which is metabolized by the cytochrome P450 pathway to form a potent antiplatelet agent.

A number of trials have studied the effect of clopidogrel as part of best medical therapy in secondary ischemic stroke prevention. The Clopidogrel vs. Aspirin in Patients at Risk for Ischemic Events (CAPRIE) study compared aspirin with clopidogrel in patients with a history of MI, stroke, or peripheral vascular disease and found that the latter may be slightly more effective than aspirin at reducing the compound risk of ischemic stroke, MI, or vascular death (RRR 8.7%) [61]. However, on subgroup analysis, the greatest benefit was in the peripheral vascular disease group (RRR 23.8%), with only a small improvement in the stroke cohort (RRR 7.3%).

Further studies have considered the merits of dual antiplatelet therapy, encouraged at least in part by the fact that the combination of aspirin and clopidogrel has a significant benefit in the management of acute coronary syndrome [62]. Evidence that dual therapy is more efficacious in inhibiting platelet function than aspirin alone in patients following ischemic stroke came from a small randomized trial [63].

The Clopidogrel for High Atherothrombotic Risk and Ischemic Stabilization, management, and Avoidance (CHARISMA) trial studied the relative benefits of clopidogrel plus aspirin against aspirin monotherapy in patients with vascular disease, including 3,837 after stroke and 1,864 after TIA, and found that combination treatment does not confer any additional protection against vascular events in patients with clinically evident cardiovascular disease or multiple risk factors, although there was a tendency to reduction of fatal and nonfatal ischemic stroke [64].

The Management of Atherothrombosis with clopidogrel in high-risk patients with recent Transient ischemic attack or isCHemic stroke (MATCH) trial noted a nonsignificant 1% absolute decrease in major vascular events in patients with recent ischemic stroke or TIA and vascular risk factors, in those treated with combination of aspirin and clopidogrel vs. clopidogrel alone – there was also a significant 1% greater absolute rate of major bleeding in the dual therapy group [65].

These latter two trials did not look specifically at large vessel ischemic stroke, and both allowed recruitment some months after a clinical event. It remains unknown whether combination of antiplatelet therapy with aspirin and clopidogrel offers specific benefit in the setting of carotid atheroembolism, compared with monotherapy, particularly in the hyperacute setting. Aggressive antiplatelet therapy may be beneficial in hyperacute carotid atheroembolism when the unstable nature of the carotid plaque renders the patient most vulnerable to early recurrent events.

Subset analysis of those groups treated early following the index event in MATCH and CHARISMA suggested improved outcome with earlier intervention [65, 66], and some supporting evidence comes from a small recent pilot study of emergency treatment of TIA/minor stroke, which was unfortunately terminated prematurely due to a failure to recruit at a prespecified level [24].

The Clopidogrel and Aspirin for Reduction of Emboli in Symptomatic carotid Stenosis (CARESS) trial [67] has explored the effect of dual antiplatelet therapy on carotid artery disease-related stroke, using transcranial Doppler signals to detect the surrogate marker of asymptomatic microemboli [68, 69]. A high density of asymptomatic microembolic signals following recently symptomatic carotid atheroembolism is associated with a greater risk of early recurrent stroke and adverse outcome [70–73]. Combination therapy with clopidogrel and aspirin was shown to significantly decrease microembolism at 7 days, compared with aspirin alone. Dual antiplatelet therapy was also associated with a trend toward reduction of recurrent stroke and TIA risk compared with monotherapy [67].

Thus, the combination may be useful in hyperacute carotid-related stroke, but there is no convincing evidence that long-term combination therapy with aspirin and clopidogrel is beneficial in the secondary prevention of large vessel ischemic stroke [74]. Confounding factors in CHARISMA might have included the high number of asymptomatic patients and patients with a remote vascular event included in the study, whereas a high proportion of patients had a lacunar stroke in the MATCH trial, who may be less likely to benefit from antiplatelets [75].

Further large-scale trials are required, looking specifically at ischemic stroke subsets, to further elucidate any useful role clopidogrel may have in this context. Although it has its advocates, on the basis of cost-benefit analysis alone, clopidogrel should not be considered first line in the long-term prevention of secondary stroke [76–79]. However, it has a useful role in aspirin intolerance, and potentially if true aspirin insensitivity is demonstrated [80]. A maintenance dose of 75 mg is standard, but some evidence exists that the antiplatelet effect is increased with a 150-mg dose. It is not clear whether this translates into a net clinical improvement [81].

Dipyridamole

Dipyridamole is another antiplatelet agent which has been in and out of vogue in the last decade or so, due to conflicting reports regarding its efficacy. It appears to work by increasing the amount of intracellular cyclic adenosine monophosphate (cAMP), via inhibition of cyclic nucleotide phosphodiesterase [82]. cAMP inhibits platelet aggregation. The large European Stroke Prevention Study 2 (ESPS2) used a double-blind randomized placebo-controlled trial to study dipyridamole against aspirin monotherapy, placebo, or combination therapy with both active agents, and the latter was shown to provide a 22% relative risk reduction over aspirin alone [60]. However, meta-analysis of four earlier trials failed to show any benefit of dipyridamole and aspirin over aspirin alone [54] and subsequent meta-analysis, taking into account the data from ESPS2, still failed to demonstrate a significant benefit of combination over aspirin [83]. However, a further large RCT, the ESPRIT study [83], which focused on dipyridamole plus aspirin following TIA/stroke of presumed arterial origin within the preceding 6 months, demonstrated a 1% per year absolute risk reduction in stroke, MI, and vascular death compared with aspirin alone (hazard ratio 0.8), akin to that seen with aspirin vs. placebo. One important difference between ESPS2 and ESPRIT and the earlier trials is that the former used a modified release preparation of dipyridamole, which has better bioavailability [2, 84]. The most recent meta-analysis, including the results of ESPRIT, now suggests that aspirin plus modified release dipyridamole have a beneficial effect in preventing adverse vascular outcomes following ischemic stroke or TIA when compared with aspirin alone. Its role in secondary prevention following CAS remains less clear.

Based on the above, current guidelines suggest that antiplatelet agents are commenced following noncardioembolic stroke to reduce risk of recurrence (I, A). Aspirin is the most cost-effective drug, but aspirin plus modified release dipyridamole, or clopidogrel in those intolerant of aspirin, are all acceptable primary therapies. The combination of aspirin and clopidogrel is not generally recommended for long-term secondary prevention due to an increased risk of hemorrhage (III, A). There is no evidence to guide the choice of medication for patients who experience a large vessel ischemic stroke whilst taking aspirin. Whether this is likely to represent aspirin resistance is unknown. However, options include switching to dipyridamole and aspirin or clopidogrel in this situation [21].

Antiplatelet Resistance

Recent attention has focused on the emerging concept of antiplatelet resistance. Whether nonresponsiveness equilibrates to resistance is a somewhat contentious issue. Some studies have demonstrated an apparent absence of a laboratory response of platelets to standard doses of aspirin in as many as 5–40% of patients [85–87], with reports suggesting a higher mortality rate in those "aspirin resistant" [88].

However, the absence of a clear dose–response curve to aspirin, and the lack of clarity regarding which measurable parameters are the best indicators of platelet function have led to debate about the true nature and extent of variable aspirin response [86, 89–91].

Increased adverse outcome has similarly been found with clopidogrel "resistance" [91, 92], although physiological response to this drug has been shown to follow a normal distribution [63]. It may be that future antiplatelet therapy is guided by assays of responsiveness to differing agents, but currently, these are not widely available and are largely of academic interest.

Periprocedural Pharmacotherapy

Anticoagulation

Heparin

Periprocedural anticoagulation is administered to reduce the risk of thromboembolism associated with indwelling vascular sheaths, catheters, and guidewires, particularly when flow may be slow because of stenotic vessels. There is wide variation in practice, but heparin is the most widely used agent and may be given solely by bolus administration or in combination with a continuous infusion. The latter is adjusted to provide an APTT of 250–300 s. The dose of heparin required is usually in the range of 75–100 units kg^{-1}; a bolus of 3,000 units of heparin provides adequate anticoagulant effect for approximately 30 min in a "typical" patient, whilst 5,000 units give about 45 min of appropriate cover. Thus, a 5,000–7,500 unit bolus administered, once arterial access is secured, should be sufficient to allow adequate anticoagulation during CAS.

Heparin, particularly the unfractionated variant, binds to various plasma and cellular proteins within the circulation, rendering it inactive. An increase in heparin-binding sites, such as occurs with raised inflammatory plasma proteins or thrombocythemia may thus reduce the effectiveness of a particular dose, and adjustment may be needed [93]. Some advocate combining initial periprocedural bolus administration with a continuous infusion of 15–20 units kg^{-1} h^{-1}, but in our unit, a heparin infusion is only started postprocedurally in the event of neurological complications, and only once intracranial hemorrhage has been excluded.

It has been shown that heparin can increase platelet aggregation in response to arachidonic acid and that this can counteract the antiplatelet effect of aspirin [82, 93, 94]. This may explain why a small proportion of patients are at risk of cardiovascular events after major vascular intervention. However, until a suitable alternative has been validated, the proaggregation risk that heparin poses during CAS is probably outweighed by the benefits.

Reports suggest that the currently unlicensed intravenous administration of low molecular weight heparin (LMWH) is significantly less likely to cause major hemorrhage than unfractionated heparin in Percutaneous coronary intervention (PCI) [95]. Furthermore, LMWHs are less proaggregatory, possibly because it has a more specific protein-binding profile than its unfractionated cousin. This increased specificity explains the more reliable dose–response characteristics of LMWH, and the general requirement for no anticoagulation level monitoring [94]. However, some reports suggest an increased risk of pericatheter thrombus formation during PCI with LMWH cover compared with UFH [96].

Heparin-induced thrombocytopenia (HIT) is an uncommon but well-known side effect of heparin administration, where an autoantibody develops against the complex of heparin and platelet factor 4. This causes platelet consumption but leads paradoxically to a prothrombotic state. Although more likely to occur with continuous infusion, it can follow bolus administration. LMWHs are less likely to cause HIT [97]. However, a prior history of HIT should prompt use of an alternative antithrombotic agent [82].

In addition to formal anticoagulation, heparinized saline (5,000 units L^{-1}) is also used to maintain guiding catheter/sheath patency and to flush catheters.

Novel Antithrombotics

More recently, novel antithrombotic agents have been developed targeting specific factors in the clotting cascade.

Fondaparinux is a synthetic specific factor Xa antagonist, which has been shown to be effective in prophylaxis and treatment of venous thromboembolism, and equivalent in management of acute coronary syndrome (ACS), when compared with LMWH, with less risk of bleeding [98]. Theoretically, it should not cause thrombocytopenia and so may be useful in the treatment of HIT [99]. However, concerns have been raised over the rates of pericatheter and wire thrombosis when used as the sole agent in PCI [98]. Oral versions are in development. It is currently not licensed for use outside of Venous thrombo-embolism (VTE) prophylaxis and treatment.

The direct thrombin inhibitors owe their existence to the medicinal leech, being a synthetic derivative of hirudin, an anticoagulant found in leech saliva [100]. Four are currently licensed for various indications with the FDA. The properties of bivalirudin suggest that this may prove a useful agent in endovascular therapy [101] and it has approval for use in PCI. In contrast to unfractionated and low molecular weight heparin, it acts on clot-bound thrombin, does not cause platelet activation or thrombocytopenia, inhibits thrombin-induced platelet activation, and has linear pharmacokinetics, with a half-life of 25 min. It has been compared with other antithrombotic regimes in low- and high-risk patients undergoing coronary intervention, with bivalirudin monotherapy offering a viable alternative to the current standard, heparin plus Gp IIb/IIIa inhibition, being noninferior in terms of ischemic outcome, but giving the additional benefit of significantly reduced rates of hemorrhage [102, 103]. Limited data exist regarding its use in the peripheral vasculature. A recent trial supported its use in carotid artery intervention [104] and it appears safe and effective in other peripheral territories [105], but more evidence is required and its use should be limited to inclusion in clinical trials or where there is contraindication to heparin, such as HIT. Other agents in this class of drug include lepirudin, desirudin, and argatroban [106]. Other oral agents are currently being developed, following the withdrawal of ximelagatran, the first to be released, which – although showing promise – led to hepatotoxicity in a proportion of patients [100].

One drawback to the newer antithrombotic agents is the lack of an antidote to their anticoagulant action. UFH can be reversed by protamine sulfate, which can also counteract about 60% of the activity of LMWH [107]. This may be an important consideration if the patient undergoing CAS is at high risk of a reperfusion bleed.

Antiplatelet Therapy

Whilst there is no compelling evidence that dual antiplatelet therapy with aspirin and clopidogrel imparts additional benefit over monotherapy in secondary prevention following ischemic stroke, a combination of aspirin and clopidogrel appears to have a significantly beneficial effect in reducing the frequency of microemboli from the recently symptomatic carotid plaque [72], and following carotid endarterectomy [108], where the freshly exposed subendothelium has thrombogenic potential [109, 110]. Arterial stenting similarly causes endothelial and intimal damage, predisposing to thrombus formation and risking embolization [111, 112]. Combination therapy with clopidogrel and aspirin, compared with aspirin alone, significantly reduces the complications of coronary intervention [113, 114]. Similarly, it appears effective in reducing the incidence of adverse neurological sequelae when compared with aspirin monotherapy following CAS, without a significant risk of increased bleeding [114–116].

Ideally, clopidogrel at a dose of 75 mg should be commenced in addition to aspirin, 5–7 days preprocedure, in order to attain adequate therapeutic effect. However, in the current climate of reducing time to carotid intervention in order to maximize benefit, an oral loading dose of 600 mg of clopidogrel may be given, at least 6 h prior to CAS. This dosage is suggested because of evidence from clopidogrel in coronary intervention, where a high loading dose (>300 mg) significantly reduces risk of nonfatal MI and death [117]. There is some evidence that a maintenance dose of 150 mg exerts a greater inhibitory effect [80], but there is no suggestion that this leads to improved clinical outcome. Most reports recommend that dual antiplatelet therapy should be continued for at least 30 days postprocedure to allow sufficient time for stent endothelialization, whereafter monotherapy can be resumed. There is no evidence to suggest that long-term dual antiplatelet agent therapy improves outcome following CAS, but the optimal duration of therapy is yet to be determined. Standard practice at our institution for uncomplicated stenting of symptomatic carotid stenoses is 4–6 weeks of combined treatment, with aspirin monotherapy thereafter in those who can tolerate it.

Other antiplatelets are available for consideration and use of these is commonplace in some centers. There is no convincing evidence to support their use during CAS, but data from coronary intervention suggest that they may be of benefit. The glycoprotein IIb/IIIa (Gp IIb/IIIa) inhibitors are potent inhibitors of platelet aggregation, by blocking the crosslinking binding of fibrinogen during thrombogenesis. Three are currently commercially available: abciximab, a mouse–human chimeric monoclonal antibody was the first to gain FDA approval in the US following evidence that it reduces complications in high-risk PCI [118, 119]; tirofiban (a synthetic tyrosine analog) and eptifibatide (another synthetic peptide) which are both derivatives of agents found in poisonous snake venom. Glycoprotein IIa/IIIb antagonists have been investigated as an adjunct to other antithrombotic drugs in the context of carotid stenting with favorable results [120, 121]. A reduction in ischemic events was noted in one study but was offset by a greater risk of bleeding [122]. However, this experience has not been shared by all authors. Use of abciximab solely as a bolus does not result in any beneficial outcome [123] and in the largest group studied so far, Wholey et al. [124] found a significantly greater incidence of adverse neurological outcomes in patients receiving Gp IIb/IIIa antagonist plus half-heparin dose (6%), than in a group assigned to periprocedural heparin alone (2.4%, both in addition to aspirin and thienopyridine). A large proportion of these complications were secondary to intracerebral hemorrhage. Despite this, some authors use Gp IIb/IIIa inhibitors routinely, with apparently low rates of complications [125]. However, the concomitant increasing utilization of cerebral embolic protection devices (EPDs) has largely supplanted use of routine adjunctive Gp IIb/IIIa inhibitors in most centers, following data to suggest that EPDs are of more benefit in preventing neuroischemic complications [126–128]. Increasing numbers of case reports indicate that there may a useful role as a rescue agent following carotid stent thrombosis [114, 129–135], but it still remains that no large-scale RCTs have been undertaken to formally evaluate the utility of Gp IIa/IIIb in the context of CAS.

Prasugrel is a newer thienopyridine whose conversion has less reliance on the cytochrome P450 enzymatic pathway than its more established cousins. It has potent antiplatelet activity, and the optimal dose has yet to be defined. It appears to reduce the number of ischemic events post MI, and incidence of stent thrombosis post-PCI, but this beneficial effect is offset by a significantly increased risk of bleeding, particularly intracranial hemorrhage compared to clopidogrel, at the dose investigated [136]. Its place in the endovascular management of carotid artery stenosis has yet to be elucidated.

Dextran is a crystalline polymer made up of repeating glucose subunits. It has had various applications in surgery over the last 60 years but is known to possess potent antiplatelet activity, inhibiting aggregation and adhesiveness. It has been shown to work rapidly to reduce symptomatic microembolism prior to carotid endarterectomy [137] and following surgery, when guided by transcranial Doppler, it decreases microembolism and stroke risk [138–141].

IV dextran therapy has also been recently used to treat symptomatic microemboli following carotid stenting [142]. Dextran therapy is known to lead to a number of complications, including hemorrhage, pulmonary edema, acute renal failure, and allergic reactions [138]. For this reason, blanket use of dextran following carotid surgery may lead to unacceptable risk [143]. However, it may have a role in treatment of neuroembolic complications resulting from CAS.

Pre-Existing Warfarin Therapy

A patient presenting with a large vessel ischemic stroke who is on warfarin introduces an interesting clinical dilemma. Combination therapy with dual antiplatelets and warfarin leads to a high risk of hemorrhage. There is no evidence that warfarin improves the outcome following CAS. Warfarin may not be protective against stent thrombosis, and may increase the risk of bleeding, particularly if combined with dual antiplatelet therapy. However, the risks of warfarin cessation vary according to the indication for treatment, and dual antiplatelets may not be as effective in protecting against the background problem. An individualized assessment should be made to delineate the optimal management in this situation, but every effort should be made to preserve dual antiplatelet therapy in the peri-stenting period.

Anticholinergic Therapy

Balloon catheter inflation in the region of the carotid sinus can induce marked baroreceptor stimulation resulting in severe bradycardia or even asystole. Anticholinergic drugs, such as atropine (0.5–1 mg), or the shorter acting glycopyrrolate (600 μg) administered via the guiding catheter/sheath prior to predilatation (or stent deployment if no predilatation is performed), block this parasympathetic reflex during carotid artery intervention, and help maintain a steady pulse rate in both patient and operator. Glycopyrrolate may be safer than atropine in patients with severe coronary artery disease, as it tends to result in less reflex tachycardia, and in our institution is the agent of choice. Self-expanding stents may exert an ongoing stimulatory effect on the carotid bulb following deployment, frequently resulting in postprocedural relative bradycardia and hypotension. However, no specific treatment is required for this in the vast majority of cases, and the pulse and blood pressure tend to return to preintervention levels over the next few days. Rarely, patients have symptomatic hypotension postprocedure, and this usually responds to conservative measures and volume expansion with intravenous fluids.

Vasodilator Agents

Arterial wall spasm is a frequent consequence of guidewire and catheter manipulation, and can also occur as a result of carotid stent deployment. It may be minimized by meticulous technique. However, should spasm occur, a slow bolus of a vasodilator, such as glyceryl trinitrate (200–300 μg to 2–3 ml of a solution of 1-mg GTN diluted in 10-ml saline), may be administered through the guiding catheter or sheath. Spasm frequently resolves on withdrawal of the cerebral protection device, guidewire, or catheter. Care should be taken to distinguish spasm from kinking of the Internal carotid artery (ICA), which may result from placement of a poorly conformable stent into a tortuous vessel. The appearances of a kinked ICA may be similar to vasospasm, and may also improve following guidewire withdrawal, but a kink may also worsen once the wire has been pulled back, and consideration should be given to further stent placement (perhaps with a more compliant device) at the site of the kink.

Summary

Patients who have experienced a recent stroke or TIA with ipsilateral high-grade carotid stenosis are at high risk of recurrent stroke and other vascular events. CAS is an evolving technique to treat symptomatic carotid disease. The adjunctive pharmacology is very important to minimize the risk of future stroke and maximize the success of the procedure. Best medical therapy should be instituted in all ischemic stroke sufferers, and comprises lifestyle modification, treatment of background medical conditions – such as hypertension, diabetes, and hyperlipidemia – and antiplatelet drugs.

Specific drugs to enable the procedure to be performed with the greatest chance of a successful result include dual antiplatelet therapy, antithrombotics, antimuscarinics, and vasodilators. More recently, other potent anticoagulants have been released and may have a role in future adjunctive pharmacotherapy. However, the institution of such drugs should be evidence based.

Key Points

- Pharmacotherapy in carotid stenting plays a major role in reducing the risk to the patient:
  - Risk of stroke/recurrent stroke
  - General cardiovascular risk
  - Procedural risk
- General vascular and stroke risk reduction strategies (= best medical therapy) should be used, including:
  - Blood pressure control
  - Use of antiplatelet agents according to local/national guidelines:
    - Aspirin
    - Clopidogrel
    - Dipyridamole
    - Combination therapy (e.g., aspirin + dipyridamole or aspirin + clopidogrel)
  - Use of lipid lowering agents:
    - Mainly statins
  - Treatment of associated conditions:
    - Diabetes
  - Lifestyle modification:
    - Smoking cessation
    - Improved diet/weight reduction
    - Increased exercise
- Specific measures to reduce the risk of the carotid stent procedure itself include:
  - Antithrombotics:
    - Heparin by infusion or bolus
    - Newer drugs:
    - Direct thrombin inhibitors – not currently licensed for CAS
    - Combination antiplatelet therapy (aspirin + clopidogrel for 30 days)
    - Other antiplatelet drugs such as abciximab, tirofiban, and eptifibatide are used by some but may increase intracranial bleeding risk:
  - Newer agents, e.g., prasugrel
  - Anticholinergics to prevent carotid sinus bradycardia and hypotension:
    - Atropine
    - Glycopyrrolate
  - Vasodilators, e.g., glyceryl trinitrate for spasm

References

1. Lovett, J.K., A.J. Coull, and P.M. Rothwell, Early risk of recurrence by subtype of ischemic stroke in population-based incidence studies. *Neurology*, 2004. 62(4): 569–573.
2. De Schryver, E.L., A. Algra, and J. van Gijn, Dipyridamole for preventing stroke and other vascular events in patients with vascular disease. *Cochrane Database Syst Rev*, 2007. 3: CD001820.
3. van Wijk, I., et al., Long-term survival and vascular event risk after transient ischaemic attack or minor ischaemic stroke: A cohort study. *Lancet*, 2005. 365(9477): 2098–2104.
4. Rothwell, P.M. and C.P. Warlow, Timing of TIAs preceding stroke: Time window for prevention is very short. *Neurology*, 2005. 64(5): 817–820.
5. Hankey, G., Impact of treatment of people with transient ischaemic attack on stroke incidence and public health. *Cerebrovasc Dis*, 1996. 6(Suppl 1): 26–33.
6. Bray, J.E., K. Coughlan, and C. Bladin, Can the ABCD Score be dichotomised to identify high-risk patients with transient ischaemic attack in the emergency department? *Emerg Med J*, 2007. 24(2): 92–95.
7. Rothwell, P.M., et al., A simple score (ABCD) to identify individuals at high early risk of stroke after transient ischaemic attack. *Lancet*, 2005. 366(9479): 29–36.
8. Johnston, S.C., et al., Validation and refinement of scores to predict very early stroke risk after transient ischaemic attack. *Lancet*, 2007. 369(9558): 283–292.

9. Purroy, F., et al., Higher risk of further vascular events among transient ischemic attack patients with diffusion-weighted imaging acute ischemic lesions. *Stroke*, 2004. 35(10): 2313–2319.
10. Eliasziw, M., et al., Early risk of stroke after a transient ischemic attack in patients with internal carotid artery disease. *Can Med Assoc J*, 2004. 170(7): 1105–1109.
11. Purroy, F., et al., Patterns and predictors of early risk of recurrence after transient ischemic attack with respect to etiologic subtypes. *Stroke*, 2007. 38(12): 3225–3229.
12. Blaser, T., et al., Risk of stroke, transient ischemic attack, and vessel occlusion before endarterectomy in patients with symptomatic severe carotid stenosis. *Stroke*, 2002. 33(4): 1057–1062.
13. Coull, A.J., J.K. Lovett, and P.M. Rothwell, Population based study of early risk of stroke after transient ischaemic attack or minor stroke: Implications for public education and organisation of services. *Br Med J*, 2004. 328(7435): 326.
14. European Carotid Surgery Trial Collaborators, Randomised trial of endarterectomy for recently symptomatic carotid stenosis: Final results of the MRC European Carotid Surgery Trial (ECST). Lancet, 1998. 351(9113): 1379–1387.
15. North American Symptomatic Carotid Endarterectomy Trial Collaborators, Beneficial effect of carotid endarterectomy in symptomatic patients with high-grade carotid stenosis. N Engl J Med, 1991. 325(7): 445–453.
16. Barnett, H.J., et al., Benefit of carotid endarterectomy in patients with symptomatic moderate or severe stenosis. North American Symptomatic Carotid Endarterectomy Trial Collaborators. *N Engl J Med*, 1998. 339(20): 1415–1425.
17. Rothwell, P.M., et al., Endarterectomy for symptomatic carotid stenosis in relation to clinical subgroups and timing of surgery. *Lancet*, 2004. 363(9413): 915–924.
18. PROGRESS Collaborative Group, Randomised trial of a perindopril-based blood-pressure-lowering regimen among 6105 individuals with previous stroke or transient ischaemic attack. Lancet, 2001. 358(9287): 1033–1041.
19. Collins, R., et al., Effects of cholesterol-lowering with simvastatin on stroke and other major vascular events in 20536 people with cerebrovascular disease or other high-risk conditions. *Lancet*, 2004. 363(9411): 757–767.
20. Adams, H.P.,Jr., et al., Guidelines for the early management of adults with ischemic stroke: A guideline from the American Heart Association/American Stroke Association Stroke Council, Clinical Cardiology Council, Cardiovascular Radiology and Intervention Council, and the Atherosclerotic Peripheral Vascular Disease and Quality of Care Outcomes in Research Interdisciplinary Working Groups: The American Academy of Neurology affirms the value of this guideline as an educational tool for neurologists. *Stroke*, 2007. 38(5): 1655–1711.
21. Sacco, R.L., et al., Guidelines for prevention of stroke in patients with ischemic stroke or transient ischemic attack: A statement for healthcare professionals from the American Heart Association/American Stroke Association Council on Stroke: Co-sponsored by the Council on Cardiovascular Radiology and Intervention: The American Academy of Neurology affirms the value of this guideline. *Stroke*, 2006. 37(2): 577–617.
22. Hackam, D.G. and J.D. Spence, Combining multiple approaches for the secondary prevention of vascular events after stroke: A quantitative modeling study. *Stroke*, 2007. 38(6): 1881–1885.
23. Rothwell, P.M., et al., Effect of urgent treatment of transient ischaemic attack and minor stroke on early recurrent stroke (EXPRESS study): A prospective population-based sequential comparison. *Lancet*, 2007. 370(9596): 1432–1442.
24. Kennedy, J., et al., Fast assessment of stroke and transient ischaemic attack to prevent early recurrence (FASTER): A randomised controlled pilot trial. *Lancet Neurol*, 2007. 6(11): 961–969.
25. Idris, I., G.A. Thomson, and J.C. Sharma, Diabetes mellitus and stroke. *Int J Clin Pract*, 2006. 60(1): 48–56.
26. Malmberg, K., et al., Randomized trial of insulin-glucose infusion followed by subcutaneous insulin treatment in diabetic patients with acute myocardial infarction (DIGAMI study): Effects on mortality at 1 year. *J Am Coll Cardiol*, 1995. 26(1): 57–65.
27. Gray, C.S., et al., Glucose–potassium–insulin infusions in the management of post-stroke hyperglycaemia: The UK Glucose Insulin in Stroke Trial (GIST-UK). *Lancet Neurol*, 2007. 6(5): 397–406.
28. Donnan, G.A. and C. Levi, Glucose and the ischaemic brain: Too much of a good thing? *Lancet Neurol*, 2007. 6(5): 380–381.
29. Bruno, A., et al., Treatment of hyperglycemia in ischemic stroke (THIS): A randomized pilot trial. *Stroke*, 2008. 39(2): 384–389.
30. Bruno, A., R.R. Shankar, and L.S. Williams, About hyperglycemia during acute stroke. *Stroke*, 2007. 38(11): e138; author reply e139.
31. Lawes, C.M., et al., Blood pressure and stroke: An overview of published reviews. *Stroke*, 2004. 35(3): 776–785.

32. Bosch, J., et al., Use of ramipril in preventing stroke: Double blind randomised trial. *Br Med J*, 2002. 324(7339): 699–702.
33. Powers, W.J., Acute hypertension after stroke: The scientific basis for treatment decisions. *Neurology*, 1993. 43(3 Pt 1): 461–467.
34. Potter, J., et al., CHHIPS (Controlling Hypertension and Hypotension Immediately Post-Stroke) Pilot Trial: Rationale and design. *J Hypertens*, 2005. 23(3): 649–655.
35. Rothwell, P.M., S.C. Howard, and J.D. Spence, Relationship between blood pressure and stroke risk in patients with symptomatic carotid occlusive disease. *Stroke*, 2003. 34(11): 2583–2590.
36. Rodgers, A., et al., Blood pressure and risk of stroke in patients with cerebrovascular disease. The United Kingdom Transient Ischaemic Attack Collaborative Group. *Br Med J*, 1996. 313(7050): 147.
37. PATS Collaborating Group, Post-stroke antihypertensive treatment study. A preliminary result. Chin Med J (Engl), 1995. 108(9): 710–717.
38. Adler, A.I., et al., Association of systolic blood pressure with macrovascular and microvascular complications of type 2 diabetes (UKPDS 36): Prospective observational study. *Br Med J*, 2000. 321(7258): 412–419.
39. Lonn, E., et al., Effects of ramipril and vitamin E on atherosclerosis: The study to evaluate carotid ultrasound changes in patients treated with ramipril and vitamin E (SECURE). *Circulation*, 2001. 103(7): 919–925.
40. Svensson, P., et al., Comparative effects of ramipril on ambulatory and office blood pressures: A HOPE Substudy. *Hypertension*, 2001. 38(6): E28–E32.
41. Paul, S.L. and A.G. Thrift, Control of hypertension 5 years after stroke in the North East Melbourne Stroke Incidence Study. *Hypertension*, 2006. 48(2): 260–265.
42. Prospective Studies Collaboration, Cholesterol, diastolic blood pressure, and stroke: 13000 strokes in 450000 people in 45 prospective cohorts. Prospective studies collaboration. Lancet, 1995. 346(8991–8992): 1647–1653.
43. Iso, H., et al., Serum cholesterol levels and six-year mortality from stroke in 350977 men screened for the multiple risk factor intervention trial. *N Engl J Med*, 1989. 320(14): 904–910.
44. Paciaroni, M., et al., Statins and stroke prevention. *Cerebrovasc Dis*, 2007. 24(2–3): 170–182.
45. Cholesterol Treatment Trialists' (CTT) Collaborators, Efficacy and safety of cholesterol-lowering treatment: Prospective meta-analysis of data from 90056 participants in 14 randomised trials of statins. Lancet, 2005. 366(9493): 1267–1278.
46. The Stroke Prevention by Aggressive Reduction in Cholesterol Levels (SPARCL) Investigators, High-dose atorvastatin after stroke or transient ischemic attack. N Engl J Med, 2006. 355(6): 549–559.
47. Mazighi, M., et al., Statin therapy and stroke prevention: What was known, what is new and what is next? *Curr Opin Lipidol*, 2007. 18(6): 622–625.
48. Coull, B.M., Statin therapy after acute ischemic stroke in the heart protection study: Is the role in recurrent stroke prevention now defined? *Stroke*, 2004. 35(9): 2233–2234.
49. Moonis, M., et al., HMG-CoA reductase inhibitors improve acute ischemic stroke outcome. *Stroke*, 2005. 36(6): 1298–1300.
50. Amarenco, P., P. Lavallee, and P.J. Touboul, Stroke prevention, blood cholesterol, and statins. *Lancet Neurol*, 2004. 3(5): 271–278.
51. Gaspardone, A. and M. Arca, Atorvastatin: Its clinical role in cerebrovascular prevention. *Drugs*, 2007. 67(Suppl 1): 55–62.
52. Sacco, R.L., et al., Comparison of warfarin versus aspirin for the prevention of recurrent stroke or death: Subgroup analyses from the Warfarin–Aspirin Recurrent Stroke Study. *Cerebrovasc Dis*, 2006. 22(1): 4–12.
53. Algra, A., et al., Oral anticoagulants versus antiplatelet therapy for preventing further vascular events after transient ischaemic attack or minor stroke of presumed arterial origin. *Cochrane Database Syst Rev*, 2006. 3: CD001342.
54. Antithrombotic Trialists Collaboration, Collaborative meta-analysis of randomised trials of antiplatelet therapy for prevention of death, myocardial infarction, and stroke in high risk patients. Br Med J, 2002. 324(7329): 71–86.
55. Chinese Acute Stroke Trial Collaborative Group, CAST: Randomised placebo-controlled trial of early aspirin use in 20,000 patients with acute ischaemic stroke. CAST (Chinese Acute Stroke Trial) Collaborative Group. Lancet, 1997. 349(9066): 1641–1649.
56. International Stroke Trial Collaborative Group, The International Stroke Trial (IST): A randomised trial of aspirin, subcutaneous heparin, both, or neither among 19435 patients with acute ischaemic stroke. Lancet, 1997. 349(9065): 1569–1581.
57. Farrell, B., et al., The United Kingdom transient ischaemic attack (UK-TIA) aspirin trial: Final results. *J Neurol Neurosurg Psychiatry*, 1991. 54(12): 1044–1054.
58. Dutch TIA Trial Study Group, A comparison of two doses of aspirin (30 mg vs. 283 mg a day) in patients after a transient ischemic attack or minor ischemic stroke. N Engl J Med, 1991. 325(18): 1261–1266.

59. SALT Collaborative Group, Swedish Aspirin Low-Dose Trial (SALT) of 75 mg aspirin as secondary prophylaxis after cerebrovascular ischaemic events. Lancet, 1991. 338(8779): 1345–1349.
60. Antiplatelet Trialists' Collaboration, Collaborative overview of randomised trials of antiplatelet therapy. I. Prevention of death, myocardial infarction, and stroke by prolonged antiplatelet therapy in various categories of patients. Br Med J, 1994. 308(6921): 81–106.
61. CAPRIE Steering Committee, A randomised, blinded, trial of clopidogrel versus aspirin in patients at risk of ischaemic events (CAPRIE). Lancet, 1996. 348(9038): 1329–1339.
62. Yusuf, S., et al., Effects of clopidogrel in addition to aspirin in patients with acute coronary syndromes without ST-segment elevation. *N Engl J Med*, 2001. 345(7): 494–502.
63. Serebruany, V.L., et al., Effects of clopidogrel and aspirin in combination versus aspirin alone on platelet activation and major receptor expression in patients after recent ischemic stroke: For the Plavix Use for Treatment of Stroke (PLUTO-Stroke) trial. *Stroke*, 2005. 36(10): 2289–2292.
64. Bhatt, D.L., et al., Clopidogrel and aspirin versus aspirin alone for the prevention of atherothrombotic events. *N Engl J Med*, 2006. 354(16): 1706–1717.
65. Diener, H.C., et al., Aspirin and clopidogrel compared with clopidogrel alone after recent ischaemic stroke or transient ischaemic attack in high-risk patients (MATCH): Randomised, double-blind, placebo-controlled trial. *Lancet*, 2004. 364(9431): 331–337.
66. Bhatt, D.L., et al., Patients with prior myocardial infarction, stroke, or symptomatic peripheral arterial disease in the CHARISMA trial. *J Am Coll Cardiol*, 2007. 49(19): 1982–1988.
67. Markus, H.S., et al., Dual antiplatelet therapy with clopidogrel and aspirin in symptomatic carotid stenosis evaluated using Doppler embolic signal detection: The Clopidogrel and Aspirin for Reduction of Emboli in Symptomatic Carotid Stenosis (CARESS) trial. *Circulation*, 2005. 111(17): 2233–2240.
68. Markus, H., A. Loh, and M.M. Brown, Detection of circulating cerebral emboli using Doppler ultrasound in a sheep model. *J Neurol Sci*, 1994. 122(1): 117–124.
69. Russell, D., et al., Detection of arterial emboli using Doppler ultrasound in rabbits. *Stroke*, 1991. 22(2): 253–258.
70. Molloy, J. and H.S. Markus, Asymptomatic embolization predicts stroke and TIA risk in patients with carotid artery stenosis. *Stroke*, 1999. 30(7): 1440–1443.
71. Siebler, M., et al., Cerebral microembolism and the risk of ischemia in asymptomatic high-grade internal carotid artery stenosis. *Stroke*, 1995. 26(11): 2184–2186.
72. Markus, H.S. and A. MacKinnon, Asymptomatic embolization detected by Doppler ultrasound predicts stroke risk in symptomatic carotid artery stenosis. *Stroke*, 2005. 36(5): 971–975.
73. Valton, L., et al., Microembolic signals and risk of early recurrence in patients with stroke or transient ischemic attack. *Stroke*, 1998. 29(10): 2125–2128.
74. Schwartz, N.E. and G.W. Albers, Is there a role for combinations of antiplatelet agents in stroke prevention? *Curr Treat Options Neurol*, 2007. 9(6): 442–450.
75. Sacco, S. and A. Carolei, CHARISMA: The antiplatelet saga continues. *Stroke*, 2007. 38(3): 854.
76. Jones, L., et al., Clinical effectiveness and cost-effectiveness of clopidogrel and modified-release dipyridamole in the secondary prevention of occlusive vascular events: A systematic review and economic evaluation. *Health Technol Assess*, 2004. 8(38): iii–iv, 1–196.
77. Norris, J.W. and H.J. Barnett, CHARISMA: The antiplatelet saga continues. *Stroke*, 2006. 37(9): 2428–2429.
78. Gorelick, P., O. Sechenova, and C.H. Hennekens, Evolving perspectives on clopidogrel in the treatment of ischemic stroke. *J Cardiovasc Pharmacol Ther*, 2006. 11(4): 245–248.
79. Hassan, A.E., et al., Drug evaluation of clopidogrel in patients with ischemic stroke. *Expert Opin Pharmacother*, 2007. 8(16): 2825–2838.
80. von Beckerath, N., et al., A double-blind, randomized study on platelet aggregation in patients treated with a daily dose of 150 or 75 mg of clopidogrel for 30 days. *Eur Heart J*, 2007. 28(15): 1814–1819.
81. Diener, H.C., et al., European Stroke Prevention Study. 2. Dipyridamole and acetylsalicylic acid in the secondary prevention of stroke. *J Neurol Sci*, 1996. 143(1–2): 1–13.
82. Mehta, R.P. and M.S. Johnson, Update on anticoagulant medications for the interventional radiologist. *J Vasc Interv Radiol*, 2006. 17(4): 597–612.
83. ESPRIT Study Group, Aspirin plus dipyridamole versus aspirin alone after cerebral ischaemia of arterial origin (ESPRIT): Randomised controlled trial. Lancet, 2006. 367(9523): 1665–1673.
84. Derendorf, H., et al., Dipyridamole bioavailability in subjects with reduced gastric acidity. *J Clin Pharmacol*, 2005. 45(7): 845–850.

85. Grundmann, K., et al., Aspirin non-responder status in patients with recurrent cerebral ischemic attacks. *J Neurol*, 2003. 250(1): 63–66.
86. Altman, R., et al., The antithrombotic profile of aspirin. Aspirin resistance, or simply failure? *Thromb J*, 2004. 2(1): 1.
87. Gum, P.A., et al., Profile and prevalence of aspirin resistance in patients with cardiovascular disease. *Am J Cardiol*, 2001. 88(3): 230–235.
88. Gum, P.A., et al., A prospective, blinded determination of the natural history of aspirin resistance among stable patients with cardiovascular disease. *J Am Coll Cardiol*, 2003. 41(6): 961–965.
89. Bhatt, D.L., Aspirin resistance: More than just a laboratory curiosity. *J Am Coll Cardiol*, 2004. 43(6): 1127–1129.
90. Johns, A., M. Fisher, and V. Knappertz, Aspirin and clopidogrel resistance: An emerging clinical entity. *Eur Heart J*, 2006. 27(14): 1754; author reply 1754–1755.
91. Myers, R.I., The variability of platelet response to aspirin and clopidogrel: Revisiting the Caprie, Cure, Credo, and Match trials. *Proc (Bayl Univ Med Cent)*, 2005. 18(4): 331–336.
92. Wang, T.H., D.L. Bhatt, and E.J. Topol, Aspirin and clopidogrel resistance: An emerging clinical entity. *Eur Heart J*, 2006. 27(6): 647–654.
93. Webster, S.E., et al., Anti-platelet effect of aspirin is substantially reduced after administration of heparin during carotid endarterectomy. *J Vasc Surg*, 2004. 40(3): 463–468.
94. Storey, R.F., J.A. May, and S. Heptinstall, Potentiation of platelet aggregation by heparin in human whole blood is attenuated by P2Y12 and P2Y1 antagonists but not aspirin. *Thromb Res*, 2005. 115(4): 301–307.
95. Dumaine, R., et al., Intravenous low-molecular-weight heparins compared with unfractionated heparin in percutaneous coronary intervention: Quantitative review of randomized trials. *Arch Intern Med*, 2007. 167(22): 2423–2430.
96. Dana, A., et al., Macroscopic thrombus formation on angioplasty equipment following antithrombin therapy with enoxaparin. *Catheter Cardiovasc Interv*, 2007. 70(6): 847–853.
97. Martel, N., J. Lee, and P.S. Wells, Risk for heparin-induced thrombocytopenia with unfractionated and low-molecular-weight heparin thromboprophylaxis: A meta-analysis. *Blood*, 2005. 106(8): 2710–2715.
98. Yusuf, S., et al., Comparison of fondaparinux and enoxaparin in acute coronary syndromes. *N Engl J Med*, 2006. 354(14): 1464–1476.
99. Lobo, B., et al., Fondaparinux for the treatment of patients with acute heparin-induced thrombocytopenia. *Thromb Haemost*, 2008. 99(1): 208–214.
100. Fields, W.S., The history of leeching and hirudin. *Haemostasis*, 1991. 21(Suppl 1): 3–10.
101. Lepor, N.E., Anticoagulation for acute coronary syndromes: From heparin to direct thrombin inhibitors. *Rev Cardiovasc Med*, 2007. 8(Suppl 3): S9–S17.
102. Lincoff, A.M., et al., Bivalirudin and provisional glycoprotein IIb/IIIa blockade compared with heparin and planned glycoprotein IIb/IIIa blockade during percutaneous coronary intervention: REPLACE-2 randomized trial. *JAMA*, 2003. 289(7): 853–863.
103. Stone, G.W., et al., Bivalirudin in patients with acute coronary syndromes undergoing percutaneous coronary intervention: A subgroup analysis from the Acute Catheterization and Urgent Intervention Triage strategy (ACUITY) trial. *Lancet*, 2007. 369(9565): 907–919.
104. Bush, R.L., et al., Routine bivalirudin use in percutaneous carotid interventions. *J Endovasc Ther*, 2005. 12(4): 521–522.
105. Katzen, B.T., et al., Bivalirudin as an anticoagulation agent: Safety and efficacy in peripheral interventions. *J Vasc Interv Radiol*, 2005. 16(9): 1183–1187; quiz 1187.
106. Lewis, B.E., Y. Rangel, and J. Fareed, The first report of successful carotid stent implant using argatroban anticoagulation in a patient with heparin-induced thrombocytopenia and thrombosis syndrome: A case report. *Angiology*, 1998. 49(1): 61–67.
107. Crowther, M.A. and T.E. Warkentin, Bleeding risk and the management of bleeding complications in patients undergoing anticoagulant therapy: Focus on new anticoagulant agents. *Blood*, 2008. 111: 4871–4879.
108. Payne, D.A., et al., Beneficial effects of clopidogrel combined with aspirin in reducing cerebral emboli in patients undergoing carotid endarterectomy. *Circulation*, 2004. 109(12): 1476–1481.
109. Stratton, J.R., R.E. Zierler, and A. Kazmers, Platelet deposition at carotid endarterectomy sites in humans. *Stroke*, 1987. 18(4): 722–727.
110. Topol, E.J. and J.S. Yadav, Recognition of the importance of embolization in atherosclerotic vascular disease. *Circulation*, 2000. 101(5): 570–580.
111. Jordan, W.D.,Jr., et al.., Microemboli detected by transcranial Doppler monitoring in patients during carotid angioplasty versus carotid endarterectomy. *Cardiovasc Surg*, 1999. 7(1): 33–38.
112. Grewe, P.H., et al., Acute and chronic tissue response to coronary stent implantation: Pathologic findings in human specimen. *J Am Coll Cardiol*, 2000. 35(1): 157–163.

113. Leon, M.B., et al., A clinical trial comparing three antithrombotic-drug regimens after coronary-artery stenting. Stent Anticoagulation Restenosis Study Investigators. *N Engl J Med*, 1998. 339(23): 1665–1671.
114. Cunningham, E.J., D. Fiorella, and T.J. Masaryk, Neurovascular rescue. *Semin Vasc Surg*, 2005. 18(2): 101–109.
115. McKevitt, F.M., et al., The benefits of combined anti-platelet treatment in carotid artery stenting. *Eur J Vasc Endovasc Surg*, 2005. 29(5): 522–527.
116. Bhatt, D.L., et al., Dual antiplatelet therapy with clopidogrel and aspirin after carotid artery stenting. *J Invasive Cardiol*, 2001. 13(12): 767–771.
117. Angiolillo, D.J. and F. Alfonso, Clopidogrel–statin interaction: Myth or reality? *J Am Coll Cardiol*, 2007. 50(4): 296–298.
118. EPIC Trial Investigators, Use of a monoclonal antibody directed against the platelet glycoprotein IIb/IIIa receptor in high-risk coronary angioplasty. The EPIC Investigation. N Engl J Med, 1994. 330(14): 956–961.
119. EPISTENT Trial Investigators, Randomised placebo-controlled and balloon-angioplasty-controlled trial to assess safety of coronary stenting with use of platelet glycoprotein-IIb/IIIa blockade. Lancet, 1998. 352(9122): 87–92.
120. Kapadia, S.R., et al., Initial experience of platelet glycoprotein IIb/IIIa inhibition with abciximab during carotid stenting: A safe and effective adjunctive therapy. *Stroke*, 2001. 32(10): 2328–2332.
121. Schneiderman, J., et al., Abciximab in carotid stenting for postsurgical carotid restenosis: Intermediate results. *J Endovasc Ther*, 2000. 7(4): 263–272.
122. Qureshi, A.I., et al., Carotid angioplasty and stent placement: A prospective analysis of perioperative complications and impact of intravenously administered abciximab. *Neurosurgery*, 2002. 50(3): 466–473; discussion 473–475.
123. Hofmann, R., et al., Abciximab bolus injection does not reduce cerebral ischemic complications of elective carotid artery stenting: A randomized study. *Stroke*, 2002. 33(3): 725–727.
124. Wholey, M.H., et al., Evaluation of glycoprotein IIb/IIIa inhibitors in carotid angioplasty and stenting. *J Endovasc Ther*, 2003. 10(1): 33–41.
125. Kramer, J., et al., Role of antiplatelets in carotid artery stenting. *Stroke*, 2007. 38(1): 14; author reply 15.
126. Chan, A.W., et al., Comparison of the safety and efficacy of emboli prevention devices versus platelet glycoprotein IIb/IIIa inhibition during carotid stenting. *Am J Cardiol*, 2005. 95(6): 791–795.
127. Kopp, C.W., et al., Abciximab reduces monocyte tissue factor in carotid angioplasty and stenting. *Stroke*, 2003. 34(11): 2560–2567.
128. Zahn, R., et al., Glycoprotein IIb/IIIa antagonists during carotid artery stenting: Results from the carotid artery stenting (CAS) registry of the Arbeitsgemeinschaft Leitende Kardiologische Krankenhausarzte (ALKK). *Clin Res Cardiol*, 2007. 96(10): 730–737.
129. Ho, D.S., et al., Intracarotid abciximab injection to abort impending ischemic stroke during carotid angioplasty. *Cerebrovasc Dis*, 2001. 11(4): 300–304.
130. Bush, R.L., et al., Transient ischemic attack due to early carotid stent thrombosis: Successful rescue with rheolytic thrombectomy and systemic abciximab. *J Endovasc Ther*, 2003. 10(5): 870–874.
131. Seo, K.D., et al., Rescue use of tirofiban for acute carotid in-stent thrombosis. *Yonsei Med J*, 2008. 49(1): 163–166.
132. Steiner-Boker, S., et al., Successful revascularization of acute carotid stent thrombosis by facilitated thrombolysis. *Am J Neuroradiol*, 2004. 25(8): 1411–1413.
133. Kittusamy, P.K., R.A. Koenigsberg, and D.J. McCormick, Abciximab for the treatment of acute distal embolization associated with internal carotid artery angioplasty. *Catheter Cardiovasc Interv*, 2001. 54(2): 221–233.
134. Green, D.W., et al., Acute thromboembolic events during carotid artery angioplasty and stenting: Etiology and a technique of neurorescue. *J Endovasc Ther*, 2005. 12(3): 360–365.
135. Tong, F.C., et al., Abciximab rescue in acute carotid stent thrombosis. *Am J Neuroradiol*, 2000. 21(9): 1750–1752.
136. Wiviott, S.D., et al., Prasugrel versus clopidogrel in patients with acute coronary syndromes. *N Engl J Med*, 2007. 357(20): 2001–2015.
137. Lennard, N.S., et al., Control of emboli in patients with recurrent or crescendo transient ischaemic attacks using preoperative transcranial Doppler-directed Dextran therapy. *Br J Surg*, 2003. 90(2): 166–170.
138. Abir, F., S. Barkhordarian, and B.E. Sumpio, Efficacy of dextran solutions in vascular surgery. *Vasc Endovasc Surg*, 2004. 38(6): 483–491.
139. Levi, C.R., et al., Dextran reduces embolic signals after carotid endarterectomy. *Ann Neurol*, 2001. 50(4): 544–547.
140. Hayes, P.D., et al., Transcranial Doppler-directed Dextran-40 therapy is a cost-effective method of preventing carotid thrombosis after carotid endarterectomy. *Eur J Vasc Endovasc Surg*, 2000. 19(1): 56–61.

141. Lennard, N., et al., Prevention of postoperative thrombotic stroke after carotid endarterectomy: The role of transcranial Doppler ultrasound. *J Vasc Surg*, 1997. 26(4): 579–584.
142. Rangi, P.S., et al., The use of intraoperative monitoring and treatment of symptomatic microemboli in carotid artery stenting: Case report and discussion. *Neuroradiology*, 2007. 49(3): 265–269.
143. Naylor, A.R., et al., Reducing the risk of carotid surgery: A 7-year audit of the role of monitoring and quality control assessment. *J Vasc Surg*, 2000. 32(4): 750–759.

10 Equipment, Basic and Advanced: An Overview

Luc Stockx

Introduction

Carotid artery stenting is a delicate intervention. Minor errors can lead to big catastrophes. A meticulous technique as well as the selection of appropriate materials are mandatory to obtain a good result and to assure the benefit of the patient.

This chapter will give an overview of the different steps of the intervention thereby highlighting the specific equipment used by most of the operators. It cannot list all the materials as new devices come onto the market everyday. Its purpose is more to serve as a guide in making an adequate choice in a specific situation. Most of the devices are produced by the major companies; some of them are mentioned because of their specific characteristics. The various embolic protection devices (EPDs) as well as the dedicated carotid artery stents will not be discussed in detail as this is the topic of other chapters in this book.

The Interventional Suite

Carotid artery stenting should be performed in a dedicated interventional suite equipped with adequate imaging and monitoring accommodation. All materials and drugs which may be necessary during the intervention should be available and present.

Imaging

Of uppermost importance is the imaging equipment. Beside optimal fluoroscopy, necessary for continuous control during the procedure, a high-quality angiographic capacity is indispensable to depict every detail of the extra- and intracranial circulation. An automatic *C*-arm, two monitors (one for live fluoroscopy and one for displaying a reference image), digital subtraction angiography (DSA), and roadmap are mandatory to perform this procedure in a safe manner.

Monitoring

During the intervention, continuous monitoring of the ECG and blood pressure are mandatory. Changes during the procedure should be detected immediately and an adequate reaction should be undertaken. An activated clotting time (ACT) should be measured to evaluate the effect of heparin, which is given after the introduction of the interventional sheath or guiding catheter. The use of EEG and TCD monitoring remain optional as these data will not have a direct influence on the intervention.

Drugs

Drugs like heparin, protamine, atropine or glycopyrrolate (in case of bradycardia), adrenaline, nitroglycerine or papaverine (in case of spasm),

S. Macdonald and G. Stansby (eds.), *Practical Carotid Artery Stenting*,
DOI: 10.1007/978-1-84800-299-9_10, © Springer-Verlag London Limited 2009

nifedipine or labetalol (in case of hypertension) have to be present in the interventional suite (see Chaps.9 and 14). Others like glycoprotein IIb–IIIa inhibitors and thrombolytic agents should be immediately available in the hospital.

Interventional Table

After analysis of the diagnostic images, all interventional materials should be prepared according to the instructions for use and put into a tray filled with heparinized saline before starting the procedure. This minimizes the time dealing with the lesion thereby reducing the chance of creating a complication.

Rescue Equipment

Although avoiding complications is much better than solving them, it is absolutely indispensable to have rescue material available (see Chap.15). A large thrombus in the internal carotid artery can be aspirated by a dedicated aspiration catheter as well as by a simple guiding catheter. Intracranial thrombolysis is performed through the microcatheters used for interventional neuroradiology procedures. With the use of dedicated clot retrievers, an attempt can be made to remove intracranial emboli.

The Procedure

Carotid artery stenting is a multistep intervention where every detail plays a major role. Before starting a carotid artery stenting program, one should be familiar with carotid artery catheterization, peripheral or coronary artery stenting, and with the use of low-profile rapid-exchange systems.

Initial Imaging

Each procedure should start with imaging of the aortic arch. This allows the operator to define the type of aortic arch, to illustrate anatomic anomalies like a bovine arch or an anomalous left carotid artery originating from the proximal innominate artery, and to demonstrate associated disease like severe atherosclerosis of the arch. Through a 4 or 5 French diagnostic sheath, under local anesthesia placed preferably in the groin, a 4 or 5 French pigtail or multiple side-hole flush catheter is introduced into the descending aorta. There, it is flushed and then advanced into the ascending arch. An angiogram of the arch and the origin of the supra-aortic vessels is performed in the left anterior oblique position.

Equipment: Arch Imaging

- Diagnostic 4–5 French sheath
- 4–5 French pigtail or flush catheter
- 0.035″ steerable hydrophilic guidewire

The next step consists of the selective catheterization of the target CCA. Most operators prefer a retrograde femoral artery approach to access the CCA; a right brachial or radial approach may facilitate access in case of a type III arch, anomalous anatomy or in patients with tortuous or obstructed aortoiliac arteries. This maneuver should be performed in a meticulous way with adapted material as it may in itself cause stroke even before the index lesion is encountered. Selection of the catheter is most dependent on the anatomy of the aortic arch. Selective catheters come in a wide range of shapes. Simple rules govern catheter choices. Most operators rely on a relatively small selection of catheters to perform all their cases. Selective catheters for carotid catheterization can be divided into two groups: those with a simple curve for easy arches and those with a more complex curve for tortuous arches or in case of an anomalous origin of the CCA. Diagnostic angiography consists of visualization of the bifurcation in several projections and of an intracranial study of the ipsilateral hemisphere.

Equipment: Selective Catheterization of the Great Vessels

- 4–5 French selective catheters:
  - Simple curves: Vertebral, Berenstein, Judkins, Headhunter, etc.
  - Complex curves: Sidewinder, Newton, VTK, Mani, etc.

Gaining Access

Once the diagnostic study is completed and the stenotic lesion is identified and analyzed, access should be established. Access to the CCA involves using either a guiding catheter or an interventional sheath and can be gained by using the exchange technique, telescopic technique, or direct probing (see Chap.11). The choice of equipment and technique is largely dependent on operator preference, although there are several anatomic factors that might favor one technique or equipment over another. The characteristics of sheaths and guiding catheters are described in Table10.1. In patients with simple arch and carotid anatomy, a 6 French interventional sheath or an 8 French guiding catheter will permit the operator to advance and retrieve the interventional equipment necessary for the procedure. When the disease process does not involve the carotid bifurcation and the external carotid artery is patent, the exchange technique can be used to introduce the interventional sheath or guiding catheter into its correct position which is in the distal CCA, a few centimeters below the bifurcation. Under roadmap control, the diagnostic catheter is advanced using a 0.035″ hydrophilic guidewire into the ipsilateral ECA. This wire is then withdrawn and replaced with a 260-cm long exchange wire (regular in case of straight anatomy, stiff or extra stiff in case of tortuous arch). The selective catheter is withdrawn and the interventional sheath or guiding catheter is advanced over the exchange wire into its desired position. If the ECA is occluded or cannot be catheterized or if the bifurcation is involved in the disease or the stenosis is located in the distal CCA, the telescopic technique is recommended to gain access. The sheath or guiding catheter is placed in the descending aorta. With the combination of a 125-cm long selective catheter and a 0.035″ steerable hydrophilic guidewire, introduced into the sheath, the CCA is catheterized. The sheath or guiding catheter is then advanced over this guidewire catheter assembly which is kept below the stenosis. In case of tortuous anatomy, the use of a stiff 0.035″ hydrophilic guidewire can increase the support and facilitate the introduction of the sheath or guiding catheter. A third technique consists of direct probing of the common carotid artery with a special shaped guiding catheter. This technique is more aggressive in relation to an atherosclerotic arch. If the common carotid artery is tortuous, placing a straight sheath or guiding catheter can aggravate this tortuosity, displace the bifurcation, and create kinks in the distal internal carotid artery. These disappear once the sheath is withdrawn but can complicate the stenting procedure. Mainly for these cases, a special curved guiding catheter (like sidewinder curve) can be used with the tip positioned in the proximal common carotid artery, thereby respecting the anatomy. This generally provides less support for the procedure. Recently guiding sheaths, combining the properties of both sheaths and guiding catheters, have been developed.

TABLE. 10.1. Characteristics of sheaths and guiding catheters.

Guiding catheter	Interventional sheath
8 French (OD)	6 French (ID)
90–100cm	100cm
Through 8 French (ID) sheath	Directly through the skin
Exchange – telescopic – direct probing	Exchange – telescopic
Straight or curved tip	Straight tip
Steerable	Nonsteerable

In case of cerebral protection by flow reversal, a specially designed double-lumen sheath has to be introduced according to the instructions for use of the specific device (see Chap.13).

Careful attention must be paid to the placement of the tip of the interventional sheath or guiding catheter to prevent spasm, thrombosis, or dissection. Continuous flushing with the use of a pressurized saline bag will prevent catheter thrombosis (see Chap.12).

Equipment Required for Establishment of Access

- 8 French guiding catheter (e.g., Cordis, Abbott, Medtronic, Balt, etc.)
- 6 French interventional sheath (e.g., Shuttle, Cook; Destination, Terumo; Arrow-flex, Arrow; Vista Brite, Cordis, etc.)
- Exchange guidewire of 260–300cm:
  - Regular for straight anatomy
  - Stiff or super stiff for tortuous anatomy (e.g., Amplatz, Supra Core, etc.)
- Pressurized bag of heparinized saline (1L)

Cerebral Protection

The use of the various EPDs is extensively described in Chap.13. All EPDs share the common goal of preventing embolic debris from reaching the intracranial circulation, leading to stroke. There are three different methods of performing cerebral embolic protection during carotid artery stenting (1) distal protection by blocking the flow distal to the lesion, (2) protection by creating flow reversal in the intracranial artery, and (3) embolic protection by filtering the blood that passes through the lesion. Although comparative studies of various EPDs have not been performed, this latter technique is most frequently used. It is desirable to deploy the EPD before any intervention is performed on the target lesion. When the internal carotid artery is tortuous or kinked, the use of an additional 0.014 rigid wire (buddy wire technique) will straighten up this segment and facilitate passage of the filter. This necessitates passage of the lesion with a soft microcatheter and a flexible 0.014 guidewire. With the tip of this microcatheter in the distal segment of the ICA, the soft microwire is exchanged for a 0.014 support wire which is left in place during the rest of the intervention. Finally, the buddy wire is retrieved just before delivery of the stent. Choosing another device like a bare wire filter system or another technique like embolic protection by flow reversal can also be an alternative. Although all EPDs appear to be able to prevent distal embolization, proper use of these devices does not ensure that this will not occur. Possible modes of failure include inability to deliver or deploy the device to the intended location, inadvertent device-induced vessel injury or embolization, cerebral ischemia due to device-induced carotid occlusion, incomplete capture or retrieval of embolic debris, or embolization into the external carotid artery that might supply collaterals to the intracranial circulation (see Chap.6):

- Buddy wire technique:
  - Microcatheter and soft microwire (interventional neuroradiology)
  - 0.014″ support wire (300cm)

Pre- and Postdilatation

Although it is less desirable to dilate the lesion before the distal circulation is protected, this may be necessary to facilitate passage of the distal EPD in case of pinpoint stenosis or heavily calcified lesion. For this unprotected predilatation, an undersized 2mm coronary angioplasty balloon should be used. After placement of the EPD, a protected predilatation using a PTA balloon with a diameter of 3–4mm can be performed to allow passage of stent delivery system. Finally, a PTA balloon with a diameter comparable to that of the normal ICA is used to postdilate the stent. Oversizing of the balloon and application of high pressure should be avoided as this can create dissections or rupture of the artery. Carotid stent operators generally do not pursue a perfect angiographic result and accept a moderate stenosis for several reasons. First, multiple and aggressive balloon inflations appear to increase the risk of complications. Second, the most common reason for moderate residual stenosis after stenting is heavy calcification of the target lesion, which generally does not respond to high pressure or repeated balloon inflations. Third, nickel–titanium alloy (nitinol) self-expanding stents have a tendency to continue to expand the lumen after the procedure. It is possible that a moderate residual stenosis immediately after intervention may remodel into a mild residual stenosis a few months later. Some operators do not perform postdilatation and this does not appear to cause problems due to stent occlusion resulting from poor throughflow.

Finally, hemodynamic perturbations such as vasovagal or vasodepressor reactions may limit the number of balloon inflations. In any case, late endothelialization of the stent will likely decrease the risk of stroke, even if a moderate residual stenosis persists:

- 0.014″-based PTA balloon:
  - 2mm coronary angioplasty balloon for unprotected predilatation
  - 4–5mm PTA balloon for protected pre- and postdilatation
- Inflation device

Stent

Several carotid artery stents are available; all are self-expanding. Balloon-expandable stents should only be used when the origin of the common carotid artery is treated. Most of the stents are made of nitinol; most of them have different designs. Conformability and scaffolding are the key characteristics while choosing the appropriate stent. Conformability, defined as the ability to conform to vessel tortuosity in the deployed state, is important especially when the anatomy is tortuous where a rigid stent would straighten the artery and create cerebral flow impairment due to a kink at the distal end of the stent. Carotid stents with an open-cell structure are more flexible and therefore conform best in tortuous lesions. Stents with a closed-cell structure like the stainless steel stents tend to be more rigid and may straighten the vessel during implantation. Scaffolding, defined as the amount of coverage and support of the vessel wall by the stent, is important when dealing with vulnerable plaque (see Chap.8). Insufficient scaffolding may be responsible for distal embolization. This can occur with nitinol stents with an open-cell structure where embolic material can be squeezed through the interstices of the stent. Radial force only plays a role in heavily calcified lesions because a stent with low radial force cannot resist the elastic recoil produced by calcified plaque. Beside straight stents, there are also tapered versions available. The tapered stents are intended to be used in bifurcation lesions and are supposed to respond better to the mismatch in diameter between the common and internal carotid artery.

Although there is a lack of proven evidence that stent selection influences the outcome and that any one stent functions better than another, it seems logical that in some cases, a particular stent design can offer advantages. This is extensively discussed in Chap.8.

Hemostatic Control

After completion angiography of both bifurcation and ipsilateral intracranial arteries, all equipment is withdrawn and hemostatic control obtained. Closure devices are of particular importance in this patient group which are treated with heparin and dual antiplatelet therapy. Their use will also allow early mobilization of the patient.

Key Points

- Meticulous technique and careful selection of appropriate materials are both vitally important to reduce the procedural hazard.
- State-of-the-art imaging equipment with DSA and roadmapping functions should be used.
- During the intervention, continuous monitoring of the ECG and blood pressure are mandatory.
- All the drugs necessary for the procedure should be in the interventional suite. Those drugs that may become necessary to deal with complications (like glycoprotein IIb–IIIa inhibitors and thrombolytic agents) should be immediately available within the hospital.
- All the interventional materials necessary for the procedure should be prepared in advance (once calibrated angiography has allowed correct sizing of the stent and protection system) to minimize the time taken for completion of the procedure and therefore the complication rate.
- Neurorescue equipment must be available in the interventional suite (see Chap.15).
- Choice of catheter for selective catheterization of the carotid artery to be treated depends on arch anatomy.
- Access technique for placement of a long sheath or guiding catheter in the common carotid artery depends on patient vascular anatomy.
- Unprotected lesion predilatation should be avoided but if necessary, should be performed after lesion crossing with a microcatheter and soft neurointerventional wire (with subsequent exchange for a support 0.014″ wire).
- Although all EPDs appear to be able to prevent distal embolization, proper use of these devices does not ensure that this will not occur.
- Choice of stent depends largely on patient vascular anatomy, lesion characteristics and to an extent, whether the patient is symptomatic or asymptomatic (see Chap.8).
- Aggressive postdilatation should be avoided. Carotid stent operators generally do not pursue a perfect angiographic result and accept a moderate stenosis for several reasons.
- Closure devices are useful in this population treated with heparin and dual antiplatelets and allow early patient mobilization, which allows earlier "resetting" of the baroreceptors (see Chap.14).

11 Difficult Access: Tips and Tricks

Peter A. Schneider

Introduction

Access to the carotid artery for the delivery of a stent must be performed safely for carotid angioplasty and stenting (CAS) to be a viable treatment option. Carotid access includes the following steps: arch assessment, carotid artery catheterization, passage of an exchange guidewire, and placement of a guiding sheath into the common carotid artery (CCA) in proximity to the target carotid bifurcation. The requirements of carotid access are that the sheath must be placed safely and, once in place, that it remain stable for the duration of the procedure. Achieving carotid sheath access may be straightforward in a patient with simple u-shaped arch, great vessels arising from the top of the arch, minimal tortuosity of the branches, and no extra lesions involving areas outside the carotid bifurcation. Unfortunately, the challenge faced in achieving access is often much greater, and is dependent on one's ability to identify, understand, and manipulate difficult anatomy. This chapter reviews anatomical consideration for carotid access, describes difficult access anatomy, and offers tips for managing the difficult carotid access.

Anatomical Considerations in Carotid Access

Anatomical considerations during CAS are a major determinant of risk (Table 11.1). Managing certain anatomical characteristics or, occasionally, avoiding them altogether, will make CAS safer [1–4]. The comparison between the medical risk of carotid endarterectomy (CEA) and the anatomical risk of CAS helps in the selection of patients for each procedure. In general, when patients are excluded from CEA, it is usually because of comorbid medical conditions; when patients are excluded from CAS it is usually because of unsuitable anatomy. When CAS is indicated, risky anatomical features, such as those which may be encountered during access, influence the planning and performance of the procedure and these features alter the risk/benefit ratio of the stent procedure.

During CEA, it is unusual that major consideration is required of anatomical features such as arch configuration and this is manifested by the infrequency with which arteriography is needed prior to CEA [5, 6]. Conversely, the arch and carotid anatomy of patients selected for CAS must be thoroughly analyzed. This increased concern about anatomical conditions in CAS vs. that required for CEA is consistent with many other situations where open surgery and endovascular surgery are competing for primacy as the treatment of choice in a given vascular bed. In open surgical approaches, the access is direct, through soft tissues or a body cavity. The pathway through the lesion itself is often less important since the conduit artery will be replaced or repaired, such as in open aortic surgery or lower extremity bypass. During endovascular repair, success is determined by the ability to negotiate the anatomical pathway to the lesion and then through it. When anatomical

S. Macdonald and G. Stansby (eds.), *Practical Carotid Artery Stenting*,
DOI: 10.1007/978-1-84800-299-9_11, © Springer-Verlag London Limited 2009

TABLE 11.1. CAS steps and how they are affected by anatomy.

Anatomical problem	Sheath placement	Lesion crossing	Filter placement	Stent placement	Filter retrieval
Aortic arch tortuosity	X				
Aortic arch variations	X				
Aortic arch disease	X				
Arch branch tortuosity	X				
Arch branch occlusive disease	X				
Carotid bifurcation lesion		X	X	X	
ECA stenosis/occlusion	X				
Tortuosity of bifurcation		X	X	X	X
Tortuosity of distal ICA			X	X	X
Disease of distal ICA			X	X	X
Stenosis of intracranial arteries			X		
Aneurysm of siphon			X		
Isolated hemisphere		X	X	X	
Contralateral CCA occlusion		X	X	X	

CAS carotid angioplasty and stenting, *ECA* external carotid artery, *ICA* internal carotid artery

factors are present during CAS, at the least they make the procedure more challenging and demand more pretreatment planning and intraoperative maneuvering; at the worst, these features increase the risk of the procedure or even prevent it from being possible. Difficult CAS access increases the stroke risk of the procedure. Many of the ongoing developments in access techniques are designed to manage these anatomical challenges.

The primary reason to perform CAS is to prevent stroke, and the most significant end point by which CAS is assessed is stroke or death. In large studies on CAS, up to 30% of the CAS-associated strokes occur in territories other than that served by the carotid artery being treated [7, 8]. Difficult access is caused by tortuous arch configuration, arch disease, anatomical variations of the arch, great vessel tortuosity, and ectopic lesions of the CCA and external carotid artery (ECA). When one or more of these anatomical factors are present and cause the access procedure to be accordingly modified, the access may be considered "difficult."

Standard Method for Carotid Sheath Access

1. After femoral guidewire placement, use vessel dilators to enlarge the arteriotomy and place a 6- or 7F standard access sheath, appropriately sized to the intended guiding sheath. Administer anticoagulation. Perform selective catheterization of the CCA using the simplest selective cerebral catheter possible [9].
2. Administer contrast through the selective catheter to roadmap the carotid bifurcation. The image intensifier should be angled to achieve the best projection of the bifurcation. Ipsilateral, steep anterior oblique projections are often the most useful. Advance a 0.035-in. steerable glidewire into the ECA. Although the ECA origin is usually located anteromedially, its branches often cross posteriorly, making it difficult to discern without a roadmap, whether the guidewire is advancing into the internal or external carotid artery.
3. In general, simple curve selective catheters, such as the H1 Headhunter, the angled taper Glidecath, and the Vert catheter, track more easily into the ECA than do the complex curve catheters such as the Simmons and the Vitek. The complex curve catheters have a secondary curve or elbow that must be straightened inside the CCA before tracking becomes easier.
4. After advancing the catheter into the ECA, perform a digital run or roadmap to see where the longest and largest branches are located for placing the guidewire to get the best anchor (Fig.11.1). Contrast usually refluxes out of the ECA and into the internal carotid artery; so do

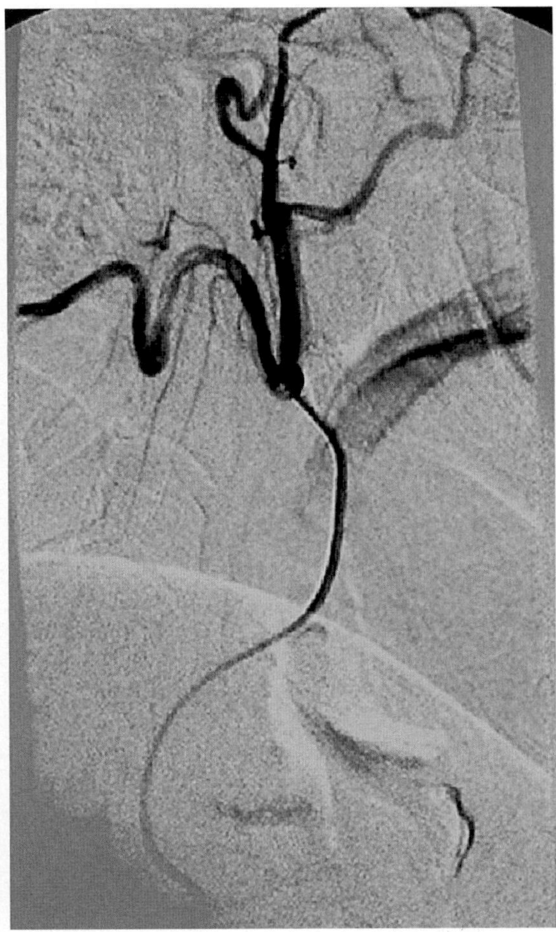

FIG. 11.1. The external carotid artery may be roadmapped in order to pick the best branch for the exchange guidewire. This is especially useful in a system with a lot of tortuosity where it is beneficial to get a longer distance of stiff guidewire distal to the last turn from the arch into the common carotid artery

not inject too forcefully. The catheter tip must be far enough into the ECA (≥2cm), so that a cough, turn of the head, or minor movement does not pop the catheter out of the ECA and into the bifurcation where its tip could cause damage.

5. After advancing the catheter into the proximal few centimeters of the ECA and roadmapping, advance the Glidewire into a distal branch of the ECA. Advance the selective catheter over the Glidewire as far as it will go. Remove the Glidewire. Make sure the catheter back-bleeds before placing the Amplatz exchange guidewire. If the catheter tip is against the wall of the ECA branch and there is no back flow, pulling the guidewire will create suction and bubbles. When the exchange guidewire is introduced to fill the lumen, air will be pushed into the system. After back-bleeding the selective catheter, place a stiff exchange guidewire. The Amplatz guidewire is 260cm in length and has a short, floppy segment at the tip. Perform fluoroscopy of the catheter tip in the distal ECA as the Amplatz guidewire is advanced. If the catheter tip begins to withdraw, stop advancing the Amplatz super-stiff guidewire. This is usually a sign that the catheter is not anchored well enough in the ECA and the Amplatz super-stiff guidewire is about to pull the catheter out of the artery. Consider exchanging for a stiffer selective cerebral catheter, such as a vertebral catheter. The Amplatz super-stiff guidewire should be advanced as far into the ECA branches as possible. Do not force the guidewire, however, as perforation of the small branch artery may occur and cause significant problems in an anticoagulated patient. The patient may complain of facial, jaw, or ear pain as the Amplatz guidewire tip is reaching its destination.
6. After the Amplatz guidewire is in place in the distal ECA, remove the selective catheter. Ensure that the guidewire tip remains in the distal ECA by using spot fluoroscopy. Remove the femoral sheath. Place the guiding sheath through the femoral access. Prior to advancing the sheath into the CCA, open and prepare the guidewire, distal protection device, and balloons intended for usage so that the procedure may proceed expeditiously once the sheath is in the CCA.
7. If there is concern about the degree of tortuosity in the system, briefly survey the course of the guidewire using fluoroscopy before advancing the sheath. There may be slack in the Amplatz super-stiff guidewire in the descending aorta or arch and this should be carefully and gently removed without withdrawing the tip of the guidewire. This may be done by focusing the fluoroscopic image on the guidewire tip and slowly withdrawing the guidewire until some sign of movement is seen in the guidewire tip. The sheath is more likely to advance smoothly

if the guidewire is in its straightest possible course.

8. Advance the guiding sheath into the CCA. The image intensifier should be positioned so that field of view includes the tip of the Amplatz guidewire in the distal ECA on the upper part of the field while the arch branch origin is visible in the lower part of the field. This permits observation of the exchange guidewire tip as the sheath turns superiorly into the arch branch (Fig.11.2). The guidewire should be pinned carefully. If the guidewire is pushed forward, it may perforate the ECA branch. As the dilator comes into view and approaches the turn into the CCA, carefully observe the shape of the dilator and sheath to see whether it is tracking over the guidewire. If the turn into the artery is too tight, the sheath may prolapse into the proximal arch and pull the guidewire out of the ECA. Sheath passage around a turn may be facilitated by having the patients take a deep breath or turn their head to help straighten this segment slightly as the sheath passes by.

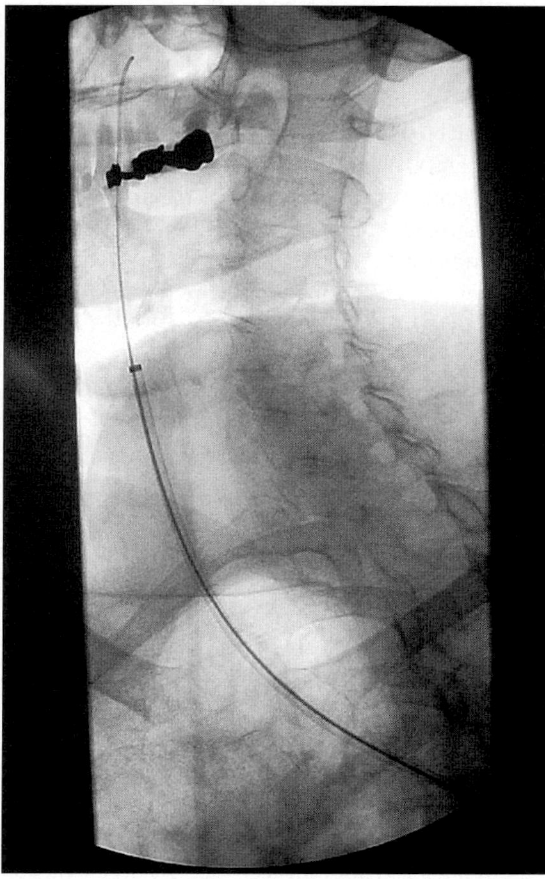

FIG. 11.2. The exchange guidewire is placed in the external carotid artery. The image intensifier is positioned so that the tip of the guidewire and the last turn from the arch into the common carotid artery are visible

9. The sheath is advanced with a steady, even, forward force while the Amplatz super-stiff guidewire is pinned and the tip of the guidewire is observed under fluoroscopy. The sheath progress cannot be observed along its entire course since the image intensifier is held stationary to observe the guidewire tip and the last turn from the arch into the CCA. If excessive resistance is met, stop pushing and pan inferiorly to see the location, angles, and course of the guidewire and the sheath. Occasionally, slack builds up along the guidewire, which must be removed. Occasionally, there is too much tortuosity for the chosen access device to cross. If there is excessive tortuosity in the abdominal aorta and iliac arteries, consider passing a larger sheath that is 45cm in length. If the intended carotid sheath is 6F, for example, pass a 7- or 8F sheath that will help to straighten some of the tortuosity and pass the 6F carotid sheath through it.
10. The tip of the dilator does not have a radiopaque marker as the end of the sheath does. However, the tip of the dilator does extend for several centimeters beyond the end of the sheath. Care must be taken to avoid mechanical dilatation of the carotid lesion with the tip of the dilator. This is especially true for focal lesions in the CCA or bifurcation lesions that begin in the CCA. The silhouette of the dilator tip can often be visualized on the magnified fluoroscopic image (small field of view).
11. Advance the sheath until the radiopaque tip is a few centimeters or more inside the CCA (Fig.11.3). This is often at the level of the clavicle or just superior. A mental note of this location should be made at the time of the arch study. If the operator is uncertain of where the relative landmarks are located to identify the origin of the CCA and the bifurcation for safe sheath tip placement, review the arch study. The tip of the sheath must be far enough inside the artery that it does not pop out into the arch, but not so far into the artery that it crosses or butts up against

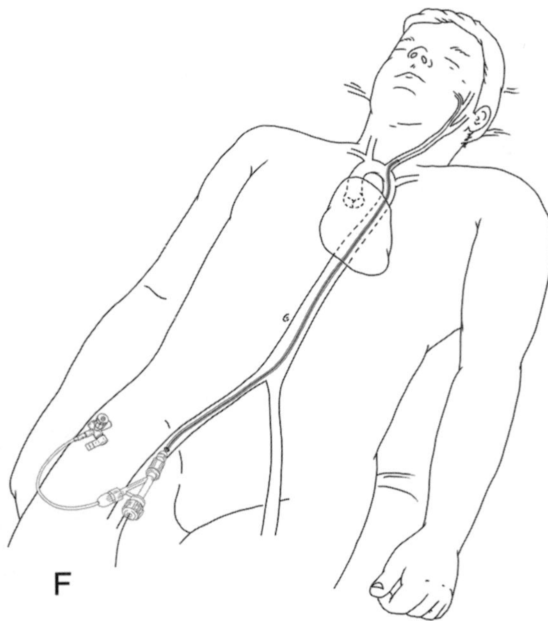

Fig. 11.3. The carotid angioplasty and stenting access sheath is placed from the femoral artery to the common carotid artery, a distance of 60–85 cm, depending on the height of the patient [9]

the lesion. The sheath tip should be placed a few centimeters or more proximal to the lesion so that there is working room for the intervention. The last few centimeters of advancement of the sheath may be achieved by holding the dilator steady and advancing the sheath over the dilator.

12. The dilator is removed. The sheath is backbled and then flushed gently, taking care to avoid bubbles. Prior to removing the Amplatz guidewire, perform a selective carotid arteriogram through the sidearm of the sheath to check sheath position, locate the lesion, and ensure that there has been no damage to the CCA during sheath passage. If the sheath must be advanced further, maintaining the stiff guidewire in place is necessary until this is completed. With each maneuver, such as sheath placement or removal of the dilator, the anatomical relationships of the carotid artery may change and tortuosity may disappear or be introduced.
13. Remove the Amplatz guidewire from the ECA. If the sheath position is tenuous or the arch anatomy was particularly challenging, the sheath may become unstable when the stiff guidewire is removed. In this case, leave the Amplatz guidewire in place as a support until the treatment guidewire is advanced into place or introduce a separate 0.014-in. buddy wire to hold the sheath steady. When the Amplatz guidewire is removed, observe with fluoroscopy to ensure that the sheath does not back up by any significant distance.
14. Technical Tips for CAS Access are described in Table 11.2.

What Makes CAS Access Difficult?

The pathologies that complicate access for CAS include tortuosity, calcification, extra lesions in inconvenient places, and anatomical variants.

Tortuosity is the most challenging anatomical pathology and may occur anywhere along the pathway from the access artery to the carotid bifurcation. Tortuosity of the approach arteries, such as the arch and its branches, makes access a challenge. Extreme tortuosity, such as arterial loops, makes access via that artery impossible. Tortuosity may be manipulated or moved but the total degree of vessel curvature cannot be reduced. If a tortuous segment is straightened with a sheath or a guidewire, that straightened segment may form a corrugated pattern of multiple contiguous curves in rapid succession. The tension may be shifted to some other segment, usually more distally, if only temporarily, and may therefore make some other part of the procedure more complicated.

Calcification may occur anywhere in the system but commonly requires consideration when it occurs in the arch. Scattered calcification poses an embolization risk. Friable lesions of the roof of the arch substantially increase the risk of catheterizing the arch and its branches. Diffuse calcification in the arch or proximal to mid arch branches is a contraindication to CAS. The arteries along the pathway from the groin to the CCA must bend to permit sheath access. In most cases the arch and its entry and exit arteries are malleable and flexible. After placement, the sheath follows a straighter course than would be predicted based on preprocedure imaging, indicating that the arch and its branches bend when stiff devices are advanced. When diffuse calcification occurs, there are no flex points

TABLE 11.2. Tips for carotid artery access for intervention.

1. Line everything up ahead of time
2. Make sure everything fits through the sheath you plan to use
3. Make sure the guidewire, balloon catheters, and stent deployment catheters are long enough to accommodate the length of the sheath you selected
4. Assess the arch by analyzing the anatomy during the planning phase of the case. Anticipate the likely level of challenge posed by the anatomy (especially the arch) in each case and be ready to perform maneuvers to enhance your likelihood of success
5. Use the lowest profile sheath possible (usually either 6- or 7F).
6. Put the sheath in warm saline bath to improve its flexibility (Be sure that your assistant does not put the Nitinol stent in the same warm saline bath.)
7. Use the external carotid artery to anchor the guidewire for sheath placement and place the Amplatz guidewire as far into the artery as possible, but do not perforate a distal branch
8. Use special maneuvers to help with sheath delivery when they are needed. These include the following: have the patient take a deep breath, turn the patient's head, take slack out of the guidewire, compress the guidewire tip along the face or scalp, use a very short floppy tip on the super-stiff guidewire, and use the push–pull technique
9. Do not perform mechanical dilation of the carotid lesion with the tip of the dilator when the sheath is advanced. Withdraw the dilator slightly if needed
10. Do not force the sheath
11. Watch the guidewire tip as the sheath is advanced so that the sheath is not permitted to pull the guidewire out of the ECA
12. Put the sheath tip a little farther than the intended location since it usually backs up a little bit when the stiff guidewire is removed

ECA external carotid artery

and passing a stiff device may cause the artery to fracture.

Tortuosity and calcification combined is a special situation. Calcification alone or the tortuosity alone may be manageable, but together they pose a substantial risk of arterial injury, sheath instability, dissection, and embolization. Tortuous and calcified arteries resist straightening and may break rather than bend.

Extra lesions in inconvenient places complicate CAS access. Occlusive disease occurs in the innominate or CCA origin and makes sheath access challenging. When these origin lesions are hemodynamically significant, they must also be stented. When they are not hemodynamically significant, they must still be crossed while avoiding injury during sheath placement. Occasionally a separate lesion is present in the CCA proximal to the bifurcation lesion. Management of these tandem stenoses may require that the proximal lesion be crossed with the exchange guidewire so that the sheath can be placed. The sheath must be deployed in a manner that avoids disruption of the proximal lesion by the tip of the sheath as it bounces up and down with the cardiac and breathing cycles. In addition, both lesions might be covered with the same stent or two separate stents may be required or if the CCA lesion is mild, no treatment may be required but disruption must be avoided.

Stenosis or occlusion of the ECA complicates sheath access because it cannot be used to anchor the exchange guidewire. The exchange guidewire tip must be maintained proximal to the bifurcation during sheath placement. The sheath is advanced over a combination of exchange guidewire and inner catheter ("telescoping technique") which provides a rail to make the turn from the arch into the CCA.

Variations in anatomy are not technically pathological entities but may function in that way in obtaining CAS access. Anatomical variation can complicate remote access, the most common one being the bovine arch [10, 11].

CAS Access Anatomy and How it Affects the Case

The arch and great vessels have features that must be negotiated and managed to achieve CAS access.

TABLE 11.3. Managing arch segments.

	Anatomy	Catheter	Considerations
Segment I	Superior to fulcrum Left side of arch	Simple curve	Straightest path to carotid Easy to maneuver Usually only subclavian is segment I
Segment II	Superior to fulcrum Right side of arch	Simple curve	Distance to right is important Width of arch is important Work over fulcrum More challenging than segment I
Segment III	Inferior to fulcrum Right side of arch	Complex curve	Distance to right is important Distance inferior to fulcrum Work over fulcrum Most challenging

Arch Configuration. The shape of the arch tends to elongate with age and this seems to accelerate with prolonged hypertension. As the arch proximal to the descending aorta becomes elongated, a peak or a focal point is created at the upper inner aspect of the arch. This point becomes a fulcrum over which the catheter must work and over which the carotid access sheath must pass to enter the CCA (Fig.11.4). To plan for CAS, the arch has been classified into segments that help anticipate the challenge of sheath access ([12]; Table 11.3).

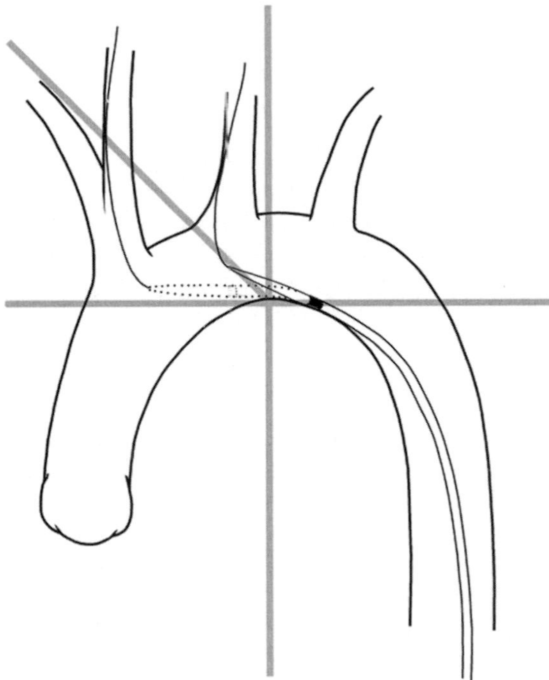

FIG. 11.4. The upper inner aspect of the arch forms a fulcrum over which the catheter and sheath must work to reach the target common carotid artery [9]

The further inferiorly and toward the patient's right side the arch branch origin is located, the more challenging the access (Fig.11.5). The trajectory from the fulcrum to the target artery determines difficulty in access. Segment I is straightforward while segment II is more difficult and segment III is usually very challenging. When the target artery originates in segment III, a stable access cannot be guaranteed. The last turn along the pathway out of the arch and into the CCA is severely angulated. When the curvature along the pathway from the beginning of the arch into the CCA adds up to more than 180°, the access is likely to be very challenging. There are other configurations where the last turn out of the arch is a hairpin, including the left CCA on a bovine arch and a retroflexed left CCA.

The more degrees of curvature in the system, the more likely that the access approach will be aided by a stiffer guidewire, a longer length of guidewire past the last turn (from the arch into the CCA), and a more flexible sheath (or even a guiding catheter).

There are many different choices of exchange guidewires. The Rosen guidewire or the Stiff Glidewire are relatively useful in a straight arch. The more tortuous arch, with the target artery originating from segment III, may require an Amplatz super-stiff guidewire or a Nitinol exchange guidewire to create a rail firm enough to advance the sheath. The exchange guidewire is anchored in a distal ECA branch if more length of guidewire is needed past the turn from the arch into the CCA.

The pathway can often be made less tortuous with the assistance of the patient. A deep inhalation

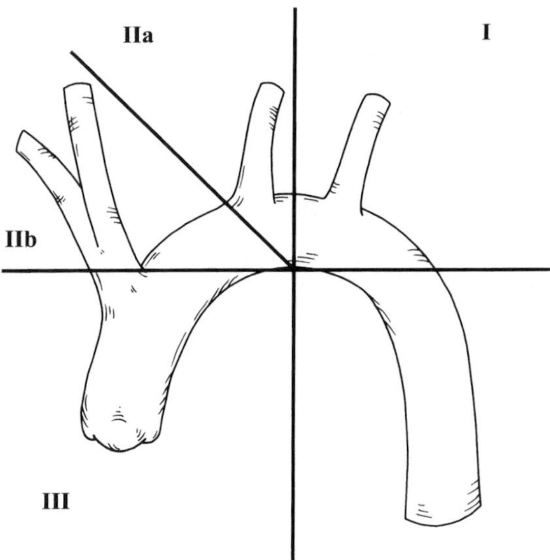

FIG. 11.5. The aortic arch may be divided into segments. A horizontal line crosses through the upper inner aspect of the arch, the fulcrum point. The arch is bisected with a vertical line. This is a quick method of assessing the potential challenge of placing an access sheath into a specific common carotid artery [12]

TABLE 11.4. Arch variations.

Common trunk, innominate/LCCA (25–30%)
LCCA origin from innominate (7%)
L vert origin from aortic arch (0.5%)
Aberrant right subclavian artery (1%)
L brachiocephalic trunk (1%)

LCCA left common carotid artery
vert vertebral

changes the angles of the arch structures. Turning the head steeply toward one side can help alleviate a kink in the proximal CCA or change its angle of origin from the arch. When placing the sheath in a tortuous arch, it is best to position the image intensifier for a left anterior oblique projection. This is the best way to visualize the turn from the arch into the CCA. As the sheath approaches the CCA during placement, the configuration of the exchange guidewire observed with fluoroscopy gives clues as to the likely success of continued sheath advancement. If the exchange guidewire becomes progressively more curved at the location of the turn from the arch into the CCA as the sheath approaches, this is a sign that the sheath will probably not make the turn and that additional adjustments will be required.

Arch Variations. There is a significant amount of anatomical variation in the aortic arch ([11]; Table 11.4). Only ~60–70% of people have classical arch anatomy with three separate brachiocephalic arteries. Arch imaging is necessary in planning for CAS access, either with arteriography or axial imaging so that the operator knows what to expect during the procedure. During carotid catheterization of the arch branches, small puffs of contrast injected by hand can be used to confirm the identity of the artery before proceeding.

The bovine arch, which occurs in ~7% of cases, poses a challenge during carotid sheath placement. In this case, the left CCA originates from the innominate artery rather than the aortic arch. A milder form of this occurs more frequently with a common trunk, where the innominate and the left common carotid arteries arise from the same trunk. The bovine variation is only important in cases where the left CCA is the target artery for CAS. The bovine left CCA presents two problems: catheterization of the left CCA is more challenging and sheath placement requires crossing a tight turn from the arch into the left CCA. Catheterization of the bovine left CCA is more complex than catheterization of standard anatomy and often requires a complex curve or reversed curve catheter [13, 14]. Simple curve catheters tend to enter the innominate and continue a trajectory into the right CCA. In the bovine configuration, the left-sided neck artery originates from the patient's right-hand side. The artery origin must, therefore, be approached from the patient's right. The complex curve catheter, with a primary and a secondary curve, permits this approach; examples of this type of catheter include the Simmons catheter and the Vitek catheter. The second problem with the bovine left CCA is that after it has been catheterized and sheath access is being obtained, the last turn from the arch into the artery is accentuated. The bovine configuration often makes the last turn a hairpin turn, making the whole pathway more tortuous. So even if the arch configuration is not particularly tortuous, a lot of curvature is introduced, just as if it were a segment III branch. In addition, the bovine left CCA may originate from the innominate at an angle that brings the artery sharply back to the patient's left side, a path that would not be an issue during CEA but makes getting there more problematic for CAS. The bovine arch can usually be managed using the same techniques as for a target artery whose branch originates in segment III, such as stiffer exchange guidewire, longer length of guidewire past the last turn into the carotid artery, and a more flexible sheath. If however, this is not possible, a right brachial approach should be considered. Coming from the right brachial artery, the pathway is often very direct into the left CCA without the need to pass through the arch.

Other variations do not necessarily affect the performance of CAS, but may make catheterization dangerous if the operator does not understand the position of the catheter. For example, one would not want to mistake a catheter placed in a left vertebral that originates from the arch and believe that it was in the left CCA.

Disease of the Aortic Arch. Significant aortic arch disease may occur in a diffuse pattern or a more focal one. The diffuse pattern may not cause significant stenosis at the origins of the branches, but it affects the roof of the arch. This is a dangerous pattern because of the risk of embolization with arch manipulation and should be avoided. If the patient requires a stent, it should be placed via direct carotid access.

Focal stenosis at the origin of the innominate or common carotid arteries is germane to the CAS procedure if it occurs along the pathway to the artery intended for CAS. These tandem lesions (arch branch origin plus carotid bifurcation) may be managed with a combination of open and endovascular surgery or with stenting alone [13]. The fact that there are two lesions in the same circuit increases the risk of whichever procedure is selected. The management option that we prefer is the following: balloon angioplasty of the CCA origin lesion on the way in to make room for the sheath; CAS with protection; then, stenting of the CCA lesion on the way out with a balloon expandable stent for an origin lesion (Table 11.5).

Tortuosity of Arch Branches. Tortuosity of the innominate and common carotid arteries provides a significant challenge in some cases. Tortuous arteries may require extra planning and take several extra steps, perhaps using a system of gradually increasing stiffness.

The innominate artery is often redundant and the segment between the distal innominate and the midright CCA is a place where kinks and loops may occur. There is often a prominent right supraclavicular pulse from this redundancy and this may be interpreted as an aneurysm. Visualization of the innominate bifurcation into proximal right common carotid and subclavian arteries usually requires a right anterior oblique projection. The innominate is usually shorter than it appears in the left anterior oblique projection since the proximal right CCA and the right subclavian artery are usually superimposed. A retroflexed left CCA, which meanders toward the left neck in an almost horizontal trajectory, makes the last turn out of the arch and into the left CCA a hairpin turn. This can mimic the effect of a bovine left CCA on the tortuosity in the system.

TABLE 11.5. Technical tips for assessing the aortic arch.

1. The initial arch aortogram is obtained in the optimum oblique projection to provide the widest arc possible to separate the arch branches
2. Factors that make sheath access a challenge include arch tortuosity, arch variations (such as bovine configuration), tortuosity of the great vessels (such as a retroflexed left carotid), and ectopic disease in the arch or great vessels
3. When planning the initial branch vessel catheterization, tortuosity of the arch and the relative complexity of the access can be estimated from the location of the vessel's origin as it relates to the fulcrum point of the arch
4. The degree of challenge increases when branches progress form segment I to segment III. Arteries that originate from segment III are the most challenging to catheterize, with the origin of the target artery inferior to the horizontal line of the arch fulcrum
5. The operator must be aware when arch variations are present so that these may be managed and inadvertent catheterization of the wrong vessel can be avoided
6. Great vessel tortuosity and extra lesions outside of the carotid bifurcation complicate catheterization and access

When a sheath is placed into a tortuous CCA and especially if the tip of the sheath is in a tortuous segment, the sheath is in an unstable position. The curvature in the innominate or CCA will attempt to "spit out" the sheath. After the dilator and exchange guidewire have been removed, the sheath relaxes and the tip of the sheath begins to back up. With the breathing cycle there is a slight intermittent straightening and recurving of the arch and branch anatomy. If the position of the sheath is unstable, it can be observed to back out of the CCA in a "wiggle worm" fashion with each breath. When there is significant tortuosity at the arch or in the arch branches, place the sheath tip farther into the CCA and closer to the bifurcation than immediately appears to be necessary. Care must be taken to avoid encountering the bifurcation lesion with the dilator as the access sheath is being placed. The sheath may be advanced over its dilator for the last few centimeters to its desired location. When the stiff dilator and guidewire are removed, the tip of the sheath will likely retract a short distance, but still be in reasonable position in the mid-CCA. If this approach is not adequate to achieve a stable sheath position, a 0.014-in. buddy wire is placed in the ECA to stabilize the sheath so that it will not be spit out. This requires that the sheath be upsized by 1F so that the stabilizing buddy wire and the stent delivery catheter may run parallel to each other within the sheath.

The proximal to mid common carotid arteries is a location where severe kinks and even full loops can occur. A severe kink may be crossed and straightened but with great caution since injury to the artery may occur during sheath placement. If any curvature is changed as a result of the procedure, possibly related to straightening one segment, a preexisting kink in another segment may become worse and impede inflow. If the kinked artery is also calcified, it may bend to the will of the exchange guidewire and sheath and may fracture. A full loop in the CCA is rare and should not be crossed with a sheath. Carotid stenting using this approach with this anatomy is contraindicated.

After the sheath is placed in a tortuous approach artery, several things can happen that must be managed. A tortuous CCA that has been forced straighter over a sheath may accordion and this might impede inflow during the stenting procedure. Impeding forward flow in the CCA may start a cascade of events that could include thrombus formation, difficulty performing the procedure due to lack of visualization in the no-flow or low-flow state, or vessel injury. If a problem does occur during the procedure, it may be impossible to tell where the defect is located in the setting of altered flow. The sheath itself may also change the anatomy at the bifurcation. By straightening the access artery, the entry and/or exit angles to the lesion itself may become more difficult to negotiate.

Occlusive Disease of the Arch Branches. Spillover plaque from the aortic arch into the innominate or left common carotid arteries must be treated in less than 5% of CAS cases [15, 16]. The most common scenario is a mild or even moderate stenosis caused by plaque at the origin of the artery. This often does not impede inflow in any significant way and does not require specific treatment but must be negotiated deliberately and safely. When the stenosis caused by the plaque is severe enough such that it causes flow limitation in an artery with planned CAS, the situation must be managed as tandem lesions, as discussed previously.

Occlusive disease may also occur proximal to the bifurcation, in the middle or distal segments of the CCA. Injury or disruption to these coincidental lesions must be avoided and, if hemodynamically significant, must be treated. These lesions may be focal or even shelflike, or may be diffuse and cover many centimeters of the approach artery. Most commonly, there is diffuse but mild stenosis with minimal hemodynamic impact. The best way to avoid disrupting these lesions during sheath placement, that are separate from the bifurcation lesion, is to place the exchange guidewire either well short of the CCA lesion, or all the way through it and well past it. Avoid having the exchange guidewire bobbing up and down through a CCA lesion during sheath placement. Likewise, the sheath tip should be placed proximal enough to a separate CCA lesion so that there is no interaction. If this is not possible because of instability of this sheath position, the sheath should be placed all the way across the lesion.

The decision must be made whether the lesion in the approach artery is severe enough that it requires stenting at the time of carotid bifurcation stent placement. When the lesion in the approach artery is significant, it should be stented at the time of CAS. If the lesion is in the distal CCA and is contiguous with the bifurcation, it should be stented along with the bifurcation, even if the degree of stenosis of the CCA itself is not severe. Avoid placing the lower end of the stent partially across the body of the lesion in the distal CCA as this may potentially transect or disrupt the lesion.

Stenosis or Occlusion of the External Carotid Artery. The ECA may have a stenosis or an occlusion that is separate from the internal carotid artery (ICA) stenosis or may be contiguous with the bifurcation lesion. The challenge of external carotid occlusive disease may present itself in several ways. External carotid artery occlusion makes this vessel unavailable as an anchor point for the exchange guidewire during sheath access, as mentioned previously. The exchange guidewire used for carotid sheath placement is placed in the CCA. If the CCA is short or the arch is tortuous, the sheath first telescoping method may be used, which is discussed below. If the ECA is occluded and the ICA lesion is critical, as the filter delivery catheter or the stent delivery catheter crosses the lesion, flow will stop. This will cause an inability to visualize the bifurcation by administering contrast since there is no flow from the CCA origin to intracranial ICA.

Alternative Methods of Achieving CAS Access

The standard method of carotid access sheath placement is described above and is performed by placing an exchange guidewire into the ECA and advancing the sheath from the groin to the neck. Sometimes this approach is not possible and an alternative must be considered. Indications for alternative access are listed in Table 11.6.

Sheath First Telescoping Method. This method is performed by advancing the sheath into the distal aortic arch first, then cannulating the CCA with an extra long catheter and advancing or telescoping the sheath over the guidewire–catheter combination. The sheath is placed in the distal arch using a standard dilator. A 125-cm selective cerebral catheter is used to cannulate the CCA that is only a few centimeters beyond the tip of the sheath. The longer cerebral catheters are required to extend beyond the 90-cm carotid guiding sheath. The selective catheter is used to roadmap the bifurcation and the exchange guidewire is advanced into the distal CCA, taking care to avoid encountering the lesion. The catheter is advanced to the mid or distal CCA over the exchange wire. The sheath is advanced the rest of the way into the CCA over the cerebral catheter–exchange-guidewire combination.

TABLE 11.6. Indications for alternative CAS access.

Method	Indication
Telescoping sheath first	Occlusion or stenosis of ECA Lesion of the distal CCA Bifurcation lesion prevents safe ECA access
Brachial or radial access	Bovine arch with left CCA target No femoral access Hostile groin Aortoiliofemoral occlusive disease Aortoiliac aneurysm Thoracic dissection Severe arch or great vessel tortuosity Where angles favor this approach
Subclavian anchor	Right CCA target with Tortuous arch or ECA occlusion or both
Direct CCA access	No femoral access Arch disease CCA tortuosity

CAS carotid artery stenting, *ECA* external carotid artery, *CCA* common carotid artery

The advantage of this approach is that the sheath has already crossed most of the distance from the femoral access site before the arch branch is engaged (Fig.11.6). The sheath can be used to support the selective cerebral catheter as it initially enters the CCA. The sheath can be advanced the short remaining distance to its desired location without catheterizing the ECA.

Subclavian Anchor. This method is performed by placing an exchange guidewire into the right subclavian artery, advancing the sheath into the innominate artery, roadmapping and catheterizing the right CCA, then advancing the sheath into the right CCA (Fig.11.7). This technique works in the uncommon but challenging scenario of a right-sided lesion with a tortuous arch and a limited distance available to place the exchange guidewire. After placement of the sheath in the innominate artery, with the exchange guidewire still present extending into the right subclavian artery, the

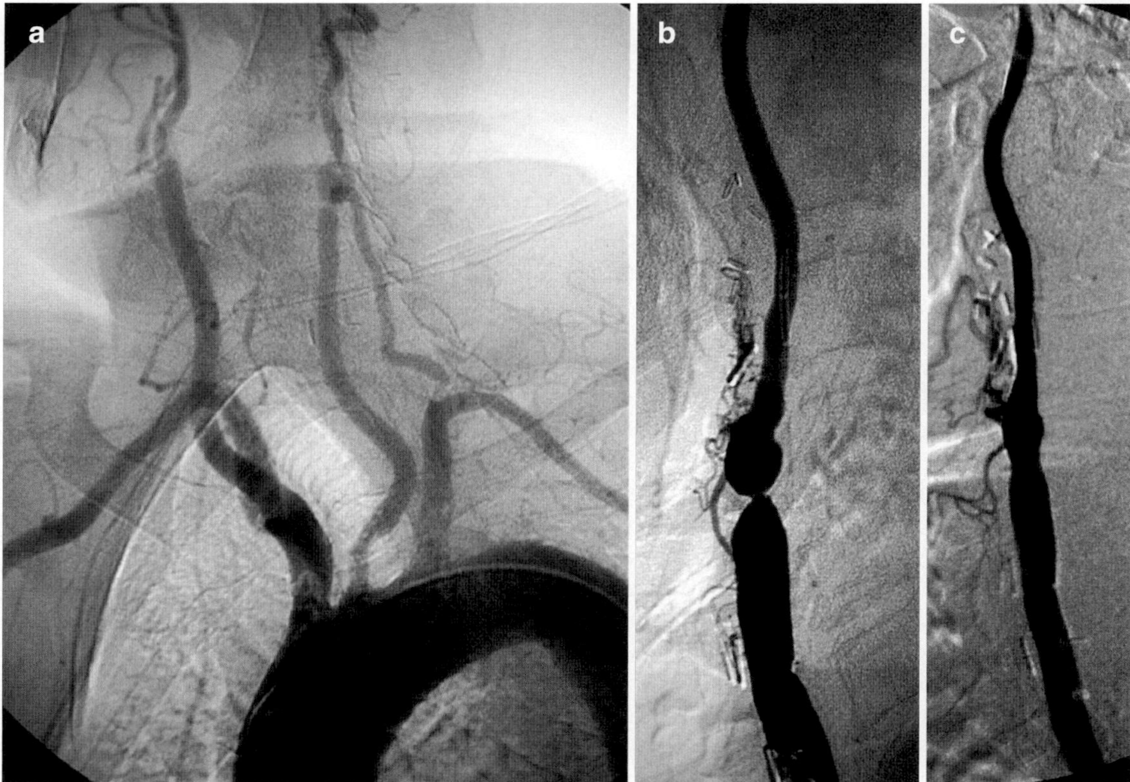

FIG. 11.6. This patient underwent carotid stenting using the sheath first telescoping technique. The external carotid artery was not usable. The sheath was advanced over the combination of the guidewire and catheter in the distal common carotid artery. (**a**) Arch aortogram. Patient has a left carotid lesion. (**b**) Lesion is present in the distal common carotid artery. (**c**) Carotid arteriogram after left carotid stent placement

sheath is used as a platform to catheterize the right CCA. A separate guidewire is advanced into the right CCA. The subclavian artery wire is removed, the dilator or a catheter is placed in the sheath over the CCA guidewire and the sheath is advanced a short distance from innominate to CCA.

Brachial or Radial Access. This method is performed by puncturing the brachial or radial artery and approaching the arch from the subclavian artery [17–19]. The selected arm is abducted on an arm board. A micropuncture set is used with a 21-gauge and a 4F dilator. After a guidewire is advanced into the axillary artery, a 4F sheath is placed. Administer nitroglycerine through the sheath and into the forearm and hand to help minimize spasm. Hold precise and continuous pressure on the arterial puncture site between exchanges to prevent the beginning of a brachial hematoma. If any diagnostic carotid arteriography is required that might change the candidacy of the patient for a stent, it can be performed with a selective cerebral catheter placed through the 4F sheath.

Which side do you puncture? If it is a right-sided lesion, almost always the right upper extremity is used for access. This avoids going into the arch altogether. If it is a bovine arch with a left carotid lesion, access the right brachial. Accessing the left CCA in a patient with standard anatomy is the least successful with this approach. Look at the entry angles from each side on preoperative imaging for clues.

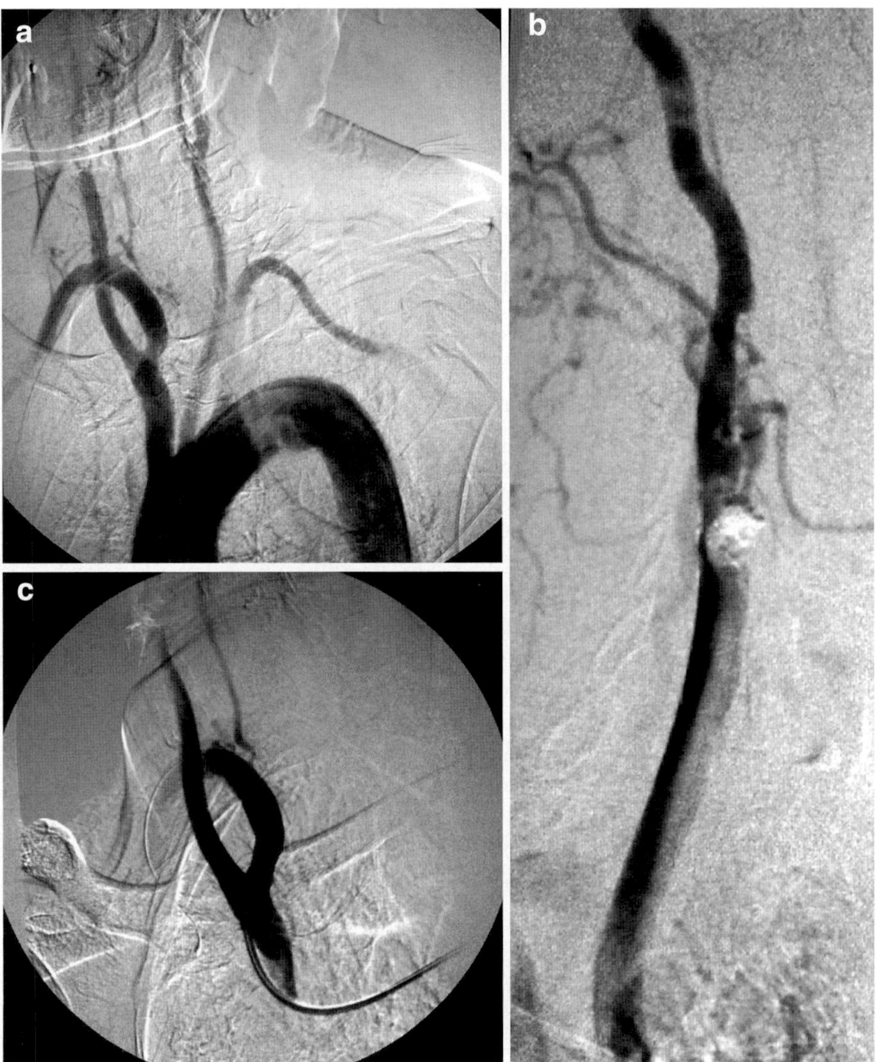

Fig. 11.7. This patient was treated with the subclavian anchor technique to obtain right carotid sheath access. (**a**) The aortogram shows that the arch is somewhat tortuous and cannulation of the right common carotid artery may be challenging. (**b**) The right carotid bifurcation stenosis adds to the challenge; the stenosis blocks access to a poor external carotid artery. (**c**) To get enough exchange guidewire purchase to advance the sheath, the guidewire is placed initially into the subclavian artery

The appropriate 6F carotid access sheath is selected. An access issue that is different about this procedure is that the tightest turn will *always* be just 10–15cm from the lesion to be treated. The challenge is to get the sheath around. The distance from the brachial puncture site to the arch is 40–55cm, depending on the size of the patient. The length of the CCA, from its origin to the desired sheath location, is 8–11cm. The sheath should be about 70cm in length for a brachial approach and 90 for a radial access.

Graduated rigid dilatation is performed prior to access sheath placement. Most of the time you are only dilating the arteriotomy with rigid dilators but in this case you are dilating the inflow brachial and radial arteries as well; so advance the dilators to the hub. If subclavian-axillary-brachial artery is tortuous, passing stiffer devices may cause it to bunch up. This can be remedied by putting the arm closer to the patient's side to stretch out the artery. Advance the tip of the sheath to just short of the major turn into the CCA. Remove the dilator for the sheath and place a diagnostic catheter;

When going from a right brachial with standard anatomy into the right carotid, use a right anterior oblique projection. When going from a right brachial with standard anatomy into the left carotid, use a left anterior oblique projection to open up the distance between innominate and left CCA. When going from a right brachial with bovine anatomy into the left carotid, use the left anterior oblique projection.

Use a hook-shaped catheter and a Roadrunner guidewire or a stiff Glidewire. Advance the catheter into the proximal to mid common carotid artery using the sheath for support. Sometimes the sheath can be advanced just slightly to give greater support to the catheter. Reposition the image intensifier to open the carotid bifurcation and roadmap the ECA. Advance the guidewire into the ECA, and then advance the catheter over the guidewire into the ECA. Place an exchange guidewire – a Supracore is a good choice. It has several centimeters of floppy tip that will make the turn into the CCA before the stiff part of the guidewire hits the turn. The sheath can be advanced over the catheter and guidewire combination or the dilator may be placed and that system advanced. The patient can also help by turning the head or extending the neck to open up the angle into the CCA. After the sheath is in place, as long as it does not kink, this is usually a fairly stable position.

Conclusion

Safe CAS access is associated with a thorough understanding of the anatomical features of the approach arteries. Several access methods are available and specific maneuvers may be performed that assist in achieving CAS access.

Key Points

- Access to the carotid artery for the delivery of a stent must be performed safely for carotid angioplasty and stenting (CAS) to be a viable treatment option.
- Managing certain anatomical characteristics or, occasionally, avoiding them altogether, will make CAS safer.
- The comparison between the medical risk of carotid endarterectomy (CEA) and the anatomical risk of CAS helps in the selection of patients for each procedure.
- In large studies of CAS, up to 30% of the CAS-associated strokes occur in territories other than that served by the carotid artery being treated; so excessive catheter/guidewire manipulation in the aortic arch can be associated with significant penalty.
- Arch imaging is necessary in planning for CAS access, either with arteriography or with axial imaging so that the operator knows what to expect during the procedure.
- The pathologies that complicate access for CAS include tortuosity, calcification, extra lesions in inconvenient places, and anatomical variants.
- If a tortuous segment is straightened with a sheath or a guidewire, that straightened segment may form a corrugated pattern of multiple contiguous curves in rapid succession. The tension may be shifted to some other segment, usually more distally, if only temporarily, and may therefore make some other part of the procedure more complicated.
- The more degrees of curvature in the system, the more likely that the access approach will be aided by a stiffer guidewire, a longer length of guidewire past the last turn (from the arch into the CCA), and a more flexible sheath (or even a guiding catheter).
- The exchange technique is the most commonly used method for gaining access to the CCA with a long sheath.
- Both the exchange technique and the "telescoping" technique can be facilitated by deep inspiration by the patient or by neck movement.
- Access may be facilitated by using a "subclavian anchor" and sheath stability may be improved by placing a 0.014-in. buddy wire in the ECA.

References

1. Lam RC, Lin SC, De Rubertis B, et al. The impact of increasing age on anatomic factors affecting carotid angioplasty and stenting. *J Vasc Surg* 2007;45: 875–880.

2. Moore WS. Extracranial cerebrovascular occlusive disease: the carotid artery. In: Vascular and Endovascular Surgery: A Comprehensive Review. Moore WS (ed.). Saunders, Philadelphia, PA, 2006, pp. 621–622.
3. Lin SC, Trocciola SM, Rhee J, et al. Analysis of anatomic factors and age in patients undergoing carotid angioplasty and stenting. *Ann Vasc Surg* 2005;19:798–804.
4. Schneider PA, Silva MB, Bohannon WT et al. Safety and efficacy of carotid arteriography in vascular surgical practice. *J Vasc Surg* 2005;41:238–245.
5. Dawson DL, Zierler RE, Strandness DE, et al. The role of duplex scanning and arteriography before carotid endarterectomy: a prospective study. *J Vasc Surg* 1993;18:673–680.
6. Deriu GP, Milite D, Damiani N, et al. Carotid endarterectomy without angiography: a prospective randomized pilot study. *Eur J Vasc Endovasc Surg* 2000;20:250–253.
7. Yadav JS, Wholey MH, Kuntz RE, et al. Protected carotid artery stenting versus endarterectomy in high risk patients. *N Engl J Med* 2004;351:1493–1501.
8. Gray WA, Hopkins LN, Yadav S, et al. Protected carotid stenting in high-surgical-risk patients: the ARCHeR results. *J Vasc Surg* 2006;44:258–269.
9. Schneider PA. Access for carotid interventions. In: Carotid Interventions. Schneider PA, Bohannon WT, Silva MB (eds). Marcel Dekker, New York, NY, 2004, pp. 93–110.
10. Osbourne A. Aortic arch and great vessels. In: Diagnostic ceveloval angiography. Osbourne A (ed) 2nd Edition. Pages 12–16. Philadelphia; London: Lippinocott-Raven, C 1999.
11. Schneider PA. Advanced cerebrovascular arteriography: Applications in carotid stenting. In: Carotid Interventions. Schneider PA, Bohannon WT, Silva MB (eds). Marcel Dekker, New York, NY, 2004, pp. 69–91.
12. Bohannon WT, Schneider PA, Silva MB. Aortic arch classification into segments facilitates carotid stenting. In: Carotid Interventions. Schneider PA, Bohannon WT, Silva MB (eds). Marcel Dekker, New York, NY, 2004, pp. 15–22.
13. Morris P. Practical Neuroangiography. Lippincott, Philadelphia, PA, 1997, pp. 63.
14. Schneider PA. Selective catheterization of the brachiocephalic arteries. In: Endovascular Skills (2nd Ed.). Schneider PA (ed.). Marcel Dekker, New York, NY, 2003, pp. 90–99.
15. Arko FR, Buckley CJ, Lee SD, et al. Combined carotid endarterectomy and transluminal angioplasty and primary stenting of the supra-aortic vessels. *J Cardiovasc Surg* 2000;41:737–742.
16. Rouleau PA, Huston J, Gilbertson J, et al. Carotid artery tandem lesions: frequency of angiographic detection and consequences for endarterectomy. *Am J Neuroradiol* 1999;20:621–625.
17. Wu CJ, Cheng CI, Hung WC, Fang CY, Yang CH, Chen CJ, Chen YH, Hang CL, Hsieh YK, Chen SM, Yip HK. Feasibility and safety of transbrachial approach for patients with severe carotid artery stenosis undergoing stenting. *Catheter Cardiovasc Interv.* 2006;67:967–971.
18. Levy EI, Kim SH, Bendok BR, Qureshi AI, Guterman LR, Hopkins LN. Transradial stenting of the cervical internal carotid artery: technical case report. *Neurosurgery* 2003;53:448–454.
19. Folmar J, Sachar R, Mann T. Transradial approach for carotid artery stenting: a feasibility study. *Catheter Cardiovasc Interv.* 2007;69:355–361.

12 Procedural Tips and Tricks

Robert Fathi

Introduction

Of all peripheral vascular interventions, carotid artery stenting (CAS) remains the procedure with the steepest learning curve and the lowest margin for error. The procedure demands a meticulous approach, advanced catheter and guidewire skills, an excellent appreciation of neuroanatomy, and the ability to manage dynamic fluctuations in hemodynamic status. Of perhaps greater importance is the decision-making and judgment necessary for appropriate patient selection.

This chapter presents a technical overview of the current approach to CAS and aims to highlight the complexities involved and safety considerations which are mandatory for successful outcomes.

Preprocedural Issues

It is of utmost importance to have an appropriately selected patient for this procedure. All referred patients are carefully screened and examined as outpatients. Carotid duplex ultrasonography results are routinely reassessed so that results for follow-up are standardized, preferably at an accredited, audited vascular laboratory. Once a patient is found to comply with the currently accepted indications for carotid stenting, the patient should also be assessed by a certified neurologist to obtain a baseline clinical report, neurological stroke scales, and at least one neuroimaging modality such as computed tomography or magnetic resonance imaging. After the decision to proceed with carotid stenting is made and informed consent obtained, the patient will be instructed to take 300 mg aspirin daily and 75 mg clopidogrel per day after a 300-mg loading dose commencing at least 3 days before the scheduled procedure date (see Chap. 9). Patients are asked to continue with all their usual medications with the exception of metformin and beta-blockers which should be withheld the day before the procedure. It may be necessary to withhold warfarin up to 5 days before the procedure. Patients with prosthetic heart valves will commonly be bridged during this period with intravenous heparin until warfarin is reinstituted and INR levels are therapeutic.

It is essential that patients are adequately volume replete prior to the procedure. They must have at least one 18-gauge or larger intravenous line. Intravenous fluids are commenced based on their preassessed left ventricular function: 1 L of normal saline at 150 mL h^{-1} for normal function (ejection fraction [EF], >50%); 100 mL h^{-1} for mild or moderate dysfunction (EF, 30–49%); 500 mL normal saline at 75 mL h^{-1} for severe dysfunction (EF, <30%) or severe aortic valve stenosis. Prior to the procedure all patients are taught to cough forcefully and repeatedly on demand. This maneuver is useful if the patient develops profound procedural hypotension or bradycardia or both. Coughing increases aortic pressures until an inotrope (e.g., 8.0 μg noradrenaline) or antimuscarinic (e.g., atropine or glycopyrrolate) can be administered. Although the routine intraprocedural administration of antimuscarinics is advocated.

S. Macdonald and G. Stansby (eds.), *Practical Carotid Artery Stenting*,
DOI: 10.1007/978-1-84800-299-9_12, © Springer-Verlag London Limited 2009

The Procedure

Efficiency of technique is paramount for successful CAS. The procedure ideally requires three persons to be scrubbed: two at the procedural table and one at the back table whose role it is to prepare the equipment. Equipment for each stage of the procedure must be prepared and available well ahead of time (see Chap. 10). Prolonged filter deployment resulting from lengthy procedures was an independent predictor associated with stroke and death in a registry of patients with severe carotid stenosis undergoing carotid stenting who were at high-risk for carotid endarterectomy [1].

Access via the common femoral artery is typically obtained using a short 5F sheath. At this point unfractionated heparin is then administered as a bolus of 70 u kg^{-1}. An activated clotting time (ACT) is checked within 5 min. A retrospective analysis of patients undergoing CAS found that the ideal ACT range for the lowest combined rate of death, stroke, or myocardial infarction was 250–299 s [2]. If the initial ACT is insufficient then further heparin boluses are administered before the procedure progresses.

In the rare patient for whom heparin use is contraindicated (e.g., heparin-induced thrombocytopenia syndrome), then bivalirudin should be considered as an alternative (see Chap. 9). Although its use has not been systematically studied in CAS, its efficacy and safety is well known for coronary artery stenting [3]. The intravenous dose of bivalirudin is 0.75 mg bolus per kg, followed by an infusion of 1.75 mg kg^{-1} h^{-1} for the duration of the procedure. In patients with significant renal impairment a lower infusion dose should be used. If the creatinine clearance is estimated to be less than 30 mL min^{-1}, the infusion rate should be reduced to 1.0 mg kg^{-1} h^{-1}. For hemodialysis patients, the infusion should be further reduced to 0.25 mg kg^{-1} h^{-1} with no alteration to the bolus dose.

Angiography

Compared to other noncoronary vascular procedures, carotid stenting is unique in the significant and rapid hemodynamic changes that can occur during the procedure (see Chap. 14). Endovascular pressure on the carotid sinus initiates the cascade of brainstem reflexes that typically lead to hypotension and bradycardia. For this reason constant direct arterial pressure measurement is essential. The preferred approach is a "closed-system" coronary manifold system, consisting of three side arms with an injection syringe at the end, in order to minimize the chances of air embolism. The side arms are the pressure manifold, the normal saline line, and finally the contrast line. This system has the advantage of continuous arterial pressure readings from the catheter tip. If the catheter is against the vessel wall, a dampened arterial waveform may be seen, which should warn the operator to adjust the catheter position and to perform cautious injection, thus minimizing the risk of vessel dissection.

Care to avoid the possibility of either air or thrombus embolization is paramount to a successful outcome. With each catheter exchange, any potential air is suctioned off with a syringe and the aspirated blood/air mix is discarded. The catheter and extension tubing are connected using a fluid-to-fluid technique, in which saline is slowly injected from the manifold as the connection is made. Care is taken not to mix blood and contrast within the manifold as the combination can cause the formation of small thrombi. The risk of air embolization is further minimized by holding the syringe at 45° angulation with the tip pointing downwards to encourage a bubble trap at the elevated end of the syringe. Prior to any injection, the syringe is tapped as slight negative pressure is applied to allow any air bubbles to rise to the top.

The procedure commences with an arch aortogram (see Chap. 10). An angled pigtail catheter is advanced over a normal J-wire to the ascending aorta and placed ~3 cm proximal to the aortic valve. The catheter is then hooked up to a pressure injector ensuring no air bubbles are trapped at the connection point. The field of view is maximized by raising the table as high as possible and by minimizing the distance between the patient and the image intensifier. The patient's head is gently rotated to the right and extended. A digital subtraction arch aortogram is then obtained in the left anterior oblique (45°) projection during a breath-hold. A power injection of 30 mL of contrast is typically administered at 15 mL s^{-1} at 900 psi.

A careful anatomical assessment of the arch is now made, paying particular attention to arch angulation, great vessel take-off and tortuosity, and any anatomical variations. Aortic arch anatomy guides the important decision on whether to use a long sheath system (for easy or medium difficulty arches – type I and II arches) or a guide catheter system (difficult arches – type III, significant proximal tortuosity, or sharp angulation of the takeoff of the internal carotid artery from the common carotid artery) (see Chap. 11).

Next, carotid angiography is done. We prefer to carry out angiography of the side *opposite* that of the index lesion, first, so that after subsequent imaging of the index side, the catheter can then be exchanged for an appropriate guide or sheath without the need to re-engage the vessel (Fig. 12.1).

To engage the great vessels from the aortic arch, the image intensifier is left in the 45° straight LAO projection so that the previous arch aortogram may be used for reference. For the majority of cases a 5F JR4 can be successfully introduced into the innominate or left common carotid arteries by counter-clockwise torque. In particularly difficult arches a reverse curved catheter such as a 5F Vitek (Cook) can be used. This catheter is taken into the descending aorta over a normal J wire. The wire is then removed and the reverse angle is formed in the descending aorta (with a simultaneous push/twist maneuver). To engage the vessels, the catheter is

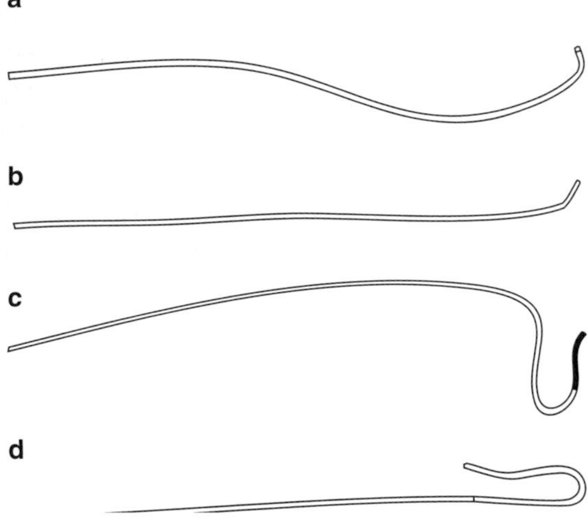

FIG. 12.1. Diagnostic catheters that are used in carotid angiography and stenting. (**a**) The most commonly used catheter is the JR4. (**b**) The angled Glide catheter can be used in simple arches. (**c**) The Vitek and (**d**) Simmons are the reverse-angled catheters that are used in difficult arches

advanced and rotated clockwise into position. To disengage a vessel, the catheter is advanced and rotated counter-clockwise. For very difficult cases (and often preferred by interventional radiologists) a 5F Simmons catheter is used, with its secondary shape most easily formed in the ascending aorta. For this reason this catheter should not be used by novices because of the risk of atheroembolization.

Once the vessel of choice is engaged with a 5F catheter, the image intensifier is moved to a 30° LAO projection. Ideally, the field of view will incorporate the top of the aortic arch up to the carotid bifurcation. A digital road-map picture is acquired using ~8 mL of contrast. This road map will then serve to guide the passage of a stiff angled hydrophilic wire, e.g. the Glidewire (Terumo), into the distal third of the common carotid artery. The second operator has an important role in controlling the wire position at this point, by ensuring that it does not either inadvertently cross the carotid bifurcation or drift caudally, in which case wire position may be lost during catheter manipulation. The primary operator slowly advances the catheter using careful counter-clockwise movements to the level of the mid common carotid artery. In difficult cases catheter advancement can be timed with patient respiration to improve the chance of success.

High-quality carotid and intracerebral angiograms are necessary for planning and are mandatory for procedural success. For the left common carotid artery, the intensifier is placed in a 30° straight LAO projection with the image centered on the mandible (the most common anatomical landmark for the carotid bifurcation). This is typically the ideal angle for separating the origins of the internal and external carotid arteries. The patient is instructed "stop breathing now, don't move, don't breathe, don't swallow." A digital subtraction angiogram is obtained. Next, the intensifier is moved to a full lateral position and a second angiogram is obtained. If the carotid bifurcation is still not well delineated then alternate views are obtained: posteroanterior or contralateral obliques (30°–60°).

Intracerebral angiography is done as follows: straight lateral digital subtraction angiogram of the cranium and finally a posteroanterior projection with ~15° of cranial angulation. For this view the anterior and posterior saggital sutures are lined up and the inferior orbital plate is lined up with the top of the ethmoid sinuses. The whole process is similarly repeated for the right common carotid artery, commencing with the 30° RAO projection, followed by the straight lateral and finally the intracerebral angiograms.

Guiding Catheter or Long Sheath?

The decision to use a guiding catheter ("guide cath" or "guide") or long sheath depends on the aortic arch angulation and proximal great vessel tortuosity. Typically for type I and II arches (see Chaps. 6 and 10) a 6F 90-cm sheath such as the Shuttle Sheath (Cook) is used (0.087-in. internal lumen, 8F outer diameter). This system has the advantages of a smooth transition between the sheath tip and the integrated dilator. The disadvantage of this system is the inability to torque the system and that it provides less support in the setting of proximal common carotid artery tortuosity. In type III arches, or cases where the internal carotid artery has a sharply angulated takeoff relative to the common carotid artery, an 8F 100-cm H1 guide cath (Cordis) should be used (0.088-in. internal lumen). The guide's secondary curve provides support during counter-clockwise rotation and advancement in a steeply angulated arch. The primary curve allows for tip orientation in difficult cases. The disadvantage of this system is the possibility of atheromatous embolization as the catheter is passed through the ostium of the common carotid artery due to the absence of a smooth transition with a dilator (Fig. 12.2).

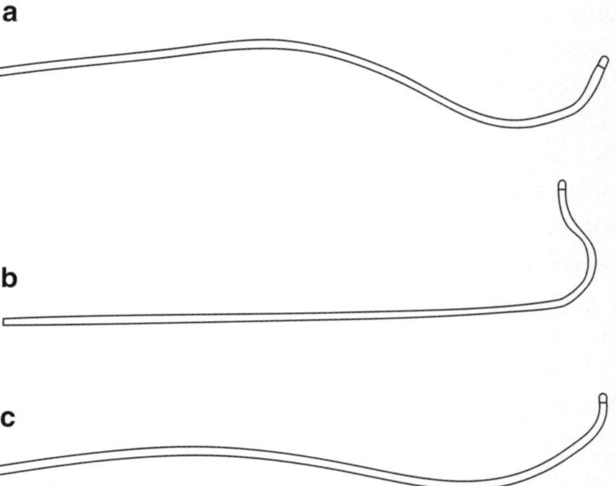

FIG. 12.2. Guide catheters commonly used for carotid stenting. (**a**) The H1 guide is most commonly used; note the sharp primary curve and gentler secondary curve. (**b**) The AL1 guide is used when only the ostium of the common carotid artery is engaged (coronary approach). (**c**) The JR4 guide is less commonly used

Techniques

Telescoping Technique

For the majority of our cases a "telescoping" technique is used. A diagnostic catheter, typically a 125-cm 5F JR4, is inserted through a 6F 90-cm Shuttle Sheath (after the dilator is removed in the descending aorta) or 8F guide cath (Fig. 12.3). Where the arch angulation is steep a 125-cm 5F Vitek catheter is used instead. This system is advanced as a unit over a standard J-wire which has been positioned in the ascending aorta. Once the diagnostic catheter portion of the "telescope" setup has reached the aortic arch the J-wire is removed.

The diagnostic catheter is used to engage the common carotid artery. The image intensifier is moved to the angle that best opened up the carotid bifurcation, typically 30° ipsilateral to the side of interest. A road map is taken with the patient being instructed not to move the position of the head. Care is taken to correctly identify the internal and external carotid arteries, remembering that the internal is typically posterior and medial to the external carotid artery. At this point a stiff angled Glidewire is carefully advanced into the external carotid artery or one of its major branches using a torquing device. The lingual branch of the external carotid artery should be carefully avoided as inadvertent wire-associated perforation of this vessel has the potential for causing rapid airways compression secondary to a tongue hematoma; bear in mind that the patient has been pretreated with a dual antiplatelet regime and has had a bolus of heparin administered. If the external carotid artery is occluded or heavily diseased then the wire is left in the distal third of the common carotid artery.

The 5F catheter is then advanced to the mid common carotid artery for type I and II arches, or into the external carotid artery if further support is needed in a type III arch. The Glidewire and diagnostic

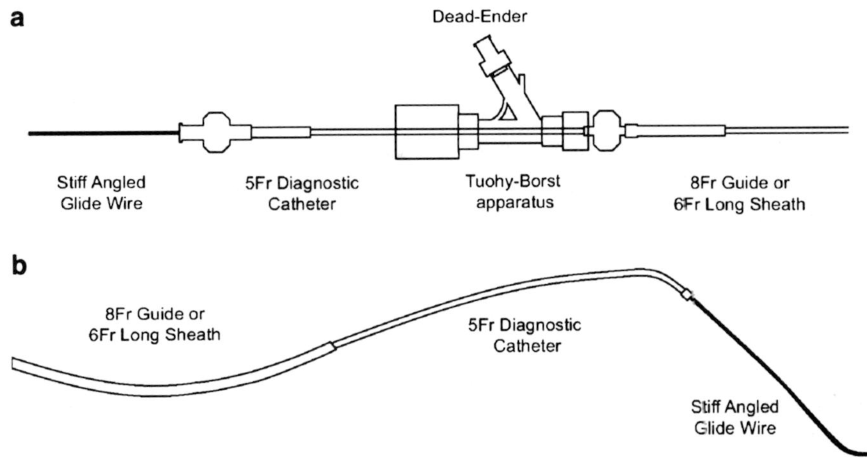

FIG. 12.3. The "telescoping technique." (**a**) The back-end consists of a 5F diagnostic catheter "telescoped" through a Tuohy-Borst apparatus and an 8F guide/6F long sheath. (**b**) The top-end of this system with a stiff angled Glidewire

catheter are held stationary as slow counter-clockwise rotation is used to advance the Shuttle Sheath or 8F guide to the distal third of the common carotid artery. When an adequate position has been obtained, the wire and diagnostic catheter are removed and the Tuohy-Borst valve is opened to allow back-bleeding before establishment of pressurized heparinized saline flushing via the side-arm of the guide/sheath.

Exchange Technique

The other common approach for advancing a selected guide or sheath into the common carotid artery as a follow-on from the diagnostic carotid angiography is the "exchange technique." While the diagnostic catheter is still engaged in the common carotid artery, a long stiff wire may be introduced over which the guide or sheath can be carefully exchanged. The "telescoping method" can also be used during any exchange, especially when a guide will be used.

This technique requires the image intensifier to be placed at 30° ipsilateral to the side of the lesion. Under road-mapping techniques a stiff angled Glidewire is advanced into the external carotid artery or one of the major branches (excluding the lingual artery). The diagnostic catheter is advanced into the external carotid artery, just proximal to the end of the wire and the Glidewire is slowly removed, ensuring that no air is entrained into the catheter. The catheter end is aspirated and an exchange length 260-cm super-stiff Amplatz wire (3-cm shapeable tip) with a preformed curve is then slowly advanced up the catheter. Importantly, the wire should never be pushed out of the catheter; instead, it should be "unsheathed," i.e., the catheter withdrawn slightly as the wire is held stationary. The patients are warned that they may experience discomfort or tension in their jaw, ears, or nose because of the presence of the stiff wire. The 5F catheter is then slowly removed under continuous fluoroscopy to ensure that the stiff wire does not migrate. After the catheter is removed the 5F short sheath is also removed while the primary operator maintains femoral hemostasis.

If a 90-cm-long sheath is to be used then it is advanced over the stiff wire with its dilator in place. Once the sheath is at the mid common carotid artery level, the dilator is broken away and the sheath advanced slowly to be ~2 cm proximal to the bifurcation. The dilator and then the stiff wire are carefully removed. Copious back-bleeding is allowed so as to ensure that no debris remains within the sheath system.

If an 8F guide is used then an 8F short sheath is placed, followed by the 8F guide. To minimize the risk of ostial great vessel dissection resulting from the relatively sharp "shoulders" of the bulky 8F guide, a telescoping technique is used. The original 125-cm 5F diagnostic catheter is "telescoped" through the guide. The guide of choice is the 8F 100-cm H1 guide (Cook). This allows for a gentler transition point from catheter to guide. The system is then advanced over the stiff wire. The diagnostic catheter is used to enter the common carotid artery and is fixed at the mid common carotid artery. This is carefully followed by the 8F guide. As the guide reaches the distal third of the common carotid artery, the wire and diagnostic catheter are slowly removed. Back-bleeding is again allowed prior to establishing continuous perfusion via a pressurized bag of heparinized saline.

Direct Guide Approach

In particularly challenging cases, such as a severely angulated arch where guide catheter advancement into the common carotid artery is not possible, or a bovine arch with the need to intervene on the left carotid artery, a direct guide or "coronary" approach may be used. For such cases an 8F AL1 guide is useful. The primary curve of the AL1 guide may be straightened using a sterile paper clip and boiling water or a heat gun. The guide is used to directly engage the ostium of the common carotid artery and perform the entire carotid stent procedure with the guide catheter sitting at the origin of the common carotid artery. To obtain extra support during the procedure, a stiff 0.014-in. coronary wire, such as an Asahi Grand Slam (Abbott Vascular) or Balance Heavyweight (Abbott Vascular), is carefully passed into the external carotid artery. This support wire is left in place until the stent is in position, and is moved to the mid common carotid artery just prior to stent deployment.

Wiring/Embolic Protection Device

The shape of the tip of the wire/emboli protection device is critical for successful lesion-crossing. For ease of passage of the wire from a large lumen vessel into a diseased and narrow vessel (as typically occurs from the common carotid artery into internal carotid artery), a double-angled tip is formed. The primary tip is formed at 45° with its length being approximately that of the width of the minimum lumen diameter of the internal carotid artery at the point of the lesion. The secondary bend is similarly at 45° with its length approximately equal to the width of the common carotid artery (Fig. 12.4). This configuration allows for the secondary bend to provide support in the common carotid artery with fine movements allowing the primary bend to negotiate the diseased internal carotid artery.

An important skill in CAS is the ability to accurately size the necessary equipment. The most reliable way to do this is by calibrated angiography. First, the operator must select an appropriate width of the embolic protection device (EPD), by measuring the distal internal carotid artery, beyond the lesion, at the "landing zone" of the distal protection device. If the EPD is undersized then insufficient wall apposition will occur and the potential arises for debris to flow around the edges of the EPD. If the EPD is oversized it is unlikely to have fully deployed and again gaps may occur between it and the vessel wall. The typical patient will have a 4–6-mm-wide prepetrous internal carotid artery. In large males a 7-mm EPD may be likely, and conversely, in small females a <4-mm EPD may occasionally be necessary.

EPDs such as the Angioguard (Cordis) are prepackaged with a single peel-away introducer. This allows for the wire tip to be passed into the guide without damaging the flexible wire tip by passage through the Tuohy-Borst apparatus. If the introducer is peeled before the wire successfully passes the lesion and the wire needs to be removed for the purposes of reshaping, then reintroduction can be difficult. In this situation a makeshift introducer needs to be fashioned. For this a 5F short sheath is

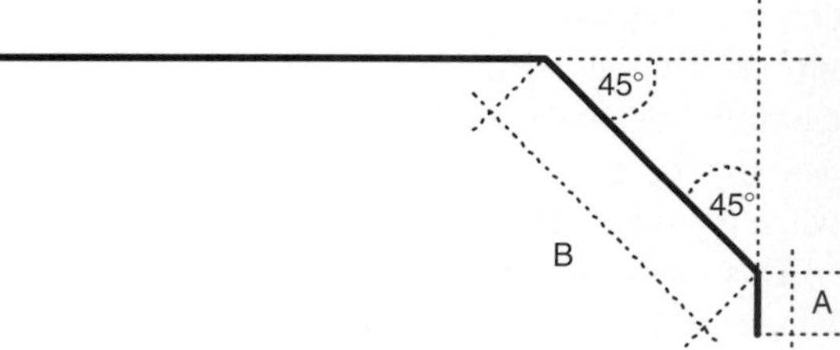

FIG. 12.4. The typical shape formed on the distal end of the wire/emboli protection device. The length "A" approximates the minimal lumen diameter of the lesion. The length "B" is equivalent to the width of the common carotid artery at its distal bifurcation

used without its dilator. The hemostatic valve portion of the sheath is cut and discarded. The remaining segment of sheath is then cut in a straight longitudinal line from end to end. This allows for the EPD to be reintroduced safely without damage to the distal end. Once it is passed, the longitudinal cut allows for the newly designed introducer to be removed. Alternatively, a separate individually packed funnel introducer such as that available from Abbott Vascular can be used.

Predilatation

The aim of balloon dilatation is to allow for the easy passage of the relatively high-profile and stiff stent-delivery system. This involves a measure of judgment, as use of too small a balloon may make no appreciable difference to the lumen, whereas an oversized balloon is known to increase the risk of atheroembolism. For the majority of cases a 0.014-in. monorail 4.0/20 coronary balloon, such as a Voyager (Abbott Vascular) or Maverick (Boston Scientific), is adequate for this task.

The low-profile monorail balloons should be meticulously prepared before loading onto the wire to minimize the possibility of air embolism resulting from balloon rupture. Although admittedly relatively rare, balloon rupture in the carotid artery would carry a much heavier penalty than such a complication in the iliac or superficial femoral artery. A three-way tap is placed at the end of the balloon. A luerlock syringe with 70% saline/30% contrast is used to trickle fluid onto the side arm of the three-way tap. The syringe is attached with the nozzle pointing downward. Negative suction is applied and the syringe is then gently tapped, allowing the space within the hypotube to be replaced by the fluid mixture. The three-way tap is then closed to air while negative suction is applied to keep the distal balloon end well deflated. A typical dilatation pressure of 6–10 atm. for 8–10 s is used.

Stent Placement

The aim of stent placement is to cover the index lesion – ideally from angiographically normal vessel at both the cranial and caudal ends. Carotid disease commonly involves the carotid bifurcation, commencing at the distal end of the common carotid artery. In the majority of cases when a stent is placed it will extend from the internal carotid into the distal common carotid artery, thus covering the ostium of the external carotid artery. Current nitinol-based carotid stents are typically between 20 and 40 mm in length, with the 30-mm ones being the most commonly used.

Before stent placement, attention should be turned to the ostium of the external carotid artery. If it is heavily diseased, stent placement over its ostium with ensuing post-stent balloon dilatation could cause sufficient plaque prolapse into this vessel to cause its occlusion. This can theoretically cause the clinical problem of jaw and tongue claudication. In clinical practice though, if the *contralateral* external carotid is widely patent, the presence of extensive collateral channels makes it unlikely that occlusion of the ipsilateral external carotid will result in significant ischemia and symptoms.

An indicator of carotid bulb sensitivity is provided by predilatation. If there is significant bradycardia or hypotension noted then a much more exaggerated response is likely to occur following stent deployment and post-stent balloon dilatation. In these cases a bolus of 200 mL of fluid is given and 0.5 mg atropine administered *before* the stent deployment.

The choice of stent width should be based on the ICA and not on the CCA width. The stent may be either tapered and allow for a natural gradation in width from the common carotid to the internal carotid arteries, such as Acculink (Abbott Vascular), or nontapered, e.g. Precise (Cordis). Because nitinol stents continue to expand in size over a number of weeks, the distal end of the stent is typically oversized by 1 mm. As an example in a 6-mm internal carotid artery, a 7.0/30 Precise stent or a tapered 7.0–10.0/30 Acculink would be deployed. This allows for the slowly expanding stent to counteract the neointimal hyperplasia that ensues.

When the stent is passed into the distal end of the guide or sheath, road-mapping and digital subtraction angiography are disabled. Instead, high frame rate cine (typically 12.5 frames per second) is then used and a cine run is obtained to show the carotid lesion. At this point boney vertebral landmarks must be selected and used as mental markers for the ideal distal and proximal ends of the stent. Taking careful note of the desired location, the stent is then passed just distal to the desired position and then pulled back. In doing this, the transmitted forces within the stent system are diffused, and as the stent is unsheathed, it is unlikely to jump forward. Stent deployment should be carried out carefully and slowly. As the first stent struts are deployed it is still possible to gently pull the stent mechanism backwards, before any further stent is opened, if the position is not considered ideal. Note that once stent deployment has commenced, however, it can no longer be advanced and its placement is committed.

In the event that the stent cannot be passed despite balloon predilatation of the lesion, there are a number of techniques that can be utilized. In order of preference these include first altering the geometry of the lesion by moving the neck – such as contralateral rotation or head extension. Often this is all that is needed to allow the passage of the stent. If this is unsuccessful then further predilatation can be done with a balloon 0.5 mm greater in diameter than initially used. Alternatively, a "buddy wire" can be used alongside the filter wire which can help to further straighten the angle between the common carotid artery and the internal carotid artery. For this purpose a heavy-bodied 0.014-in. coronary wire, such as an Asahi Grand Slam (Abbott Vascular) or Balance Heavyweight (Abbott Vascular), can be used. In particularly difficult situations, and as a last resort, an assistant places firm digital pressure just below the angle of the mandible, again altering the local geometry while attempting to pass the stent. Adequate collimation of the X-ray beam will ensure that the assistant's hands are not directly irradiated.

Post-Stent Dilatation

Post-stent dilatation is routinely used to ensure adequate stent-wall apposition. It is also the segment of the procedure with the highest risk of plaque embolization. For post-stent deployment balloon dilatation a 0.014-in. monorail peripheral balloon such as a Viatrac (Guidant) or Aviator (Cordis) is used. Typically, this balloon is 1.5 mm narrower than the deployed stent width. It should also be shorter than the stent if possible so that the balloon dilatation occurs only within stented segment and does not damage uncovered native intima, thereby minimizing the risk of restenosis. The patients are warned that they may feel an uncomfortable pressure in their neck. For this purpose a balloon pressure of 6–8 atm. is often used typically for 10–15 s. To reduce the risk of embolization during postdilatation, lower inflation pressures are deliberately used and balloon deflation is done gradually. A residual stenosis of 20% after dilatation is generally acceptable.

Retrieval Catheter

When postdilatation has been carried out and angiography reveals a satisfactory result, the EPD needs to be retrieved. It is not uncommon when the EPD retrieval sheath is passed for it to catch on the proximal edge of the stent struts. It is imperative if this occurs that attempts are not made to force the retrieval catheter forward. This may result in the EPD being dragged proximally while still open and potentially lead to the expulsion of captured debris. Excessive force can also cause the retrieval catheter to raise stent struts.

Instead, it is best to attempt movement of the patient's head and neck – for example, contralateral rotation, or head extension so that the angulation of the EPD wire is sufficiently altered as to allow smooth passage of the catheter. If a guiding catheter has been used, it can be torqued to alter the distal orientation. Alternatively, some retrieval catheters can be removed and the tip fashioned into a gentle curve using your fingers. This curve may be all that is necessary to successfully negotiate any stent struts that are impeding passage. If such maneuvers are unsuccessful then the catheter can be withdrawn 10 mm proximal to the stent struts and as the catheter is advanced the EPD wire is gently pulled backwards. Performing these two maneuvers simultaneously often allows the retrieval catheter to smoothly cross stent struts.

The retrieval catheter should then be gently advanced towards the EPD under fluoroscopic guidance. As the proximal end of the EPD is approached, extra care is taken as the EPD is kept in position and the sheath slowly advanced over it, causing the EPD to collapse. Once this has occurred, the sheath and EPD wire are slowly withdrawn as a single unit. During this process firm negative traction is placed on the wire, relative to the capture sheath so as to ensure that as the EPD is removed it does not accidentally open, releasing its debris. After the EPD is withdrawn the Tuohy-Borst is allowed to freely back-bleed to remove any particulate matter that may be within the guiding catheter or sheath. Final carotid and cerebral angiography is now done to assess the final result and to exclude any distal embolization.

Postprocedural Management

After ensuring adequate vascular access site hemostasis, all patients are transferred to our step-down telemetry unit for monitoring. They are prescribed bed rest until the following morning. All patients are reviewed by a staff neurologist the following day for an objective assessment of neurological status, including the National Institutes of Health Stroke Scale.

The typical antiplatelet regimen after carotid stenting consists of 300 mg aspirin daily for 30 days, followed by 100–300 mg per day lifelong (see Chap. 9). For the first month we also treat with clopidogrel (75 mg per day). If there are no other indications for continuing clopidogrel therapy, such as drug-coated cardiac stents, the drug is ceased at 30 days as stent endothelialization is likely to have occurred. For patients with an indication for warfarin therapy a typical regimen consists of warfarin, aiming for an INR of 2.0–2.5, 100 mg aspirin per day lifelong, and 75 mg clopidogrel per day for 1 month only. If the patient has a need for high INR levels, such as for mechanical valves or recurrent pulmonary emboli, then the treating cardiologist or physician should be consulted *prior* to the procedure. In the rare circumstance where a patient has a proven allergy to clopidogrel, then 250 mg ticlopidine twice daily is used in lieu of clopidogrel.

In the majority of cases the issues of hypotension associated with CAS are resolved by the end of the procedure. In the infrequent patient who continues to have significant symptomatic hypotension (<90 mmHg systolic) then a low dose dopamine infusion (5.0 $\mu g\ kg^{-1} min^{-1}$) may be used overnight (see Chap. 14). Furthermore, oral pseudoephedrine up to 60 mg every 4–5 h may provide useful pressor support until the blood pressure has stabilized.

A potentially devastating postprocedural complication is that of the hyperfusion syndrome (HPS) in which chronic low flow distal to a severe carotid artery stenosis results in an autoregulatory disturbance of the cerebral vascular bed in which the maximally dilated distal vessels fail to increase vascular resistance with increased blood flow after revascularization. This increased and uncontrolled cerebral blood flow after revascularization can lead to intracranial hemorrhage (ICH). Postrevascularization HPS has been well described in the carotid endarterectomy literature [4] and typically occurs between the third and fifth days after revascularization [5]. Abou-Chebl and colleagues [6] recently described the incidence of HPS in a cohort of 450 patients undergoing carotid stenting to be 0.44%, with the incidence of intracranial hemorrhage as 0.67% (combined incidence, 1.1%). Intracranial hemorrhage was uniformly associated with a poor clinical outcome. HPS is heralded by the presence of a throbbing frontal, temporal, or retroorbital headache on the same side as the treated vessel. It may progress to focal seizure activity or focal neurological deficits. Untreated, it can progress to frank intracerebral hemorrhage. Clinical factors associated with HPS include high-grade contralateral stenosis or obstruction, critical stenosis of the treated lesion, and hypertension [5].

To minimize this risk, all patients after CAS will have their systolic blood pressure aggressively controlled in hospital. The primary class of choice for this indication is beta-blockade, and we will commonly prescribe either boluses of metoprolol or labetalol or infusions of these medications. If beta-blockers are not tolerated by the patient we will then typically use a nitroglycerine infusion acknowledging that this agent may precipitate a headache which can then make an assessment of the HPS difficult. Agents that can paradoxically increase cerebral flow, such as hydralazine, must be avoided. After discharge all patients are mandated to obtain a home blood pressure recording device to check their blood pressures twice daily for a duration of 4 weeks. With two consecutively elevated readings (typically 140/90) patients contact the interventionalist to adjust blood pressure medications as necessary.

Conclusion

Carotid stenting requires advanced catheter and wiring skills. It is inherently different from the typical coronary and peripheral interventions. The operator must be initially competent to carry out complete carotid and cerebral angiography. The critical component of this procedure is the appreciation of the aortic arch and its inherent complexities. This allows for the proper selection of equipment to maximize the chances of success and minimize the length of the procedure. Operators must be able to perform the telescoping and exchange techniques as they are commonly utilized. The use of EPDs needs to be mastered to minimize the devastating risk of stroke. Finally, a number of mental algorithms must be present to deal with the various technical issues that invariably arise during the carotid case.

Key Points

- Adequately trained support staff is vital for procedural success.
- It is vital to avoid both the entrainment of micro air emboli during the procedure and microthrombi within sheaths and equipment.
  - A "closed-system" coronary manifold system, comprising three side arms with an injection syringe at the end, will mitigate microemboli of particulate and gaseous nature.
  - A fluid-to-fluid interface must be maintained at each injection of heparinized saline or contrast in order to prevent embolization.
  - Syringes must be held at a 45° angle to further reduce the risk of air embolism.
  - Pre- and postdilatation balloons should be carefully prepared in order to minimize the risk of air embolism should they burst on inflation.

For lesion-crossing with the 0.014-in. wire integral to many distal protection systems a double-angled tip is formed manually in order to negotiate a lesion commonly sited between a relatively large vessel (CCA) and a narrow diseased vessel (ICA).

Lesion-crossing should be carried out in a "no touch" fashion wherever possible, preferably using the "road-map" function.

Ideal stent positioning (after initial placement by road-mapping) may be achieved by contrast injections and utilization of bony landmarks.

If there is difficulty advancing the stent, the patient can help by changing the neck/jaw position, or a "buddy" wire (0.014 in.) can be passed alongside the "working" 0.014-in. wire in order to straighten out any curvature in the path.

Enthusiastic postdilation should be avoided; a pressure of 6 atm. should be sufficient with care taken to deflate the balloons in a gradual rather than sudden fashion to avoid promoting plaque fracture.

In the event that the retrieval catheter of the delivery system will not pass beyond the trailing stent struts of the stent, patient neck movement may sufficiently alter the geometry as to allow the catheter to pass.

References

1. Safian RD, Bresnahan JF, Jaff MR, Foster M, Bacharach JM, Maini B et al. Protected carotid stenting in high-risk patients with severe carotid artery stenosis. *J Am Coll Cardiol* 2006; 47(12):2384–2389.
2. Saw J, Bajzer C, Casserly IP, Exaire E, Haery C, Sachar R et al. Evaluating the optimal activated clotting time during carotid artery stenting. *Am J Cardiol* 2006; 97(11):1657–1660.
3. Lincoff AM, Kleiman NS, Kereiakes DJ, Feit F, Bittl JA, Jackman JD et al. Long-term efficacy of bivalirudin and provisional glycoprotein IIb/IIIa blockade vs heparin and planned glycoprotein IIb/IIIa blockade during percutaneous coronary revascularization: REPLACE-2 randomized trial. *JAMA* 2004; 292(6):696–703.
4. Solomon RA, Loftus CM, Quest DO, Correll JW. Incidence and etiology of intracerebral hemorrhage following carotid endarterectomy. *J Neurosurg* 1986; 64(1):29–34.
5. Ouriel K, Shortell CK, Illig KA, Greenberg RK, Green RM. Intracerebral hemorrhage after carotid endarterectomy: incidence, contribution to neurologic morbidity, and predictive factors. *J Vasc Surg* 1999; 29(1):82–87.
6. Abou-Chebl A, Yadav JS, Reginelli JP, Bajzer C, Bhatt D, Krieger DW. Intracranial hemorrhage and hyperperfusion syndrome following carotid artery stenting: risk factors, prevention, and treatment. *J Am Coll Cardiol* 2004; 43(9):1596–1601.

13 Embolic Containment Devices and How to Avoid Disaster

Alberto Cremonesi, Giancarlo Biamino, Armando Liso, Shane Gieowarsingh, and Fausto Castriota

Introduction

Carotid artery stenting (CAS) is emerging as an alternative therapy to surgical carotid endarterectomy (CEA) for the treatment of extracranial carotid stenosis [1–3]. The common goal of both procedures is the prevention of stroke, and the efficacy of the procedure depends highly on the periprocedural complication rates. Despite the routine application of stents, advanced stenting techniques, and dual antiplatelet therapy, embolization of debris into the cerebral circulation occurs invariably during CAS. Obstructive carotid artery lesions are known to contain friable, ulcerated, and thrombotic material [4] that can embolize during the intervention, as shown in histopathologic analysis in both ex vivo [5] and in vivo [6] studies, and also demonstrated in transcranial Doppler studies. In addition, it has been shown that microembolization occurs considerably more frequently during CAS than during CEA [7].

To minimize the risk of embolic neurological events, a number of neuroprotection strategies have been introduced into the carotid stenting procedure. A reduction of the Doppler-defined embolic load by means of a protection device has been shown [8]; and preliminary results indicate that with the refinement of stenting techniques and the increasing experience of the interventionist, along with the routine use of cerebral protection devices, the results of CAS are comparable with those of the best surgical series [3, 9, 10]. Histopathologic analysis of the debris collected using various protection systems has demonstrated that this debris comprises fragments of the atheromatous plaque dislodged during carotid stenting [6]. According to the size, embolic particles can be classified as either macroemboli (>100 μm) or microemboli (<100 μm). Macroemboli, especially those >200 μm, are usually associated with clinically evident neurological damage ranging from transient ischemic attack (TIA) to major stroke. On the contrary, the effects of microembolization are not well known and may include subtle changes in neurocognitive function rather than motor or sensory manifestations.

Protected Carotid Stenting: Clinical Results

At the moment there is no randomized clinical trial comparing the efficacy of protected with unprotected CAS, and it is difficult to imagine that such a randomized controlled study will ever be conducted on a sufficient number of patients. The published data regarding cerebral protection during CAS indicate some interesting points:

- Visible debris, mainly represented by atheromatous plaque material, was observed in 60% of cases of filter-protected CAS by Sprouse et al. [11] and in 66.8% by our group [12], with particles >2 mm in 9% of cases.
- In the German registry, the use of an embolic protection device was associated with a significantly

S. Macdonald and G. Stansby (eds.), *Practical Carotid Artery Stenting*,
DOI: 10.1007/978-1-84800-299-9_13,

lower rate of ipsilateral stroke (1.7% vs. 4.1%; $P = 0.007$) [13].

- We have reported a 79% reduction in the rate of embolic complications with the use of cerebral protection [14].
- In the early phase of the EVA-3S study, unprotected CAS was associated with a 3.9 times higher stroke rate at 30 days, compared with the rate associated with CAS done under cerebral protection [15].
- A 2003 review of the global carotid artery stent registry found that the rates of stroke and death were 5.2% for unprotected CAS and 2.2% for protected CAS [16].

Kastrup et al. [9], in a systematic review of the literature regarding the early outcome of CAS with and without cerebral protection devices, analyzed studies published between January 1990 and June 2002 by means of a PubMed search and a cumulative review of reference lists of all relevant publications. In 2,357 patients a total of 2,537 CAS procedures were done without protection devices, and in 839 patients 896 CAS procedures were done with protection devices. Both groups were similar in age, sex distribution, cerebrovascular risk factors, and indications for CAS. The combined stroke and death rate within 30 days in both symptomatic and asymptomatic patients was 1.8% in patients treated with cerebral protection devices, compared with 5.5% in patients treated without cerebral protection devices ($\chi^2 = 19.7$, $P < 0.001$). This effect was mainly due to a decrease in the occurrence of minor strokes (3.7% without cerebral protection vs. 0.5% with cerebral protection; $\chi^2 = 22.4$, $P < 0.001$) and major strokes (1.1% without cerebral protection vs. 0.3% with cerebral protection; $\chi^2 = 4.3$, $P < 0.05$), whereas death rates were almost identical (~0.8%; $\chi^2 = 0.3$, $P = 0.6$). On the basis of this analysis of single-center studies, the conclusion must be that the use of cerebral protection devices appears to reduce thromboembolic complications during CAS.

Distal Protection Devices

Distal protection devices work by interrupting or filtering blood flow in the internal carotid artery (ICA). They are placed beyond the carotid lesion in a straight portion of the carotid artery ("landing zone"). The first protection system widely used was the distal occlusion balloon. Nowadays, filter-type devices are more commonly used (up to 90% of cases).

Filter neuroprotection systems are able to entrap embolic debris from medium to large size, i.e., particles more than 100 μm in diameter. Filter performances are related to "crossing profile" and "capturing capability."

The crossing profile is an important technical characteristic related to the fact that the wire and the filter, constrained in the delivery system, must pass the embologenic lesion without detaching atheromatous plaque. The capturing capability of the filter is related to the amount of embolic load, produced during the procedure, which can be actually captured and removed. This technical performance is strictly related to both filter wall apposition and membrane pore size.

Characteristics of Principal Distal Neuroprotection Systems

Percusurge GuardWire

The best-known distal occlusion device is the Percusurge GuardWire (Medtronic), which consists of a simple balloon mounted on a 0.014-in. wire. The advantage of this device is mostly related to its low crossing profile (0.036 in.).

Wire-Mounted Filters

Angioguard XP

The Angioguard XP filter (Cordis) consists of a polyurethane concentric filter affixed to a guidewire with a soft atraumatic tip. The filter is kept open by a cage of eight nitinol struts. The pore size of the filter is 100 μm, and the system has a crossing profile between 3.2 and 3.9F. The filter is available in different sizes ranging from 4 to 7 mm in diameter.

FilterWire EZ

The FilterWire EZ (Boston Scientific) is an eccentric polyurethane filter with a proximal radiopaque nitinol loop. The pore size of the filter is 110 μm and the crossing profile of the delivery system is 3.2F. The proximal loop can fit all arteries between 3.5 and 5.5 mm in diameter.

RX Accunet

The RX Accunet (Abbott Vascular) is a concentric polyurethane filter which achieves vessel wall apposition by a stent-like nitinol structure. Embolic debris is captured by the membrane, which has a pore size of 125 μm. The filter is available in four sizes: 4.5, 5.5, 6.5, and 7.5 mm. The crossing profiles range between 3.5 and 3.7F.

Bare-Wire Filter Systems

Emboshield Pro

The Emboshield Pro (Abbott Vascular) is a nylon membrane concentric filter (120 μm pore size). The nylon membrane is treated by a hydrophilic coating with antithrombogenic properties (low absorption of plasma proteins and reduced platelet activation).

Emboshield Pro is a bare wire system, which means that the lesion is crossed by a high-quality 0.014-in. guidewire and the filter subsequently loaded. The wire, which is packaged with the filter, has a 0.018-in. bead 3 cm down from the platinum tip of the wire. The filter is 0.014 in. compatible, and the 0.018-in. bead serves to prevent the filter from migrating off the end of the wire and into the cerebral circulation. Clearly, therefore, it is vitally important to use the wire that is packaged with the filter and not just any 0.014-in. wire available. The system is 6F sheath compatible.

The filter is available in two sizes:

- Small – 2.5–4.8 mm vessel diameter
- Large – 4.0–7.0 mm vessel diameter

The crossing profiles for the small and the large devices are 2.8F and 3.2F respectively. This is the only filter system that allows the operator to leave the 0.014-in. wire across the lesion after removal of the filter.

Spider (ev3)

The Spider filter is characterized by a windsock-like nitinol mesh basket, with variable pore size from the proximal end up to the distal tip. The filter captures debris as small as 50 μm.

The Spider system differs from the other distal filters in that the lesion can be crossed with any 0.014-in. guidewire of the operator's choice. After lesion-crossing, the 2.9F delivery catheter is advanced over the 0.014-in. wire distal to the lesion. The initial 0.014-in. guidewire can be removed and the Spider basket is advanced and released at the landing zone. The system then becomes a standard wire-mounted system and the filter must be removed with the guidewire at completion of the CAS procedure. The crossing profile of the delivery system is 2.9F for the entire range of filter sizes (3–7 mm).

Distal Filters: Comparative Outcomes

A recent retrospective analysis [17] was carried out on 701 patients who underwent carotid angioplasty and stenting under cerebral protection. The study was conducted to identify patient and procedural parameters, including type of distal filters, that negatively impact the 30-day rates for stroke, death, and transient ischemic attack (TIA) after CAS. In this investigation of a dual-center CAS database, a subset of patient-related, lesion-related, or procedure-related variables (age ≥ 80, left-sided lesion, symptomatic, nicotine abuse, hypertension, diabetes mellitus, other peripheral vascular disease, hypercholesterolemia, embolic protection devices usage, predilation, ulcerated lesion, echolucent plaque, restenosis after surgery) were analyzed for association with occurrence of stroke, death, or TIA ≤30 days after CAS. In terms of distal filters, eccentric devices such as FilterWire EX/EZ (62.8% of cases) and SpiderFX/SpiderRX (11.4% of cases) were compared with concentric filters such as Angioguard XP (10.6% of cases) and Emboshield (3.9% of cases). Subgroup analysis of the 304 symptomatic patients (43%) showed that open-cell stent designs and concentric EPD designs yielded an OR of 4.1 (95% CI, 1.4–12; P = 0.0136) and 3.3 (95% CI, 1.016–10; P = 0.0525), respectively, for 30-day stroke/death/TIA within this database. Analysis of open-cell stent designs and concentric EPD designs in patients with echolucent lesions yielded an OR of 3.1 (95% CI, 1.2–8.2; $P = 0.0343$) and 3.7 (95% CI, 1.3–10; $P = 0.0174$), respectively, for 30-day stroke/death/TIA. The authors concluded that, particularly in symptomatic patients or those with echolucent lesions, the combination of closed-cell design stents and eccentric filters seems superior. Nevertheless, it is important to highlight some important limitations of this study, including the retrospective nature of the analysis, the voluntary data submission, self-audit, and the increased operator experience with eccentric filters than concentric ones.

Limitations of Distal Protection Devices

Distal occlusion devices are limited by the fact that lesion-crossing is unprotected, and, despite being able to block microemboli by occluding the ICA, can lead to cerebral embolization through collaterals from the external carotid to the middle cerebral artery (retinal and cerebral infarcts through large periorbital and occipital collaterals have been reported) [8, 18]. Moreover, about 5–8% of patients develop intolerance due to this form of "endovascular clamping" [19].

Filter-type devices also have some drawbacks:

- They are not effective in trapping microemboli, since the pore size ranges from 100 to 140 μm.
- The lesion must be crossed by the wire and the filter before deployment, with the risk of unopposed embolization, especially in tight lesions.
- Even macroemboli may pass in the case of incomplete vessel wall apposition (tortuous landing zone or large artery).
- Emboli that were originally captured may be dislodged during the retrieval of filters (squeezing effect – like squeezing toothpaste out of a tube).

Finally, both distal filters and balloons may be an embolic source themselves, because of intimal damage at the level of the ICA landing zone [20]. In some studies using transcranial Doppler, the use of distal filters was even associated with a greater microembolization (Micro Embolic Signal count), compared with unprotected stenting, although this did not translate into a clinically evident difference [21].

Proximal Protection Devices

Proximal protection devices work by interrupting or reversing blood flow in the ICA. Compared with filters, they offer the advantage of protected lesion-crossing, use of the guidewire of the operator's choice, and capture of both macro- and microemboli irrespective of size. Moreover, it is not necessary to navigate any part of the device in the distal ICA, thus reducing the risk of intimal damage, spasm, or dissection. Currently, there are two such devices available: the neuroprotection system (NPS, Gore), which is derived from the Parodi antiembolic system (PAES, ArteriA), and the Mo.Ma system (Invatec).

Neuroprotection System

This system allows complete arrest of ICA flow, continuous passive ICA flow reversal plus/minus augmented active ICA flow reversal. This is achieved by endovascular clamping of the common carotid artery, by inflating an elastomeric balloon located at the tip of a 9F sheath (the "balloon catheter"), and of the external carotid artery, by inflating an independent elastomeric balloon on a 0.014-in. wire (the "balloon wire") which is advanced through the sheath. At this point there is flow arrest in the ICA to be treated. Once the back of the "balloon-sheath" is connected to a 6F sheath in the contralateral femoral vein via an interposed extracorporeal filter, there is reversed flow in the ICA to be treated, driven by cerebral backpressure (passive flow) or actively aspirated by a syringe.

The extracorporeal filter has pores of 180 μm and this collects debris before the blood reenters the venous system, in order to avoid the risk of paradoxical embolism in case of a patent foramen ovale.

Once the system is working, the lesion can be crossed with a guidewire under protection and angiographic guidance, since the contrast medium is cleared by backflow; then, conventional stenting and postdilatation are carried out. After each stage of the procedure, particularly those associated with the greatest risk of embolization, 10 mL of blood is actively, but gently, aspirated; then the balloons are deflated while active aspiration is applied to retrieve any particle contiguous to the balloon occluder in the common carotid artery.

Mo.Ma

The Mo.Ma system consists of a 100-cm, 8–9F catheter with a 5–6F working channel and two distal, independently inflatable balloons placed at a distance of 7.2 cm. The distal balloon occludes the external carotid artery up to a diameter of 6 mm, whereas the proximal balloon occludes the common carotid artery up to a diameter of 13 mm, achieving a static blood column at the carotid bifurcation. At this point the stenting procedure can be done by crossing the lesion under protection with the selected materials; after postdilatation, at least three 20-mL syringes of blood are actively aspirated and checked for debris before deflating the balloons.

Proximal Protection During CAS: Clinical Outcomes

Most of the clinical data on the NPS were obtained with the first version, i.e. the PAES. In the first series of 100 patients reported by Parodi in 2001, no embolic stroke was observed, but clamping intolerance occurred in 8% [22]. Other small, non-randomized studies confirmed the efficacy of PAES in preventing embolic complications [23, 24]. In 2005, Parodi reported on the first 200 patients treated; in this series, the technical success rate was 98.5%, the 30-day stroke and death rate was 1.5%, and perioperative clamping intolerance was observed in six patients (3%) [25]. The first clinical experience with the Mo.Ma system was reported by Diederich et al. [26], wherein 42 patients were treated (26.2% with symptomatic carotid artery disease), with an overall technical success of 97.6%. Mean clamping time was 10.6 ± 6.5 min, and transient clamping intolerance occurred in 12% of patients. Macroscopic debris was collected in 76.1% of cases. Two patients had neurological deficits that lasted 2 and 12 h respectively, and two other patients (4.7%) had a minor stroke.

In the PRIAMUS multicenter registry [27], 416 patients (63.4% with symptomatic carotid artery disease) underwent CAS with the Mo.Ma device. Technical success was achieved in 99% of cases. Mean clamping time was 4.91 ± 1.1 min, and transient clamping intolerance was observed in 5.76%, whereas macroscopic debris was retrieved in about 60% of patients. At 30-day follow-up, the cumulative incidence of adverse events was 4.56%, with a 0.72% rate of major strokes and deaths.

The efficacy of the Mo.Ma device in preventing microembolization was assessed in a comparative study with a distal filter (E.P.I. FilterWire, Boston Scientific) by detecting microembolic signals with transcranial Doppler during the CAS procedure [28]. The Authors identified five different procedural steps:

1. Positioning of the protection system
2. Passage of the stenosis
3. Stent deployment
4. Balloon dilatation
5. Retrieval of the protection system

The number of MES was significantly lower in steps 2–4 with the Mo.Ma, compared with the filter, whereas no significant differences were observed during the first and last phases. MES detection is a surrogate marker of cerebral microembolization which can be hampered by technical limitations, such as the inability to differentiate between solid and gaseous emboli [29]; nevertheless, the association of a high MES count with neurological complications was established in the Antonius CAS registry [9].

Limitations of Proximal Protection Devices

The drawbacks of proximal protection devices include their large size, the occurrence of clamping intolerance, and the fact that they cannot be used in patients with severe disease of the external or of the common carotid artery, although contralateral ICA occlusion is not necessarily a contraindication.

The need for large femoral sheaths may preclude the insertion of the devices in patients with severe peripheral arterial disease and could theoretically be associated with an increase in vascular access site complications. Yet, with the first version of the Mo.Ma device, requiring a 10F femoral sheath, in the PRIAMUS registry [13] the rate of local complications was 4.08%, none of which required surgical repair or blood transfusions. Higher complication rates were reported by Rabe et al. [30] with the PAES, but given the current availability of

9F size for both the Mo.Ma and the NPS device, it is reasonable to expect a lower rate of clinically significant access site complications in the future.

Clamping intolerance may occur in a portion of patients (up to 8%) following interruption of cerebral perfusion during the intervention and is generally associated with severe contralateral disease or poorly developed cerebral collateral circulation. An intraprocedural parameter predictive of tolerance is represented by a backpressure >30 mmHg. Another key factor is overall clamping time, which has progressively shortened with the increased experience of operators (from 10 min in the study of Diederich et al. [26] to 5 min in the PRIAMUS registry [27], with a parallel decline in the rate of clamping intolerance from 12% to about 6% [11, 31]. The same holds true for the PAES/NPS device, since the rate of clamping intolerance dropped from 8% in 2001 to 3% in 2005. However, the occurrence of clamping intolerance does not represent an absolute contraindication for continuing the procedure. Indeed, three strategies can be adopted: timely completion of the procedure, in order to restore perfusion as soon as possible; positioning under protection through flow reversal/arrest a distal filter and then deflating the balloons and allowing antegrade perfusion ("seat-belt and air-bag" technique) [32]; and performing intermittent flow reversal/flow arrest in which the balloons are inflated and deflated at each procedural step. Finally, for both proximal protection devices two potential drawbacks have to be considered:

1) A nonocclusive balloon or a sizeable superior thyroid artery originating proximal to the ECA balloon may lead to continuous antegrade flow in the target vessel during clamping.
2) At the end of the procedure, the balloon in the ECA, usually "jailed" by the stent, must be removed and, at least theoretically, might be entrapped in the struts of an open-cell geometry stent.

When to Use Proximal or Distal Protection in CAS

At the current time large clinical studies comparing proximal with distal protection are lacking, and so device selection is quite empirical. In challenging anatomies, with angulated ICA-CCA takeoff and/or lack of a suitable ICA landing zone for distal protection, the use of proximal protection is strongly recommended. The same holds true for lesions with high embolic risk, since proximal protection devices seem to be more effective than filters in avoiding distal embolization, especially in the procedural steps at higher risk, irrespective of debris size. Therefore, noninvasive characterization of the carotid plaque in order to quantify its embolic potential ("vulnerable plaque") represents a very important issue when planning the CAS procedure. In practice many factors should be assessed and integrated in order to predict the embolic risk of a specific carotid lesion during CAS. If this risk is estimated to be high and there are no anatomical contraindications, proximal protection would probably represent the safest approach for the patient.

Both long lesions and clinically unstable plaques (i.e. recurrent TIAs) define a high-risk lesion subset, because of high plaque burden and inflammatory activation, respectively. Indeed, Krapf et al. [33] reported that the risk of new cerebral ischemic lesions at diffusion-weighted MRI after CAS was related to the length of the lesion as assessed by B-mode echography, whereas preprocedural leucocyte count was found to be associated with increased microembolization during CAS [34]. The vulnerable plaque, as opposed to the stable, fibrous plaque, is made of a large lipid pool covered by a thin fibrous cap. A study in 200 CEA specimens showed that plaque phenotype correlated with embolization during CEA, since vulnerable plaques were more prone to cause perioperative microembolization when compared with fibrous plaques [35]. Fatty, vulnerable plaques are less echogenic, and this pattern can be quantified by the Grey Scale Median (GSM) method. In the ICAROS study [36], the risk of CAS-related stroke was 7.1% in lesions with GSM <25 and 1.5% in lesions with GSM >25 (see Chap. 8).

Potential Complications Related to Protection Devices

The feasibility, safety, and the clinical efficacy of protection devices have been addressed in several studies. However, few registries give more detailed information regarding incidence, type, and the outcome of complications that could be related to the use of protection devices [3, 31, 37]. Most frequently, transient complications with distal protection devices are distal spasm and slow flow, with a described incidence of up to 3.6 and 7.2% respectively [37]. Distal spasm generally resolves spontaneously a few minutes after the removal of a distal protection device, or if blood pressure allows, following the administration of intraarterial nitrates. Slow flow may occur when using distal filters and is due to partial or complete occlusion of the filter pores with debris and, according to the literature, is related to neurological events. Slow flow disappears following removal of the filter.

Dissections of the distal ICA, at the site of placement of distal protection devices, may occur and have been described in 0.5–0.9% of cases [3, 31]. These dissections were managed with balloon angioplasty, additional stent implantation, or no treatment at all [3, 31]. All described dissections were without clinical complications. One occlusive dissection which could not be recanalized has been described but thankfully was without clinical sequelae [31]. In another single case, failure to remove the filter necessitated surgical extraction [31]. Endovascular management of displaced filters has been described [38, 39]. Care must always be taken to avoid entrapment of the leading end of rapid exchange balloons or stent delivery systems and the trailing end of the filtration element. This complication has been reported and dealt with endovascularly [40].

Possible complications related to occlusive protection systems, distal or proximal, are mostly related to intolerance of the patients to the interruption of blood flow. In the recently completed Mo.Ma registry, intolerance to flow blockage was observed in 7.1% of patients [41]. In 5.1% the procedure could be accomplished without modifying the technique, in 1.9% patients intermittent balloon deflation was necessary to complete the procedure, and in 0.6% a distal filter was subsequently used for cerebral protection. In all patients presenting with occlusion intolerance, stent implantation was successfully done through the sheath of the Mo.Ma device and without in-hospital and 30-days neurological complications. Intolerance for distal balloon occlusion systems varies between 5.3 and 9.0% and is equally related to poor collateralization of the cerebral vessels [3, 42].

Key Points

- Carotid stenting generates emboli by the endovascular manipulation of atheromatous plaque. It has been shown that microembolization occurs considerably more frequently during CAS than during CEA.
- The neurological effects of macroemboli are clearly evident. The neurological effects of microembolization may be clinically covert; indeed they may perhaps only be evident on robust cognitive function testing of the patient.
- While there is no randomized trial evidence to support the use of protection systems, the available literature (levels III and IV) suggest benefit.
- Protection systems may be broadly subdivided into distal (including distal balloon occlusion and distal filters) or proximal (including flow arrest (the Mo.Ma) and flow reversal (Gore NPS).
- Filters are the most commonly used protection system currently. The technical factors that are important to consider while using them are crossing profile (as the lesion must be crossed with this protection system while flow is antegrade; i.e., lesion-crossing is *unprotected*) and filter efficacy (which is related to pore size and wall apposition).
- No single system is capable of optimal management of the embolic burden associated with each lesion, each anatomy, and each patient. There are trade-offs for each system. For example, the benefits of constant cerebral perfusion when filters are used must be balanced against an acceptance of subtotal protection with these systems.
- Particularly vulnerable lesions or patients with tortuous distal internal carotid arteries (that would comprise the landing zone for filters) are probably best protected by means of "proximal systems," i.e., either flow arrest (Mo.Ma) or flow reversal (Gore NPS).
- Protection systems themselves may be the cause of neurological complications and their use is associated with a unique learning curve as these devices are infrequently used for other endovascular interventions.

Tips and Tricks

Tip 1: Individual Treatment Strategy

Although carotid angioplasty and stenting (CAS) is becoming more widely performed for the treatment of severe carotid obstructive disease, no data are actually available about the correct use of specific devices.

Each protection device and stent has its own technical features. Our experience of more than 2,200 procedures since 1997 has led us to believe that carotid stenting equipment should be selected according to predefined logical indications rather than by chance. This recommendation comes from the consideration that nothing can be defined as "perfect" in carotid stenting: neither protection devices nor stents. With respect to protection devices, no single system allows a fully protected procedure. Embolic events are frequently related to aortic arch manipulation during supraaortic trunk engagement, and they occur in a phase that is unprotected by definition. There are no conclusive scientific data to indicate superiority of either proximal protection devices or distal filters. With respect to stent platforms, a universally applicable stent (appropriate to all lesions and all anatomies) does not exist, and plaque coverage, vessel conformability, and shape adaptability appear to be conflicting physical parameters.

Another crucial point, frequently neglected, is the fact that the stent frame, with its specific design and radial force, exerts an intrinsic antiembolic activity, and stent struts of some stent systems are better at preventing future embolization of ruptured plaque than others.

Taking these two considerations into account, the interventionist wishing to do carotid stenting safely should have the following:

1. A sound understanding of *patient variables*, i.e., clinical and neurological status, vascular anatomy, carotid plaque characteristics
2. *Advanced knowledge of the technical features of the materials used*: guiding catheters and sheaths, wires, balloon, stents, embolic protection devices, etc.

The optimum means of avoiding disaster is the "individual treatment strategy." In the face of different types of embolic protection devices and stents, the CAS strategy should always consist of a process of tailoring the endovascular procedure to a specific patient and to a specific carotid lesion and vascular anatomy.

Tip 2: Safe CAS and the "Protected Procedure" Concept

The current major source of CAS complications is related to the problem of distal embolization, either intraprocedural or postprocedural.

Generally speaking, most operators think that the safety of CAS is dependent on the effective reduction of the embolic risk during the stenting procedure. That is true, but it does not mean that we can achieve protection only by use of a cerebral protection device.

In reality, we have to put into practice two protection strategies, the former regarding the entire procedure (which includes consideration of the indication for CAS) and the latter related specifically to the use of neuroprotection devices.

Active Protection

- Any method and/or work strategy that minimises generation of sizeable particles of embolic material during the endovascular procedure
- Appropriate patient and lesion selection
- Meticulous device selection and interventional technique

Passive Protection

- Devices that allow the operator to capture and remove embolic material generated during the procedure

Some embolic events may occur hours or days after the stent implantation. Despite the routine application of stents, advanced stenting techniques, and combined antiplatelet therapy with aspirin and clopidogrel or ticlopidine, embolic neurological events may occur within 30 days of the procedure.

The mechanisms involved in late embolic events are complex and still under investigation, but these events tend to occur in the postprocedure period, between stent implantation and its complete reendothelization (3–4 weeks). The most likely explanation is that these late symptomatic embolic events are due to prolapsed soft tissue as well as platelet microaggregates/thrombi detached from the stent metallic frame.

In light of the considerations about late embolic events, it is clear that the stent frame (and its design) plays an important role in terms of scaffolding and plaque coverage: the stent has the potential to exert a specific intrinsic antiembolic action, dependent on its design.

Tip 3: Applicability of Tailored Carotid Stenting in Daily Practice

If we accept the fact that neither the ideal neuroprotection device nor the ideal stent exists at the moment, individual treatment strategy is currently the only logical answer for treating standard as well as complex carotid lesions and anatomies.

All the following clinical cases were selected for teaching purposes to demonstrate how to put into practice tailored carotid stenting: the materials (stents, embolic protection devices, guiding catheters, balloons, wires, etc.) were chosen in order to marry the technical features of the devices with specific lesion and/or vessel anatomy.

From a clinical stand point, all the presented cases were from patients treated for symptomatic carotid lesions (TIA, or minor stroke within 6 months of intervention).

Case 1

Angled soft ulcerated plaque associated with anatomic complexity (Fig. 13.1)
Technical issues:

- Difficult angled ICA anatomy which may preclude the use of distal protection devices
- High-grade, asymmetric ulcerated soft plaque at the origin of RICA

Solution:

- Proximal system
- Stent: high scaffolding closed cell design (braided mesh frame)

Strategy endpoints:

- Prevention of massive distal embolization
- Respect of original anatomy
- Prevention of plaque prolapse (postprocedural)

Procedure

Over a long, stiff 0.035 in. wire (Supracore, Guidant), the proximal stop flow blockage system (Mo.Ma) is advanced until the distal tip is properly placed in

Type of stent	Hybrid mesh frame, tapered 7–10/40 mm (Cristallo Ideale, Invatec)
Type of embolic protection	Proximal endovascular clamping (Mo.Ma, Invatec)

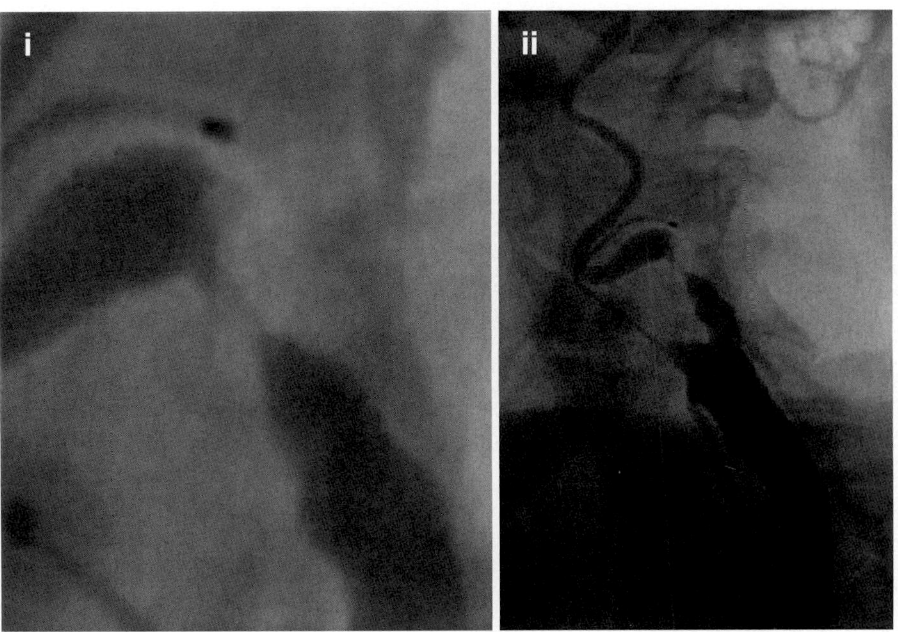

FIG. 13.1. Angled soft ulcerated plaque associated with anatomic complexity (extreme post-stenosis tortuosity)

the origin of the external carotid artery (Fig. 13.1). Distal occlusive balloon is inflated (arrow).

The complete stop flow blockage is achieved by inflating the proximal elastomeric balloon in the common carotid artery. Under flow blockage, a 0.014-in. hydrophilic wire (Choice PT, Boston Scientific) is advanced across the lesion.

Once predilated with a 3.5/30-mm coronary balloon (Maveric, Boston Scientific), a hybrid stent tapered 7–10/40 mm is delivered at the lesion site and postdilated with a 5.5/20 mm balloon (Maveric) (Fig. 13.2).

Case 2

Right carotid artery high-grade stenosis with ultrasound features of a vulnerable plaque associated with a marked proximal common carotid artery bend (Fig. 13.3)

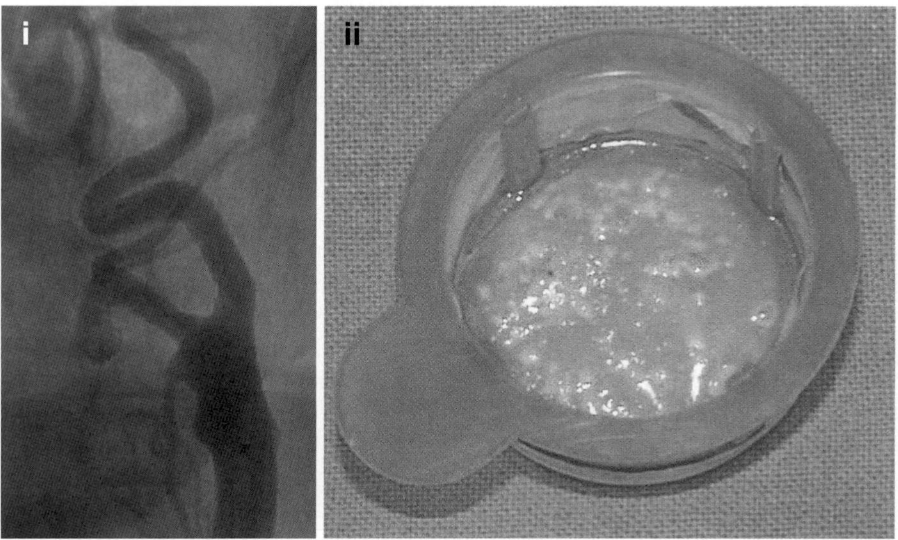

Fig. 13.2. Final result and plaque debris collected by aspiration of 60 cm^3 of blood (*arrow*)

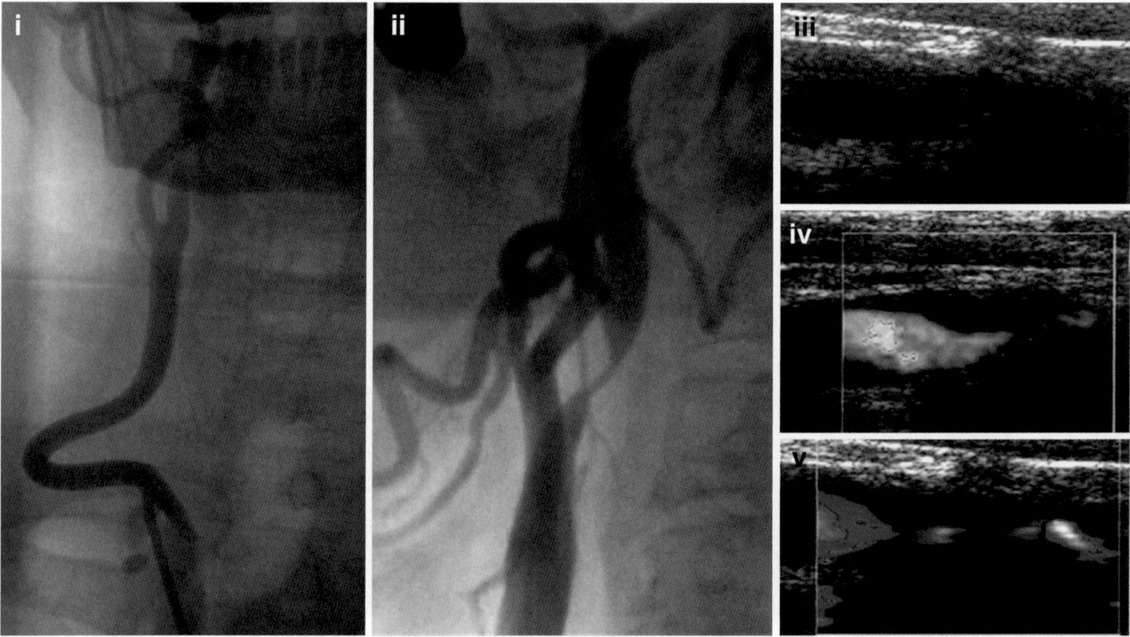

Fig. 13.3. Angiographic and echo-Doppler evaluation

Technical issues:

- Difficult angulated common carotid anatomy which may preclude the use of proximal protection devices
- High-grade, symmetric soft plaque at the origin of RICA

Solution:

- Buddy wire technique to straighten the angled anatomy of common carotid artery
- Guiding catheter with a long, soft, and steerable tip
- Distal filter with high capturing capabilities

Strategy endpoints:

- Secure engagement of guiding catheter in right CCA (buddy wire technique)
- Prevention of significant distal embolization
- Prevention of plaque prolapse (late events)

Type of stent	Nitinol, closed cell 20 mm, cylindrical (XAct, Abbott)
Type of embolic protection	Distal filter (Emboshield, Abbott)

Procedure

Over a standard soft 0.035-in. hydrophilic wire (Glidewire, Terumo), the 8F multipurpose 40° guiding catheter (Boston Scientific) is advanced up to the proximal bend of right common carotid artery (Fig. 13.4a).

A second 0.014-in. hydrophilic wire (Choice PT, Boston Scientific) is then placed in the external carotid artery, in order to gently straighten the common carotid artery and to stabilize the guiding catheter (buddy wire technique). The 0.035-in. wire is retrieved and the distal protection device (Emboshield 6 mm) is advanced across the internal carotid lesion and deployed at the prepetrous part of right ICA (Fig. 13.4b).

Lesion predilatation is achieved by inflation of a 2.5/20-mm coronary balloon. Under angiographic control, a short cylindrical nitinol closed cell stent (XAct 8/20 mm) is deployed at the lesion site (Fig. 13.5a) and postdilated with a 5.5/20 balloon (Maveric) (Fig. 13.5b). After stent postdilatation, the distal filter is retrieved and completion angiograms in two orthogonal

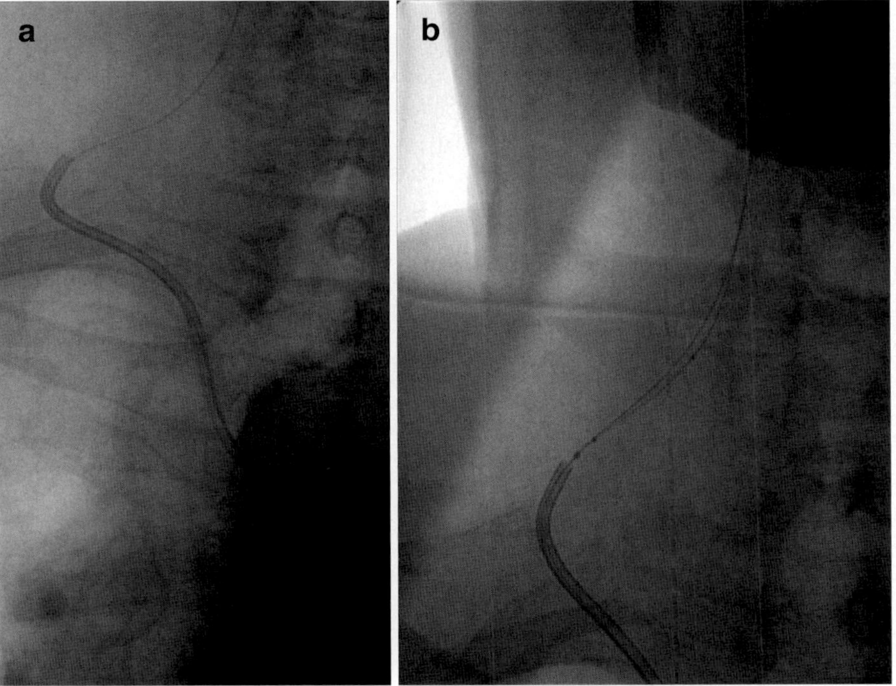

Fig. 13.4. (**a**) Guiding catheter placement. (**b**) "Buddy wire" technique: two wires for straightening the common carotid artery kink

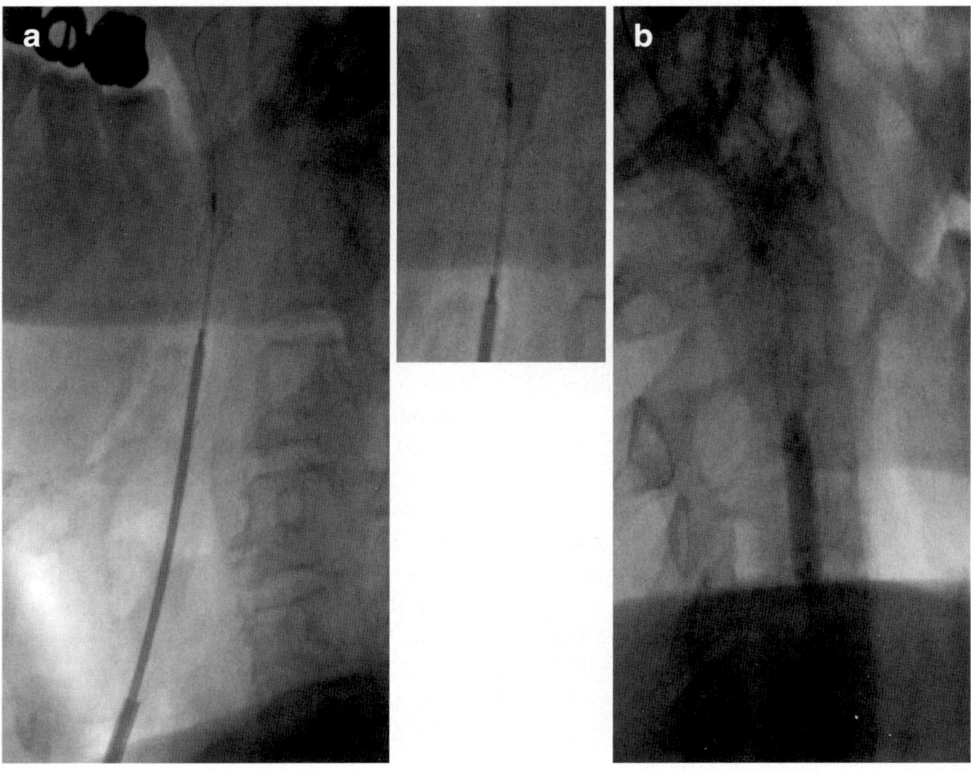

FIG. 13.5. (**a**) XAct closed cell stent. (**b**) Stent postdilatation

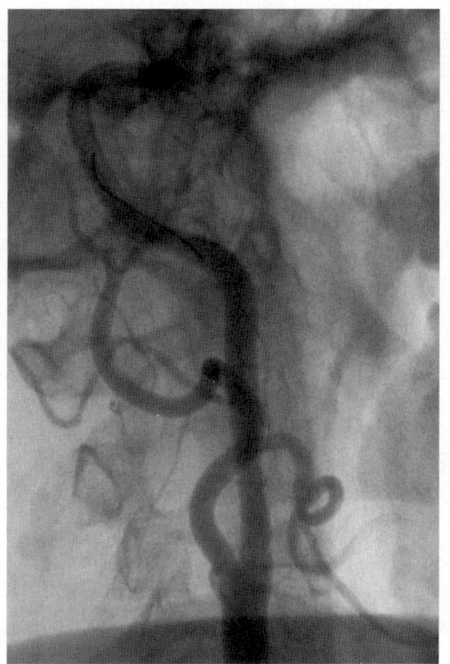

FIG. 13.6. Final angiographic result

projections are taken, demonstrating a good final result (Fig. 13.6).

Case 3

Right carotid high-grade soft ulcerated lesion, type I/II aortic arch, left common and ICA occluded (Fig. 13.7)

Technical issues:

- High-grade ulcerated soft plaque at the origin of RICA, at high risk for intraprocedural cerebral embolization
- Diffuse long thrombosis of left common and ICA, a situation which may preclude the use of a

Type of stent	Braided mesh, closed cell 30 mm (Carotid Wallstent, Boston Scientific)
Type of embolic protection	Proximal endovascular clamping (Mo.Ma, Invatec)
	Distal filter (EPI filter EZ, Boston Scientific)

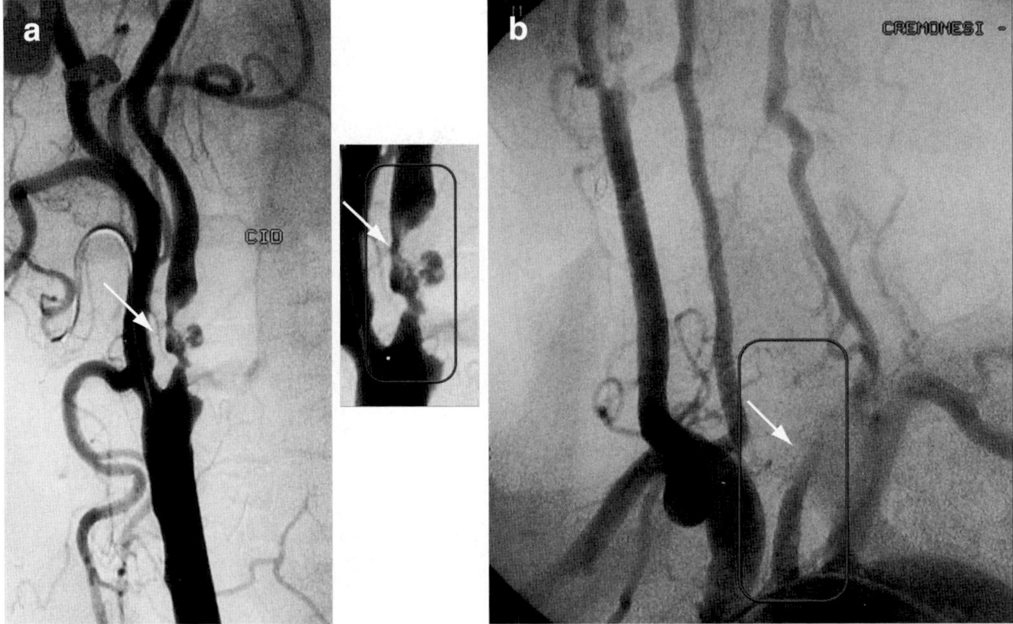

FIG 13.7. (**a**) Right carotid high-grade soft ulcerated lesion (*arrow*). (**b**) Left common and internal carotid artery occluded (*arrow*)

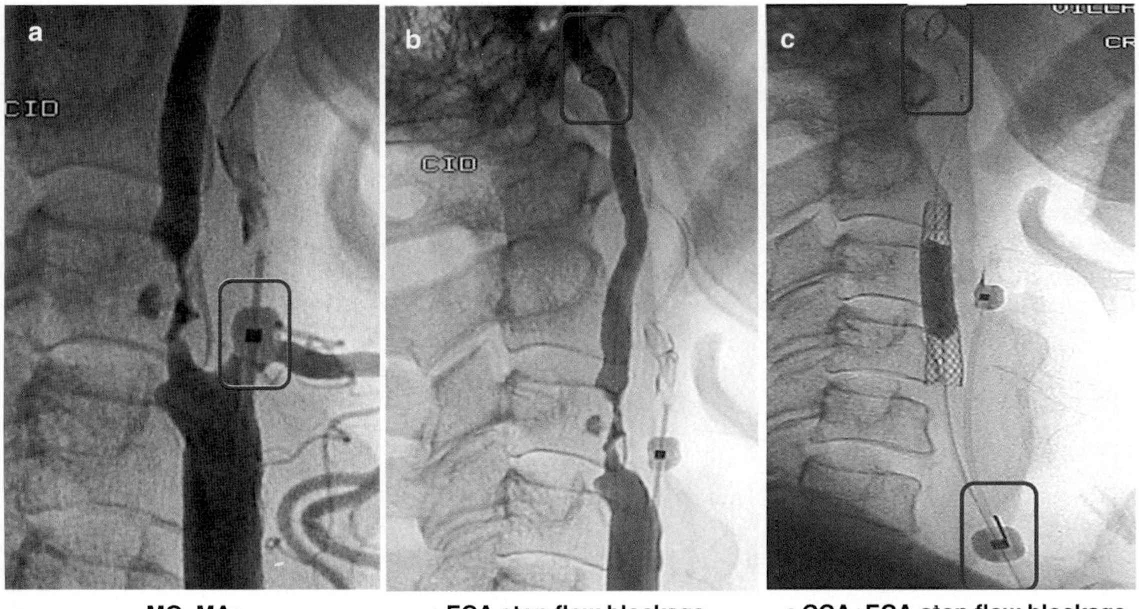

FIG. 13.8. (**a**) ECA flow blockage (*arrow*). (**b**) EPI filter EZ in distal ICA (*arrow*). (**c**) Carotid Wallstent 9/30 post-dilatation (*arrow*) under proximal and distal protection

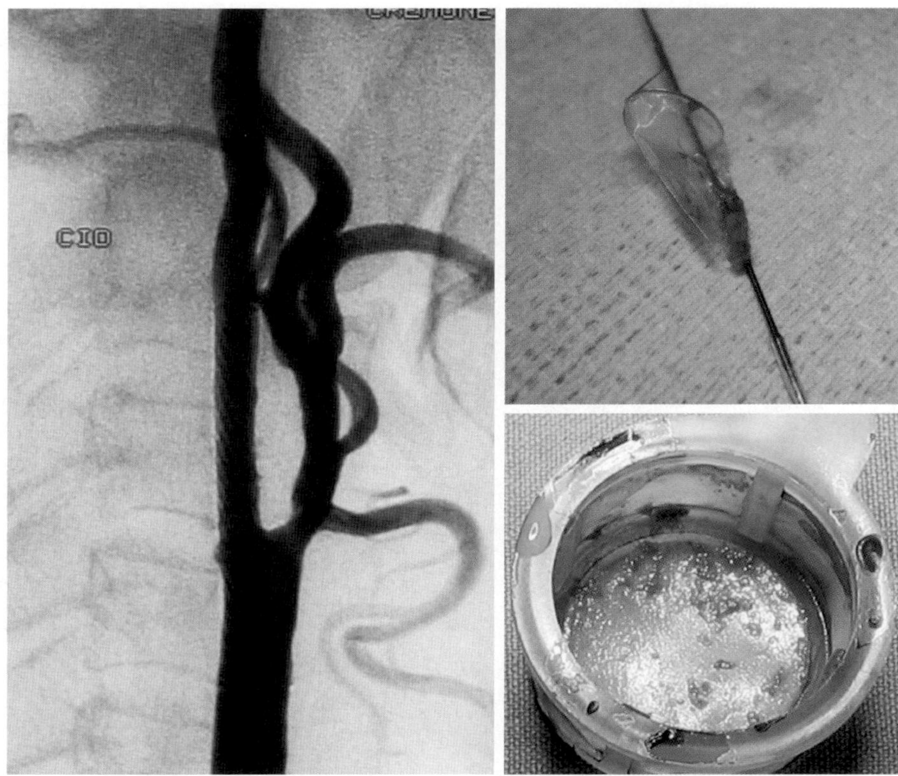

Total occlusion time 72 seconds

FIG. 13.9. Final angiographic result and visible debris collected in both proximal protection system and distal filter

proximal protection system (because of intraprocedural neurological intolerance)

Solution:

- Double cerebral protection (proximal protection and distal filtration)
- Closed cell design carotid stent with high scaffolding and wall coverage performances

Strategy endpoints:

- Prevention and management of significant distal embolization
- Prevention of plaque prolapse (late events)

Procedure

Over a long, stiff 0.035-in. wire (Supracore, Guidant), the proximal stop flow blockage system (Mo.Ma) is advanced until the distal tip is properly placed in the origin of the external carotid artery. The distal occlusive balloon in the ECA is then inflated (Fig. 13.8a).

The 0.035-in. stiff wire is retrieved and the distal protection device (EPI filter EZ) is advanced across the internal carotid lesion and deployed at the prepetrous part of right ICA (Fig. 13.8b).

Lesion predilatation is done under distal filtration, by using a 2.5/20-mm coronary balloon. Under angiographic control, a 9/30-mm Carotid Wallstent is deployed at the lesion site. Complete flow arrest (Fig. 13.8c) is achieved by inflating the proximal elastomeric balloon in the common carotid artery. Under flow arrest, the closed cell stent is postdilated with a 5.5/20 balloon (Maveric) (arrow) (Fig. 13.8c).

After stent postdilatation, 60 cm^3 of blood is aspirated. The proximal elastomeric balloon in common carotid artery is deflated and the antegrade cerebral flow restored. The distal filter is finally retrieved and completion angiograms are taken, demonstrating a good final result (Fig. 13.9).

References

1. Roubin SG, New G, Iyer SS, et al. Immediate and late clinical outcomes of carotid artery stenting in patients with symptomatic and asymptomatic carotid artery stenosis. A 5-year prospective analysis. *Circulation* 2001;103:532–7.
2. Endovascular versus surgical treatment in patients with carotid stenosis in the carotid and vertebral artery transluminal angioplasty study (CAVATAS): a randomised trial. *Lancet* 2001;357:1729–37.
3. Reimers B, Schlüter M, Castriota F, et al.. Routine use of cerebral protection during carotid artery stenting: results of a multicenter registry of 753 patients. *Am J Med* 2004;116:217–22.
4. Imparato AM, Riles TS, Gorstein F. The carotid bifurcation plaque: pathologic findings associated with cerebral ischemia. *Stroke* 1979;10:238–45.
5. Ohki T, Roubin GS, Veith FJ, et al. Efficacy of a filter device in the prevention of embolic events during carotid angioplasty and stenting: an ex vivo analysis. *J Vasc Surg* 1999;30:1034–44.
6. Angelini A, Reimers B, Dalla Barbera M, et al. Cerebral protection during carotid artery stenting: collection and histopathologic analysis of embolized debris. *Stroke* 2002;33:456–61.
7. Crawley F, Clifton A, Buckenham T, et al. Comparison of hemodynamic cerebral ischemia and microembolic signals detected during carotid endarterectomy and carotid angioplasty. *Stroke* 1997;28:2460–4.
8. Al-Mubarak N, Roubin GS, Vitek JJ, Iyer S, New G, Leon MB. Effect of the distal-balloon protection system on microembolization during carotid stenting. *Circulation* 2001;104:1999–2002.
9. Kastrup A, Groschel K, Krapf H, et al. Early outcome of carotid angioplasty and stenting with and without cerebral protection devices: a systematic review of the literature. *Stroke* 2003;34:1936–41.
10. Brooks WH, McClure RR, Jones MR, et al. Carotid angioplasty and stenting versus carotid endarterectomy: randomized trial in a community hospital. *J Am Coll Cardiol* 2001;38:1589–95.
11. Sprouse LR, II, Peeters P, Bosiers M. The capture of visible debris by distal cerebral protection filters during carotid artery stenting: is it predictable? *J Vasc Surg* 2005;41:950–5.
12. Cremonesi A, Setacci C, Manetti R, De Donato G, Setacci F, Balestra G, Borghesi I, Bianchi P, Castriota F. Carotid angioplasty and stenting: lesion related treatment strategies. *Eurointervention* 2005;1:289–95.
13. Zahn R, Mark B, Niedermier N, Zeymer U, Limbourg P, Ischinger T, Haerten K, Hauptmann KE, Leitner ER, Kasper W, Tebbe U, Senges J. Embolic protection devices for carotid artery stenting: better results than stenting without protection? *Eur Heart J* 2004;25:1550–8.
14. Castriota F, Cremonesi A, Manetti R, Liso A, Oshoala K, Ricci E, Balestra G. Impact of cerebral protection devices on early outcome of carotid stenting. *J Endovasc Ther* 2002;9:786–92.
15. Mas JL, Chatellier G, Beyssen B; EVA-3S Investigators. Carotid angioplasty and stenting with and without cerebral protection: clinical alert from the Endarterectomy versus Angioplasty in Patients with Symptomatic Severe Carotid Stenosis (EVA-3S) trial. *Stroke* 2004;35:e18–e20.
16. Wholey MH, Al-Mubarek N, Wholey MH. Updated review of the global carotid artery stent registry. *Catheter Cardiovasc Interv* 2003;60:259–66.
17. Hart JP, Peeters P, Verbist J, Deloose K, Bosiers M. Do device characteristics impact outcome in carotid artery stenting? *J Vasc Surg* 2006;44(4):725–30.
18. Mames RN, Snady-McCoy L, Guy J. Central retinal and posterior ciliary artery occlusion after particle embolization of the external carotid artery system. *Ophthalmology* 1991;98:527–31.
19. Whitlow PL, Lylyk P, Pondero H, Mendiz OA, Mahias K, Jaeger H, Parodi J, Schönholz C, Milei J. Carotid artery stenting protected with an emboli containment system. *Stroke* 2002;33:1308–14.
20. Müller-Hülsbeck S, Stolzmann P, Liess C, Hedderich J, Paulsen F, Jahnke T, Heller M. Vessel wall damage caused by cerebral protection devices: ex vivo evaluation in porcine carotid arteries. *Radiology* 2005;235:454–60.
21. Vos JA, van den Berg JC, Ernst SM, Suttorp MJ, Overtoom TT, Mauser HW, Vogels OJ, van Hessewijk HP, Moll FL, van der Graaf Y, Mali WP, Ackerstaff RG. Carotid angioplasty and stent placement: comparison of transcranial Doppler US data and clinical outcome with and without filtering cerebral protection devices in 509 patients. *Radiology* 2005;234:493–9.
22. Parodi JC, Schönholz C, Ferreira M, Mendaro E, D'Agostino H. Parodi antiembolism system in carotid stenting: the first 100 patients. Presented at Society of Interventional Radiology 27th Annual Scientific Meeting, Baltimore, MD, 2002, April 6–11.
23. Adami CA, Scuro A, Spinamano L, Galvagni E, Antoniucci D, Farello G, Maglione F, Manfrini S, Mangialardi N, Mansueto G, Mascoli F, Nardelli E, Tealdi D. Use of the Parodi anti-embolism system in carotid stenting: Italian trial results. *J Endovasc Ther* 2002;9:147–54.
24. Bates MC, Molano J, Pauley ME. Internal carotid artery flow arrest/reversal cerebral protection techniques. *W V Med J* 2004;100:60–3.

25. Parodi JC, Ferriera LM, Lamura R, Sicard G. Results of the first 200 cases of carotid stents using the ArteriA device. Presented at the International Congress of Endovascular Interventions XVII, Scottsdale, AZ, 2005, February 13–17.
26. Diederich KW, Scheinert D, Shmidt A, Scheinert S, Reimers B, Sievert H, Rabe K, Coppi G, Moratto R, Hoffmann FJ, Schuler GC, Biamino G. First clinical experiences with an endovascular clamping system for neuroprotection during carotid stenting. *Eur J Vasc Endovasc Surg* 2004;28:629–33.
27. Coppi G, Moratto R, Silingardi R, Rubino P, Sarropago G, Salemme L, Cremonesi A, Castriota F, Manetti R, Sacca S, Reimers B. Proximal flow blockage cerebral protection during carotid stenting (PRIAMUS). *J Cardiovasc Surg* 2005;46:219–27.
28. Schmidt A, Diederich KW, Scheinert S, Bräunlich S, Olenburger T, Biamino G, Schuler G, Scheinert D. Effect of two different neuroprotection systems on microembolization during carotid artery stenting. *J Am Coll Cardiol* 2004;44:1966–9.
29. Markus HS. Monitoring embolism in real time. *Circulation* 2000;102:826–8.
30. Rabe K, Sugita J, Gödel H, Sievert H. Flow-reversal device for cerebral protection during carotid artery stenting – acute and long-term results. *J Interv Cardiol* 2006;19:55–62.
31. Cremonesi A, Manetti R, Setacci F, Setacci C, Castriota F. Protected carotid stenting: clinical advantages and complications of embolic protection devices in 442 consecutive patients. *Stroke* 2003;34(8):1936–41.
32. Parodi J, Schönholz C, Ferreira L, Mendaro E, Ohki T. "Seat belt and air bag" technique for cerebral protection during carotid stenting. *J Endovasc Ther* 2002;9:20–4.
33. Krapf H, Nagele T, Kastrup A, Buhring U, Gronewaller E, Skalej M, Kuker W. Risk factors for periprocedural complications in carotid artery stenting without filter protection. A serial diffusion-weighted imaging. *AJNE Am J Neuroradiol* 2005;26:376–84.
34. Aronow HD, Shishehbor M, Davis DA, Katzan IL, Bhatt DL, Bajzer CT, Abou-Chebl A, Derk KW, Whithlow PL, Yadav JS. Leukocyte count predicts microembolis Doppler signals during carotid stenting: a link between inflammation and embolization. *Stroke* 2005;36:1910–4.
35. Verhoeven BA, de Vries JP, Pasterkamp G, Ackerstaff RG, Schoneveld AH, Velema E, de Kleijn DP, Moll FL. Carotid atherosclerotic plaque characteristics are associated with mcroembolization during carotid endarterectomy and procedural outcome. *Stroke* 2005;36:1735–40.
36. Biasi GM, Froio A, Diethrich EB, Deleo G, Galimberti S, Mingazzini P, Nicolaides AN, Griffin M, Raithel D, Reid DB, Valsecchi MG. Carotid plaque echolucency increases the risk of stroke in carotid stenting. The ICAROS study. *Circulation* 2004;110:756–62.
37. Reimers B, Corvaja N, Moshiri S, et al. Cerebral protection with filter devices during carotid artery stenting. *Circulation* 2001;104:12–5.
38. Baril DT, Wholey MH. Endovascular salvage of a displaced carotid filter. *Endovascular Today. Challenging Cases and Great Saves*. January 2008.
39. Chane M, Ballard A, Vanpatten A, et al. Management of detached accunet embolic protection filter during percutaneous carotid artery intervention. *Vasc Dis Manag* 2006;3:218–22.
40. Campbell JE, Bates MC, Elmore M. Endovascular rescue of a fused monorail balloon and cerebral protection device. *J Endovasc Ther* 2007;14:600–4.
41. Reimers B, Sievert H, Schuler GC, et al. Proximal endovascular flow blockage for cerebral protection during carotid artery stenting: results from a prospective multicenter registry. *J Endovasc Ther* 2005;12(2):156–65.
42. Schlüter M, Tübler T, Mathey DG, Schofer J. Feasibility and efficacy of balloon-based neuroprotection during carotid artery stenting in a single-center setting. *J Am Coll Cardiol* 2002;40:890–5.

14 Relevance of Periprocedural Hemodynamics

Sumaira Macdonald

Mechanisms of brain injury during carotid artery stenting (CAS) include embolic and hemodynamic events, acute carotid occlusions occurring through a variety of means, and the relatively rare contrast-induced encephalopathy. Impaired clearance of emboli due to relative hypoperfusion may exacerbate their clinical relevance and thus embolic and hemodynamic causes of stroke may be closely linked.

Hemodynamic injury may result from hemodynamic depression and hypoperfusion (which may result in watershed infarction) (Fig. 14.1) or the hyperperfusion syndrome, which may, if severe, result in hemorrhagic stroke. While most interventionists are very cognisant of embolic causes of stroke, hemodynamic instability is often under-recognized as an important cause of periprocedural neurological and sometimes cardiac complications. There is much that can be done to avoid and manage such complications.

Hemodynamic Depression

Hemodynamic instability during CAS is commonplace and is baroreceptor-mediated. During the recruitment phase of the CAVATAS trial, the hemodynamic responses to carotid angioplasty (stents were placed in only 26% of cases) and endarterectomy (CEA) were compared [1]. Hypotension was defined as a fall in systolic blood pressure (BP) >3 mmHg, compared with preintervention values. In the first 24 h after the procedure, episodes of hypotension occurred in 75% of the CEA group and 76% of the endovascular group. There was a significant fall in BP in both groups at 1 h, but this was only sustained in the endovascular group. Systolic BP was significantly lower at 1 and 6 months in the surgical group.

Carotid stents have the potential for a more profound impact on the carotid baroreceptors than does angioplasty alone. More prolonged hypotension and bradycardia occur with balloon-expandable stents with high radial force but these have largely fallen from favor in the carotid territory because of their propensity to deform. Nitinol (nickel–titanium alloy) self-expanding stents exert continued expansion forces for some 24 h postimplantation and there is anecdotal evidence that suggests that hypotensive effects may be more marked after placement of stents with higher radial force. Performing CAS under general anesthetic does not reduce the incidence of hemodynamic instability [2].

The literature indicates that without anticholinergic prophylaxis, the incidence of intraprocedural bradycardia ranges from 28 to 71% and intraprocedural hypotension from 17 to 22%. Some caution must be exercised in the interpretation of these figures as there is substantial heterogeneity in populations treated and variable definitions of bradycardia and hypotension.

Procedural vital signs were recorded in 741 patients undergoing CAS with atropine prophylaxis [3]. Severe hypotension was defined as a systolic BP of <8 mmHg and bradycardia as a heart rate of <50 beats per minute. Thirty-four patients (7%) had

S. Macdonald and G. Stansby (eds.), *Practical Carotid Artery Stenting*,
DOI: 10.1007/978-1-84800-299-9_14, © Springer-Verlag London Limited 2009

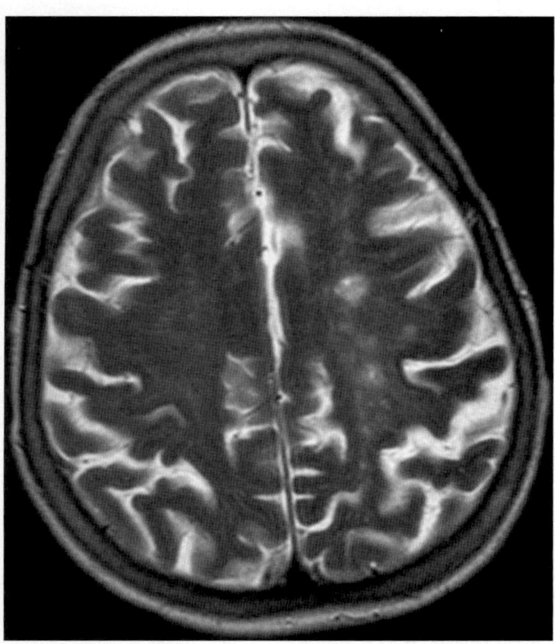

Fig. 14.1. Here there is a left-sided "internal" watershed infarction, between medullary arteries arising from the superficial pial plexus and deep penetrating arteries arising from the basal cerebral arteries. The tissue at risk is the white matter tracts of the corona radiata and centrum semiovale (as demonstrated)

severe hypotension ($n = 23$), bradycardia ($n = 2$), or both ($n = 9$) despite atropine and adequate preprocedure fluid balance. Intravenous catecholamines (dopamine) were necessary in eight patients with prolonged hypotension. Age >77 years (OR, 6.40; 95% CI, 1.80–22.78; $p = 0.004$) and coronary artery disease (OR, 2.81; 95% CI, 1.29–6.14; $p = 0.010$) were associated with an increased adjusted risk of hypotension or bradycardia.

Older patients may have impaired cerebral autoregulatory responses to hypotension and bradycardia. Similarly, those with compromised cardiac reserve, possibly due to chronic structural and functional myocardial impairment may be more vulnerable to procedural hemodynamic instability.

A retrospective analysis of 500 consecutive CAS procedures sought to evaluate the rate, predictors, and consequences of hemodynamic depression after CAS [4].

In this review, hemodynamic depression was defined as periprocedural hypotension (systolic BP <90 mmHg) or bradycardia (heart rate <60 beats per minute). Hemodynamic depression occurred in 210 procedures (42%) and was persistent in a further 84 procedures (17%). Features that independently predicted hemodynamic instability included lesions involving the carotid bulb (OR, 2.18; $P < 0.0001$) or the presence of a calcified plaque (OR, 1.89; $P < 0.002$). Prior ipsilateral CEA was associated with reduced risk of hemodynamic instability (OR, 0.35; $P < 0.0001$), presumably because of prior surgical denervation of the carotid baroreceptors. Patients with persistent hemodynamic instability were at significantly increased risk of stroke (OR, 3.34; $p < 0.03$). Previous work from the same unit on a dataset of 404 CAS procedures indicated that those with hemodynamic instability had, in addition, increased risk of myocardial infarction (OR, 4.5; 95% CI, 1.2–16.9) and death (OR, 3.6; 95% CI, 1.0–7.6) [5].

That patients with post-CEA restenosis are less hemodynamically labile was also demonstrated in a study on 86 patients [6]. In this study, patients given prophylactic atropine had a reduced incidence of intraoperative bradycardia, as expected (9% vs. 50%, $p < 0.001$), but also a lower perioperative cardiac morbidity (0% vs. 15%, $p < 0.05$).

There is a linear correlation between the intraprocedural magnitude of drop in systolic BP and the severity of any ensuing neurological event [7]. In a cohort of 60 patients, the mean systolic BP change during or after stenting in 55 cases without neurological events was 34 ± 14 mmHg, while patients with transient or permanent neurological events had significantly greater changes in systolic BP (107 ± 3 mmHg, $p < 0.003$; and 134 ± 1 mmHg, $p < 0.001$, respectively). Patients with neurological sequelae had significantly higher systolic BP before the procedure than those without complications (203 ± 30 vs. 165 ± 2 mmHg; $p < 0.001$). There were no neurological events in patients with a <50-mmHg change in systolic BP. The authors concluded that patients with severely elevated baseline systolic BP, i.e., >180 mmHg, were at higher risk of hemodynamic instability and neurological events during CAS.

Impaired Clearance of Emboli: The Link Between Hypoperfusion, Emboli, and Ischemic Stroke

Hypoperfusion and embolism often coexist and the clinical sequelae of each are interactive [8]. Hypoperfusion limits clearance of emboli and reduces available blood flow to regions rendered ischemic by embolic events. The border zones are a favored destination for emboli that are not "washed out."

Patients with critical carotid stenosis have several factors, including age, hypertension, and/or diabetes, that could jeopardize the microcirculation and increase the vulnerability of the brain to ischemic injury from microemboli. These patients also are likely to have had previous microembolic episodes that would reduce the available microcirculation collaterals and further increase the potential risk. If a shower of microemboli are liberated during CAS that are of a size that would pass through available cerebral protection devices of the filter-type, i.e., <80 µm, neurological injury is not necessarily guaranteed if the patient has good cerebral reserve and collateral circulation. In an elderly patient or one with reduced reserve/collaterals this otherwise innocuous shower may assume more clinical relevance. If the patient suffers intraprocedural hypotension and a microembolic shower, the potential for clinical sequelae due to reduced "wash-out" of these microemboli increases.

Pharmacotherapy and Avoidance of Hemodynamic Depression

Atropine, from deadly nightshade, is a competitive inhibitor of muscarinic acetylcholine receptors. Its parasympathetic antagonistic effects prevent baroreceptor-induced bradycardia during CAS. Atropine sulphate is usually administered at doses of 600 µg – 1.2 mg intravenously or into the arterial sheath. If administered into the arterial sheath there will be unilateral dilatation of the pupil, a feature that should be explained to the nurses and junior doctors looking after the patient on the ward following CAS as it may otherwise be a cause for concern. Glycopyrronium bromide (glycopyrrolate), given in 200-µg aliquots, is a synthetic derivative of atropine and has less cardioaccelerator effects than the latter. It also has less central nervous system effects than atropine in the elderly, which may include amnesia, confusion, and excitation. It is therefore preferred in older patients and in those with significant coronary artery disease.

I know of at least two patients (who were awaiting urgent coronary artery bypass grafting) who suffered ventricular fibrillation during CAS after the administration of atropine. Since glycopyrrolate became the standard of care at my institute, there have been no more cases of life-threatening cardiac arrhythmia.

Of course, neither atropine nor glycopyrrolate will prevent procedural hypotension. Relative postprocedural hypotension (e.g., 90–10 mmHg systolic) due to endovascular carotid sinus manipulation is commonplace but clinically irrelevant in the majority. Patients with significant coronary artery disease and reduced myocardial reserve, however, may not tolerate hypotension of this degree. While there may be concerns about acute carotid thrombosis following CEA, this is not a major concern following CAS, perhaps because of the stringent antiplatelet and anticoagulation regimens, but in a symptomatic patient, intravenous fluids may be indicated. Vasopressors or inotropes may be required to maintain systolic BP above 80 mmHg. The beta-adrenergic agonist isoprenaline was evaluated in a retrospective study [9]. Patients undergoing CAS with isoprenaline prophylaxis were compared with historical controls treated with atropine prophylaxis. Compared with atropine, isoprenaline was associated with a reduction in the occurrence of bradycardia, asystole, and hypotension. Isoprenaline, working on both the heart rate and contractility by stimulating cardiac beta-1 receptors, is given intravenously usually as an infusion of 2–4 µg min^{-1} because of its short duration of action.

In an analysis of patients requiring vasopressor support either in the short-term (<24 h) or for a more prolonged period (>24 h), it was concluded that older females were most likely to need prolonged support while patients of either sex with a history of prior myocardial infarction were more likely to require short-term support. A recent study evaluated the use of vasopressors in the critical care unit (CCU) for treatment of persistent post-CAS hypotension in 623 patients [10]. The authors concluded that compared with the use of the mixed alpha-/beta-agonist dopamine, the more selective alpha-agonists norepenephrine and phenylephrine were associated with a shorter infusion time and consequently reduced CCU length of stay and fewer major adverse events.

Regardless of whether expectant or "active" management of hypotension has been instituted, patients should be monitored for 24 h and care taken in case vasovagal syncope occurs. Baroreceptors may "reset" earlier if the patient is mobilized sooner [11], and routine use of a puncture-site closure device during CAS supports this initiative, but caution should be exercised and graded, supervised mobilization is appropriate. While the timing of complications suggests that day-case CAS may be feasible [12, 13], patients with postprocedural BP derangements clearly need careful monitoring. In addition to procedural management of the BP, it may also be necessary to reduce or discontinue the patient's antihypertensives temporarily on discharge until the BP returns to preinterventional levels.

Hyperperfusion Syndrome and Intracranial Hemorrhage: Definitions and Pathophysiology

Cerebral hyperperfusion syndrome is defined as a cerebral blood flow that exceeds the metabolic requirements of brain tissue and/or an increase in cerebral perfusion of more than 100% compared to preinterventional values. The concept of "normal perfusion pressure break-through" was described by Spetzler in 1978 in the setting of the resection of a cerebral arteriovenous malformation. Spetzler theorized that intracranial hemorrhage (ICH) occurred because of loss of autoregulation in the surrounding normal brain parenchyma. In 1981 Sundt related the phenomenon to CEA, describing a triad of complications to include ipsilateral throbbing headache (often frontal and including ipsilateral face and eye pain), transient focal seizures, and ICH [14]. The pathophysiology of hyperperfusion syndrome is complex. It is thought to be due to prevailing hypoperfusion, resulting from a significant carotid stenosis in conjunction with impaired reserve due to poor collaterals, culminating in compensatory dilatation of the distal cerebral vasculature as part of the cerebral autoregulatory mechanism. Upon restoration of flow following CEA or CAS, there is a momentary loss of autoregulation, leading to hyperperfusion in previously underperfused areas. The capillaries of the previously protected capillary bed are then more prone to rupture, culminating in hemorrhagic infarct.

The literature provides support for the concept of exhausted cerebral reserve capacity [15, 16]. It is worth noting that a carotid stenosis does not reach hemodynamic significance until it is ≥75% [17].

Hyperperfusion During and After CAS: Clinical Outcomes

Large clinical series on CEA have shown that the overall incidence of ICH complicating the procedure is of the order of 0.2–0.7% [18–21]. A total of 54 cases of CAS-associated ICH have been reported. A pooled analysis of these cases indicates that the incidence of ICH in the setting of CAS is 0.63% (95% CI, 0.38–0.97%) in studies consisting of >100 cases, which is significantly lower ($p < 0.0001$) than that of case series consisting of <100 cases (2.69%; 95% CI, 1.75–3.94%) [22]. Symptomatic lesions, severe stenosis (≥90%), maximal stenosis in the internal carotid artery distal to the bifurcation, and preexisting cerebral infarction were predisposing factors. The incidence of ICH is 2.01% (9/448; 95% CI, 0.98–3.65%) in patients treated with glycoprotein IIb/IIIa inhibitors [22]. The interval between carotid angioplasty or CAS and ICH ranges from immediately after the procedure to 6 days. In 33 of 47 reported cases (70%) the interval was ≤24 h; in 13 cases, the interval was ≤1 h. In two cases described in the literature, a sustained hypotension prior to hemorrhage was reported, contrary to expectation, and in 9–21 patients (43%) there were no prodromal symptoms.

Some workers postulate a spectrum of hyperperfusion entities following CAS that is not easily defined by the original description of the hyperperfusion syndrome [23, 24]. The literature on

CAS-associated ICH reveals many instances of acute or hyperacute ICH, i.e., within hours of CAS wherein hemorrhage occurred in the basal ganglia. In these cases there was no preexisting evidence of focal basal ganglia ischemia and classical prodromal symptoms were absent [14, 24]. Preexisting hypertension, evidence of microangiopathy, treatment of a high-grade stenosis, and localization of hemorrhage to the basal ganglia seemed to be recurring themes. The authors postulated that there were two types of pathophysiology. The first, described as "classical," resulted from primary cerebral edema giving rise to the classical triad of symptoms (accepting that ICH is not an inevitable consequence of this entity), and the second entity, a hyperacute and often fatal primary ICH resulting in basal ganglia hemorrhage from weak anterior perforating arteries. It was hypothesized that the former is more commonly encountered in the context of CEA, and the latter, perhaps potentiated by the powerful mandatory antiplatelet regime, is more commonly seen during CAS. Clearly, there is an overlap between these two entities and both have common predisposing factors.

In contradistinction to CEA, ICH in the setting of CAS seems to occur at shorter intervals and often presents as subarachnoid hemorrhage. This form of extraaxial bleeding has not been described following CEA (Fig. 14.2).

Evaluation of Cerebral Reserve in Patients at Risk of Hyperperfusion

Exhausted reserve capacity may be evaluated pre-CAS in patients thought to be at risk of hyperperfusion by acetazolamide magnetic resonance perfusion studies [25, 26]. Cerebrovascular reserve may be objectively quantified so that appropriate steps (e.g., lowering periprocedural BP perhaps to subnormal levels) can be taken.

Hyperperfusion Injury: Pharmacotherapy and Strategies for Avoidance and Control

There is no available level-1 evidence to support practice. Intracranial hemorrhage during carotid interventions is associated with a poor prognosis. Following CEA, ICH carries a 37–80% mortality and a 20–37% risk of poor recovery in survivors [19, 27]. Following CAS there may be a 75% mortality, which usually occurs within days of the procedure.

Prevention is therefore critical, and vigilance is of vital importance. In the periprocedural period, aggressive monitoring and control of systemic BP may mean the difference between a favorable and a

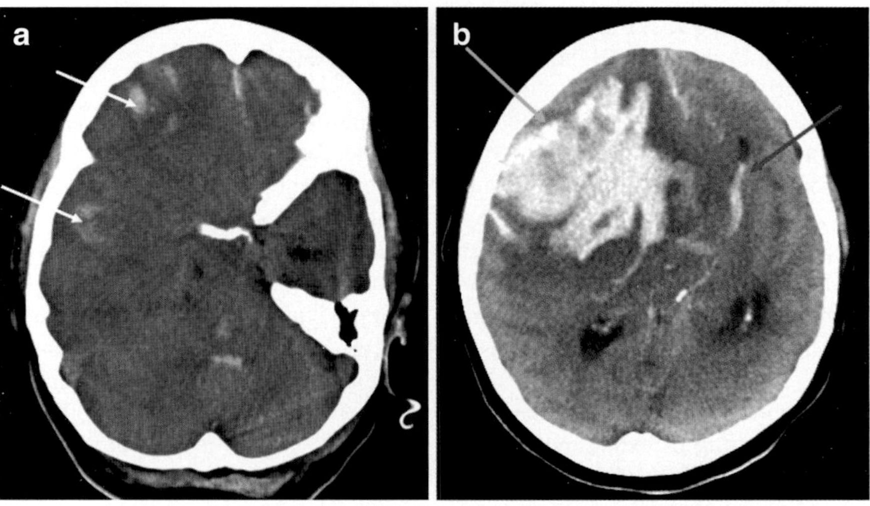

Fig. 14.2. (**a**,**b**) Extensive subarachnoid (*white arrows*), parenchymal (*green arrow*), and intraventricular hemorrhage (*pink arrows*) 24 h after uncomplicated carotid stenting. There were no prodromal symptoms, and no prior risk factors were evident. This patient died

disastrous outcome. Junior medical staff and ward nurses may be unfamiliar with caring for patients after CAS, although they are usually familiar with the care of patients undergoing CEA. An educational program for nurses and junior doctors can reap many rewards. In patients with postprocedural sustained hypertension (i.e., >20% above systolic baseline for >1 h), the aim should be to lower the BP to 10–20% below baseline, i.e., below preinterventional values, although it has also been suggested that BP in at-risk groups with BPs in the normal range should be lowered to subnormal values. Beta-blockers such as labetolol or the ultrashort acting esmolol have several advantages over other antihypertensive agents, although they may induce relative bradyarrythmias. Hydralazine may further increase cerebral blood flow, leading to a counterproductive effect and nitrates may cause headache [28].

A recent report evaluated the efficacy of a comprehensive BP management protocol in reducing ICH following CAS [29]. A total of 836 patients were included in this study; 266 prior to institution of a BP protocol and 570 patients treated subsequently. The BP of all patients in the latter group was lowered to 140/90 mmHg; those with a treated stenosis ≥90%, contralateral ICA stenosis ≥80%, and baseline hypertension was more strictly controlled (aiming for a BP of <120/80 mmHg). Patients who developed the hyperperfusion syndrome received parenteral beta-blockers or nitrates. The incidence of hyperperfusion syndrome/ICH was 5/266 (1.9%) prior to the institution of the strict BP control program and 3/570 (0.5%) thereafter. The incidence of ICH was 3/266 (1.1%) and 0/570 respectively (p = 0.0032). In high-risk patients both hyperperfusion syndrome and ICH were significantly reduced from 29.4 to 4.2% (p = 0.0006) and 17.6%–0% (p = 0.006) respectively. There were no complications attributable to the hypotensive regimen, and the length of stay was not significantly increased after institution of the hypotensive regimen (2.6 vs. 2.1 days, p = 0.18).

Relative intracerebral vasoconstriction may protect the brain in the setting of exhausted cerebral reserve and this may be achieved by hyperbaric ventilation. This of course mandates sedation, intubation, and artificial ventilation. The 5-HT receptor agonist sumatriptan has had beneficial effects in experimentally induced cerebral hyperperfusion, without effect on blood flow at normal flow volumes but this strategy has not yet been formally assessed in the setting of either CEA or CAS.

Additional efforts to reduce the risk of ICH in patients at risk may include limiting the duration of balloon inflation during pre- and postdilatation stages, which may help to minimize procedural brain ischemia and thus reduce the likelihood of hyperperfusion syndrome and ICH. Some workers would advocate withholding antiplatelet agents in symptomatic patients with a documented increase in mean MCA velocities until their symptoms have resolved and their BP is controlled. Clearly, this represents a balance of risk and benefit with, on the one hand, the specter of ICH and on the other, potential stent thrombosis and the potential for platelet-rich showers of emboli [30]. Others advocate deliberate underdilatation or no postdilatation after stent placement in at-risk patients, although the theoretical trade-off in these circumstances would again be the risk of acute stent thrombosis due to suboptimal stent through-flow.

Monitoring of BP should continue after discharge for at least 2 weeks following CAS, either by self-monitoring in a motivated patient or through the patient's family practitioner. Patients should be advised to return immediately to the treating center should severe headache develop within the first few weeks of intervention.

Key Points

- Generally, there is a lack of appreciation of nonembolic causes of neurological injury and there is much that can be done to control these factors.
- Hemodynamic instability is an important but underrecognized cause of procedural stroke.
- Hemodynamic instability, commonplace during CAS, is not abolished by atropine but is reduced by its routine prophylactic administration.
- Baseline systolic BP >180 mmHg is an independent risk factor for hemodynamic compromise – and may result in postprocedural hypotension and hypertension.
- Regarding procedural hypotension, the degree of drop in BP correlates linearly with the severity of subsequent neurological insult.

- Postprocedural relative hypotension is common but usually benign and treatment is reserved for symptomatic patients.
- Earlier mobilization, facilitated by routine use of puncture-site closure devices, may promote timely "resetting" of the baroreceptors, but graded supervised mobilization is advised.
- Pharmacotherapy for hemodynamic depression occurring during the procedure centers on antimuscarinic and/or selective alpha agonist prophylaxis.
- Careful postprocedural monitoring is vital, and the patient's usual antihypertensive regimen may need to be temporarily or permanently rationalized.
- Pharmacotherapy for hyperperfusion, preferably by short-acting beta-blockers, is centered on groups considered to be at high risk and, as ICH is often devastating, on aggressive BP control in these patients.
- Institution of an aggressive BP control program will reduce the incidence of hyperperfusion syndrome and ICH.
- BP monitoring should continue after discharge for at least 2 weeks following CAS, and patients should be advised to return immediately to the treating center should severe headache develop within the first few weeks of intervention.

References

1. McKevitt FM, Sivaguru A, Venables GS, Cleveland TJ, Gaines PA, Beard JD, Channer KS. Effect of treatment of carotid artery stenosis on blood pressure: a comparison of hemodynamic disturbances after carotid endarterectomy and endovascular treatment. Stroke 2003;34:2576–2581.
2. Dangas G, Laird JR, Jr, Satler LF et al. Postprocedural hypotension after carotid artery stent placement: predictors and short- and long-term clinical outcomes. Radiology 2000;215:677–683.
3. Mlekusch W, Schillinger M, Sabeit S, Nachtmann T, Lang W, Ahmadi R, Minar E. Hypotension and bradycardia after elective carotid stenting: frequency and risk factors. J Endovasc Ther 2003;10: 851–859.
4. Gupta R, Abou-Chebl A, Bajzer CT, Schumacher HC, Yadav JS. Rate, predictors and consequences of hemodynamic depression after carotid artery stenting. J Am Coll Cardiol. 2006;47:1538–1543.
5. Abou-Chebl A, Gupta R, Bajzer H, Scumacher C, Yadav J. Consequences of hemodynamic instability after carotid artery stenting. J Am Coll Cardiol 2004;43 (Suppl 1):A20–A21.
6. Cayne NS, Fairies PL, Trocciola SM, Slatzberg SS, Dyal RD, Clair D, Rockman CB et al. Carotid angioplasty and stent-induced bradycardia and hypotension: impact of prophylactic atropine administration and prior carotid endarterectomy. J Vasc Surg 2005;41:956–961.
7. Howell M, Krajcer Z, Dougherty K, Strickman N, Skolkin M, Toombs B, Paniaqua D. Correlation of periprocedural systolic blood pressure changes with neurological events in high-risk carotid stent patients. J Endovasc Ther 2002;9:810–816.
8. Caplan LR, Hennerici M. Impaired clearnace of emboli (washout) is an important link between hypoperfusion, embolism and ischemic stroke. Arch Neurol 1998;55:1475–1482.
9. van Sambeek M, Hendriks JM, van Dijk LC, Koudstaal P, van Urk H. Hemodynamic changes during CAS cause half of the complications: how can they be prevented? Presented at the 32nd Annual Vascular and Endovascular Issues, Techniques and Horizons; Veith Symposium, New York, November 2005.
10. Nandalur MR, Cooper H, Satler LF. Vasopressor use in the critical care unit for treatment of persistent post-carotid artery stent induced hypotension. Neurocrit Care 2007;7:232–237.
11. Al-Mubarak N, Roubin GS, Vitek JJ, New G, Iyer SS. Procedural safety and short-term outcome of ambulatory carotid stenting. Stroke 2001;32:2305–2309.
12. Tan KT, Cleveland TJ, Berczi V, McKevitt FM, Venables GS, Gaines PA. Timing and frequency of complications after carotid artery stenting: what is the optimal period of observation? J Vasc Surg 2003;38:236–243.
13. Spetzler RF, Wilson CB, Weinstein P, Mehdom M, Townsend J, Telles D. Normal perfusion pressure breakthrough theory. Clin Neurosurg 1978;25: 651–672.
14. Sundt TM, Sharbrough FW, Piepgras DG. Correlation of cerebral blood flow and electroencephalographic changes during carotid endarterectomy with results of surgery and hemodynamics of cerebral ischemia. Mayo Clin Proc 1981;56:533–543.
15. Waltz AG. 1968;Effect of blood pressure on blood flow in ischaemic and nonischaemic cerebral cortex. Neurology18:613–621.
16. Bernstein M, Fleming JFR, Deck JH. Cerebral hyperperfusion after carotid endarterectomy: a cause of cerebral haemorrhage. Neurosurgery 1984;15: 50–56.
17. Archie JP, Jr, Feldtman RW. Critical stenosis of the internal carotid artery. Surgery 1981;89:67–72.

18. Solomon RA, Loftus CM, Quest DO, Correl JW. Incidence and etiology of intracerebral hemorrhage following carotid endarterectomy. J Neurosurg 1986;64:29–34.
19. Piepgras DG, Morgan MK, Sundt TM, Jr, Yanagihara T, Mussman LM. 1988Intracerebral hemorrhage after carotid endarterectomy. J Neurosurg ;68: 532–536.
20. Pomposelli FB, Lamparello PJ, Riles TS, Craighead CC, Giangola G, Imparato AM. Intracranial hemorrhage after carotid endarterectomy. J Vasc Surg 1988;7:248–255.
21. Wilson PV, Ammar AD. The incidence of ischemic stroke versus intracerebral hemorrhage after carotid endarterectomy: a review of 2452 cases. Ann Vasc Surg 2005;19:1–4.
22. Hyun-Seung K, Han MH, Kwon O-Ki, Kwon BJ et al. Intracranial hemorrhage after carotid angioplasty: a pooled analysis. J Endovasc Ther 2007;14:77–85.
23. Coutts S, Hill MD, Hu WY, Sutherland GR. Hyperperfusion syndrome: toward a stricter definition. Neurosurgery 2003;53:1053–1060.
24. Buhk JH, Cepek L, Knauth M. Hyperacute intracerebal hemorrhage complicating carotid stenting should be distinguished from hyperperfusion syndrome. AJNR 2006;27:1508–1513.
25. Griffiths PD, Gaines P, Cleveland T, Beard J, Venables G, Wilkinson ID. Assessment of cerebral haemodynamics and vascular reserve in patients with symptomatic carotid artery occlusion: an integrated MR method. Neuroradiology 2005;47:175–182.
26. Macdonald S. Strategies for avoidance of non-embolic stroke during carotid artery stenting. J Cardiovasc Surg (Torino) 2007;48:27–37.
27. Connolly ES. 200:Hyperperfusion syndrome following carotid endarterectomy. In: Loftus CM, Editor. Carotid Artery Surgery. New York, NY: Thieme Medical, 493–500.
28. Penn AA, Scomer DF, Steinberg GK. Imaging studies of cerebral hyperperfusion after carotid endarterectomy. Case report. J Neurosurg 1995;83:133–137.
29. Abou-Chebl A, Reginelli J, Bajzer CT, Yadav JS, . Intensive treatment of hypertension decreases the risk of hypersperfusion and intracerebral hemorrhage following carotid artery stenting catheter cardiovasc interv. 2007;69:690–696.
30. Abou-Chebl A, Yadav JS, Reginelli JP, Bajzer C, Bhatt D, Krieger DW. Intracranial hemorrhage and hyperperfusion syndrome following carotid artery stenting. J Am Coll Cardiol 2004;43: 1596–1601.

15 Dealing with Complications: Neurorescue

Claudio Schönholz, Renan Uflacker, and Juan C. Parodi

Recent reports in the literature show that carotid angioplasty and stenting is an acceptable alternative to carotid endarterectomy in the treatment of carotid artery stenosis in a specific population. The procedure, however, has some possible complications, and distal embolization can occur and may cause stroke or even death [1]. In the past decade, several different techniques and devices have been developed to prevent cerebral damage associated with accidental embolization. The principal types of cerebral protection devices (CPD) are proximal and distal occlusion balloons, distal filters, and reversal-of-flow mechanisms [2]. Transcranial Doppler studies carried out during carotid artery stenting (CAS) procedures have shown that high-intensity transient signals consistent with microembolization occur during simple manipulation of the guidewire across the lesion [3] and throughout the procedure unless flow reversal is applied.

The devices that provide proximal occlusion with or without reversal of flow activate cerebral protection before interaction with the lesion and collect all released particles [4, 5]. This represents an important advantage over distal protection devices, since *ex vitro* studies found that 15% of the particles released during CAS are related to crossing the lesion before protection can be initiated [6].

Despite the use of meticulous techniques and cerebral protection devices, the incidence of neurological complications due to thromboembolic events may be still 3–5% [1]. When a stroke occurs during CAS, an angiogram of the intracranial circulation in AP and lateral views should be obtained and compared with those obtained before treatment in order to assess angiographic evidence of an embolic event [7]. If the angiogram fails to show intracranial vessel occlusion, the patient will most likely develop a minor stroke or a TIA and can be treated with heparin and GP-IIb/IIIa inhibitors. The presence of intracranial vessel occlusion could be associated with progression to a major stroke if left untreated. Severity and characteristics of deficit will depend upon the localization of the occlusion. Therefore, in such cases, heparinization, intraarterial fibrinolytic agents, GP-IIb/IIIa inhibitors, and mechanical disruption and thrombectomy should be implemented in order to establish antegrade flow in the occluded vessels (Fig. 15.1).

GP-IIb/IIIa Inhibitors

Abciximab (ReoPro) is the Fab fragment of a chimeric (human/murine) monoclonal antibody that binds to the GP-IIb/IIIa receptor, the final pathway for platelet aggregation. Abciximab binds to the GP-IIb/IIIa receptor in its resting state and hinders its ability to bind fibrinogen [8]. Abrupt vessel closure after CAS is seen in some cases despite the concomitant use of heparin and aspirin, and platelet aggregation plays a pivotal role in thrombus formation and propagation [9]. Regardless of the stimulus, the final common pathway of platelet aggregation involves the surface GP-IIb/IIIa receptors [10]. Receptors on activated

S. Macdonald and G. Stansby (eds.), *Practical Carotid Artery Stenting*,
DOI: 10.1007/978-1-84800-299-9_15,

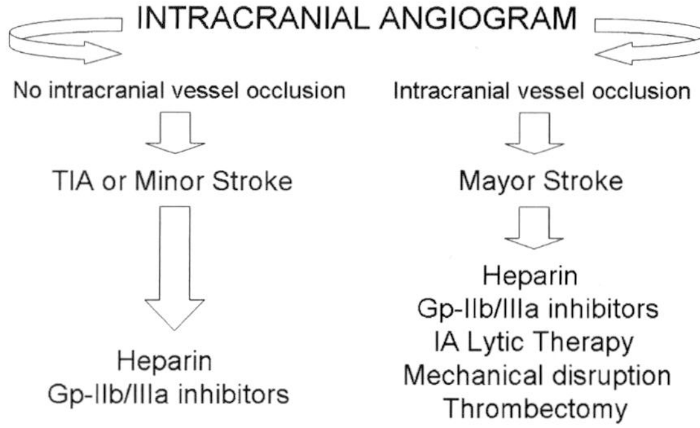

FIG. 15.1. Management of complications during carotid stenting

platelets couple with adjacent platelet GP-IIb/IIIa receptors by an interposed fibrinogen molecule. Unlike aspirin, which blocks only the arachidonic acid–thromboxane pathway of platelet activity, and ticlopidine and clopidogrel, which block the platelet ADP receptors, the GP-IIb/IIIa receptor antagonists markedly inhibit platelet aggregation regardless of the pathway or stimulus. The GP-IIb/IIIa receptors on platelets are believed to be the only platelet adhesion receptor for fibrinogen and therefore the use of selective and potent antagonists to GP-IIb/IIIa receptors will not only prevent platelet aggregation, but may lead to dissolution of formed fibrinogen bridging in platelet aggregation [11]. However, Abciximab is not currently FDA approved for use in acute cerebral ischemic stroke or for the use as a rescue agent in acute cerebral embolization during CAS. The only current indication for abciximab is for the prevention of ischemic complications in patients undergoing percutaneous coronary interventions.

Carotid artery branch occlusion should be expected to behave in a similar way as does coronary lesions, where the lessons learned in coronary interventional trials could be extrapolated [12]. Concerns of excessive intracranial hemorrhage risk in patients with stroke have limited the use of GP-IIb/IIIa inhibitors. However, there have been successful reports on the use of abciximab as a rescue agent in dissolving thrombus in intracranial vessels. Ho et al. [13] described three patients who experienced ischemic cerebrovascular events with symptoms involving the middle cerebral artery territory while undergoing percutaneous angioplasty and stenting to their internal carotid arteries. Abciximab was administered to each patient within 10 min of symptom onset as a bolus (0.25 mg kg^{-1}) into the ipsilateral common carotid artery, followed by continuous intravenous infusion (9 μg min^{-1}) for 12 h. All patients' symptoms resolved completely (by 25 min, 40 min, and 5 h, respectively), with no further neurological complications. Qureshi et al. [14] reported a case of complete occlusion of the right vertebral artery after angioplasty with complete recanalization after 24 h of abciximab infusion. Tong et al. [15] reported that an acute carotid stent thrombosis resolved completely after 20 min of administration of abciximab.

Nevertheless, different groups have evaluated the use of GP-IIb/IIIa inhibitors as prophylactic and adjunctive therapy for carotid angioplasty and stent placement [14, 16–20]. In all series the incidence of intracerebral bleeding was greater with the administration of GP-IIb/IIIa inhibitors. Therefore, GP-IIb/IIIa inhibitors should not be used routinely in carotid stenting.

Intraarterial Thrombolysis

Thrombolytic therapy plays an important role in the reopening of intracranial branches occluded by a clot embolus [21, 22]. A microcatheter should be navigated through the guide catheter into and across the thrombus. Urokinase or recombinant t-PA can be infused through the microcatheter in amounts of 200,000–1,300,000 IU or 5–40 mg, respectively. Slow infusion of the thrombolytic agent, at rates of 5,000–20,000 IU min^{-1} for urokinase and 0.5–2.0 mg min^{-1} for recombinant t-PA, is preferred. Usually, 500,000 IU of urokinase is administered initially [23] (Fig. 15.2). If no recanalization is achieved, mechanical disruption using a wire or catheter or balloon angioplasty can be done, followed by additional urokinase administration. Mechanical clot disruption or angioplasty can be effective if pharmacological recanalization alone is initially ineffective [24]. Sorimachi et al. described different techniques of mechanical embolus disruption in conjunction with intraarterial thrombolysis, showing a high incidence of recanalization and

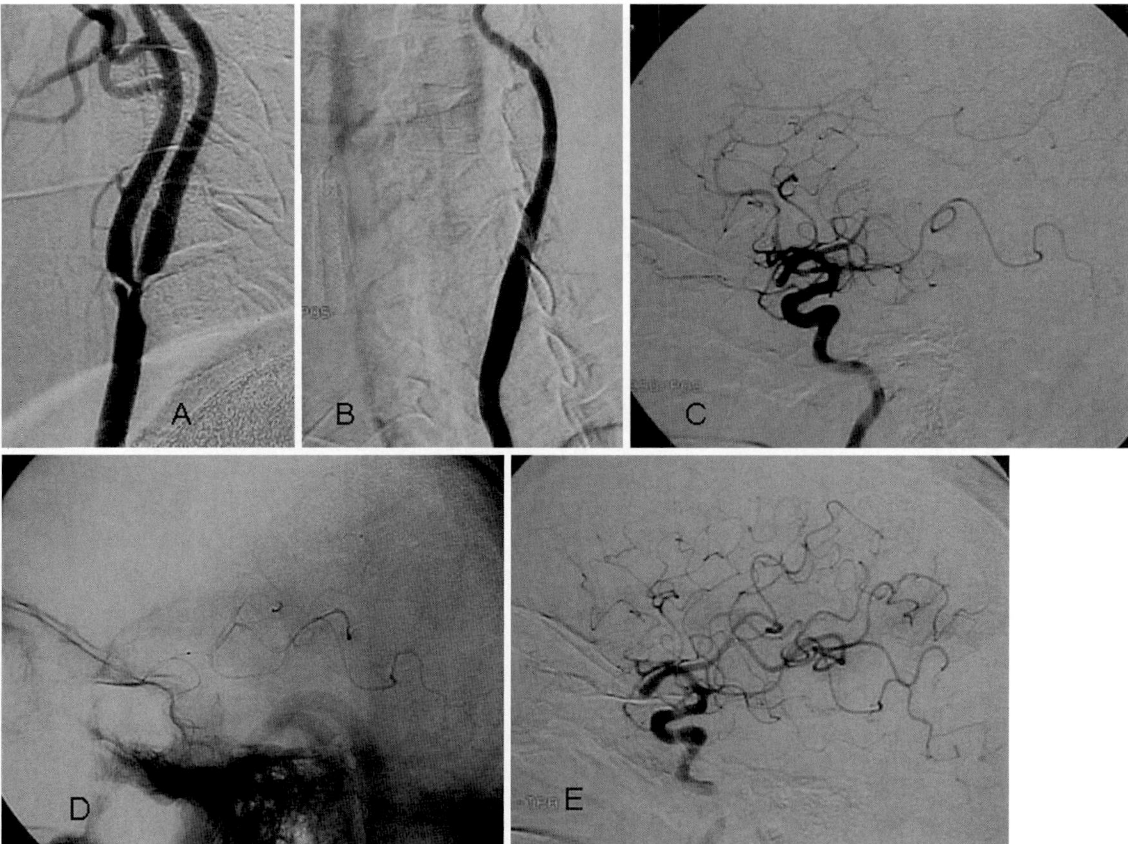

FIG. 15.2.

clinical improvement in patients with acute occlusion of the distal internal carotid artery and middle cerebral artery [25].

Prourokinase was evaluated in phase II and III trials and exhibited good success in recanalization for middle cerebral artery occlusion of less than 6 h [26, 27]. Intraarterially administered prourokinase, at doses of 6–9 mg, can be used instead of urokinase or recombinant t-PA. Heparinization during thrombolysis may enhance the thrombolytic efficacy of urokinase or recombinant t-PA [28]. The intravenous administration of a heparin bolus (70 units kg^{-1}) before thrombolysis, to maintain the ACT between 250 and 300 s, may be considered. Postthrombolytic use of heparin to prevent reocclusion is recommended for patients with partial recanalization, arterial dissection, or persistent distal emboli not amenable to selective thrombolysis. Intravenous heparin administration should be titrated to maintain a PTT of 1.5–2.3 times the control values. For quick action, arterial access should be maintained for 12–24 h for patients at high risk. In addition, patients should be closely monitored in a neuro intensive care unit environment.

There are multiples of reports in the literature showing successful recanalization using lytic therapy [27–30, 52–53]. Although these studies showed positive results when strict selective criteria were used, the risk of hemorrhagic transformation was increased, possibly because of the fibrinolytic agent action [31] (Fig. 15.3). Ischemic signs on the baseline CT prove to be a significant predictor of intracranial bleeding after thrombolysis [32]. Intracranial bleeding was observed in 7–38% [32, 33] of the patients with acute stroke who received intraarterial thrombolysis.

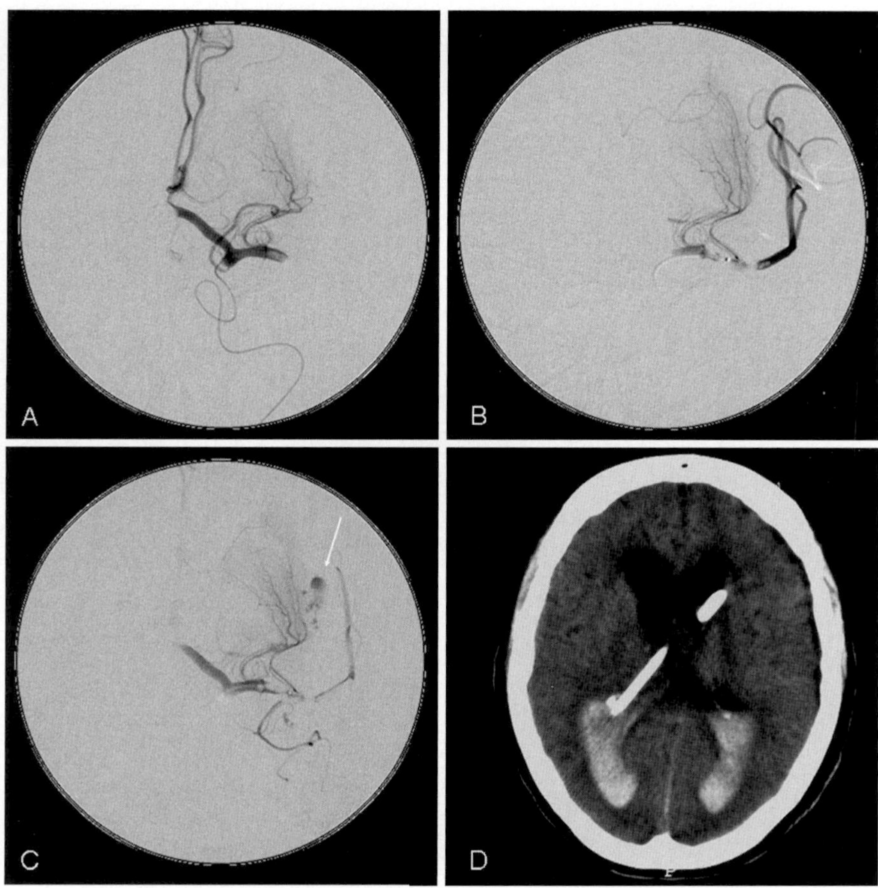

Fig. 15.3.

Mechanical Thrombectomy

Intracranial thrombectomy involves the extraction of the thrombus through a catheter and should provide rapid recanalization and reduce the risk of distal embolic complications seen with mechanical clot disruption. This method may be used as a stand-alone technique or in conjunction with a markedly reduced dose of a thrombolytic drug. The technical challenges of thrombectomy include intracranial navigation of these devices, capture of occlusive material within the tortuous and branched cerebral vasculature, and safety issues such as vessel wall damage or perforation [34].

In cases with "in stent thrombus formation" the vessel can be catheterized with a 7F guiding catheter (Brite-tip; Cordis, Miami, FL) that is navigated over a guidewire into the proximal third of the thrombus. A 60-mL syringe is used to aspirate the thrombus. Aspiration is done by moving the catheter in and out of the thrombus several times; it is continued for ~10 s each time. The guide catheter is slowly withdrawn to allow more complete removal of the thrombus. Aspiration is stopped when the catheter is pulled out of the occluded artery [35].

The Merci Retrieval System

The Merci Retrieval System (Concentric Medical Inc., Mountain View, CA) consists of the Merci Retriever, the Merci Balloon Guide Catheter (BGC), and the Merci microcatheter. The BGC is a 9F catheter with a large 2.1-mm lumen and a balloon located at its distal tip. The Merci Retriever is a tapered wire with five helical loops of decreasing

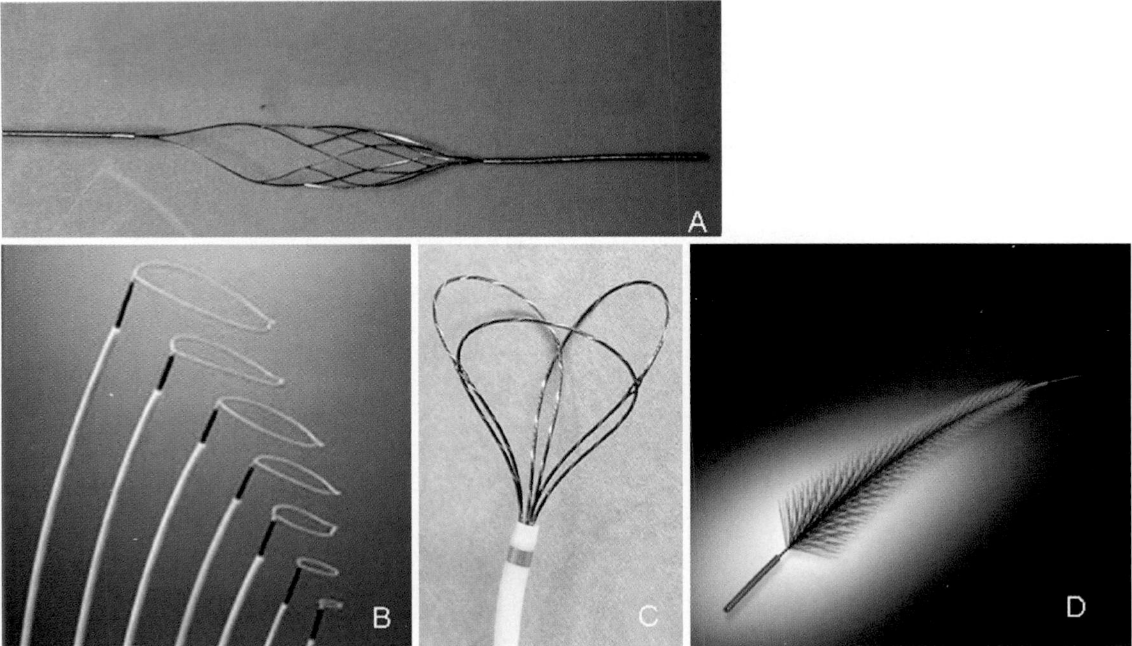

FIG. 15.4.

diameter (from 2.8 to 1.1 mm) at its distal end. The Merci Retriever is advanced through the microcatheter in its straight configuration and resumes its preformed helical shape once it is delivered into the occluded intracranial artery in order to ensnare the thrombus. The BGC is placed into the common or internal carotid artery for anterior circulation proximal occlusion, or the subclavian artery for posterior circulation occlusion. Using standard cerebral catheterization techniques, the microcatheter is guided into the occluded vessel and passed beyond the thrombus. A selective angiogram is taken distal to the thrombus to evaluate the size and tortuosity of the distal arteries, where the Merci Retriever is to be deployed. The Merci Retriever is then advanced through the microcatheter and 2–3 helical loops are deployed beyond the thrombus. It is then retracted to contact the thrombus, and the proximal loops are then deployed within the thrombus. The BGC balloon is inflated to control intracranial blood flow during removal of the thrombus and five clockwise rotations are applied to the Merci Retriever to further ensnare the thrombus. The Merci Retriever with the ensnared thrombus, and the microcatheter, are withdrawn together into the BGC lumen, during continuous aspiration to the BGC, to ensure complete evacuation of the thrombus. The balloon of the BGC is deflated to reestablish the flow. Upon confirmation

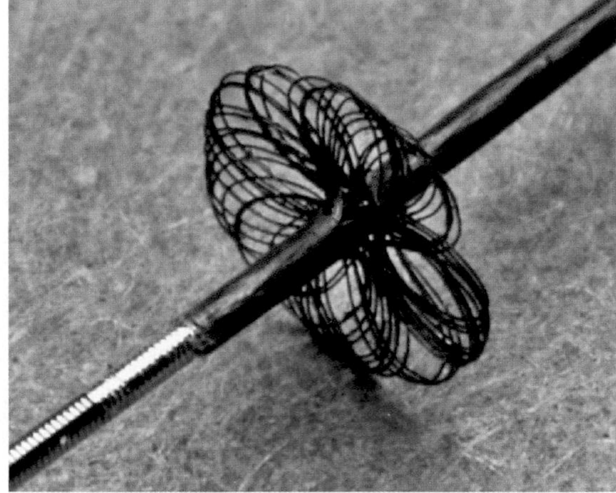

FIG. 15.5. The distal end of the GORE neuro thrombectomy device in its expanded state

of complete evacuation of the thrombus (brisk reflux of blood), another angiogram is taken (Fig. 15.6). If the occlusion persisted, then the procedure is repeated up to six passes [36].

The MERCI trial (Mechanical Embolus Removal in Cerebral Ischemia trial) was designed to evaluate the safety of the Concentric Retriever™ System in the treatment of neurovascular thromboembolic occlusions. Recanalization was achieved in 46% (69/151) of patients on intention to treat analysis, and in 48% (68/141) of patients in whom the device was deployed [37, 38].

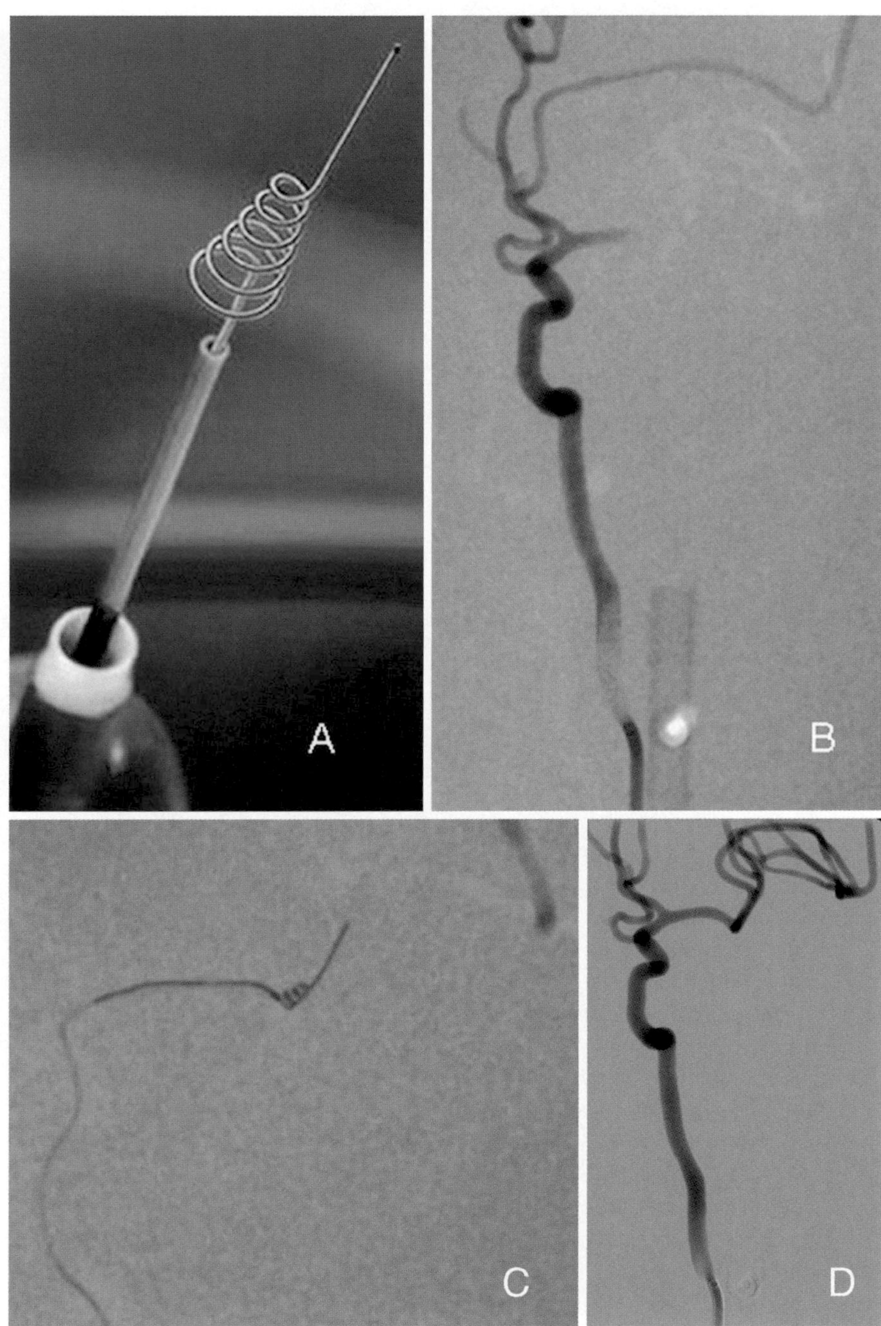

Fig. 15.6.

Guidant Neuronet

This microguidewire-based device consists of a laser-cut nitinol basket that can be pushed through a standard microcatheter. The self-expanding basket has more struts distally than proximally and is attached to the microwire excentrically to load the thrombus. The technique for deployment consists of passing the microcatheter ~2 cm beyond the occlusion and then advancing the device to the tip, followed by unsheathing the device by pulling back the microcatheter. The device is then withdrawn to capture the embolus but requires no resheathing [34, 39, 40].

Gooseneck Snare

The gooseneck snare uses a nickel–titanium (nitinol) wire oriented at a right angle to the catheter tip. The radiopaque loop of the microsnare is available in 2-, 4-, and 7-mm diameters of 175-cm cable length and can be placed through any standard 0.018-in. microcatheter. This device is approved for coil retrieval but has been used for treatment in patients with acute stroke [41]. The loop of the snare is pushed out of the microcatheter just enough for it to open fully and take its built-in shape perpendicular to the catheter and the vessel. The microcatheter is then pushed together with the snare into the embolus, and a minor buckling of the loop can often be seen. After this, the snare is pulled back slightly into the microcatheter so that only a small eye can be seen outside the catheter tip on fluoroscopy. Then, the microcatheter and snare are pulled out a few centimeters. A control angiogram is cautiously obtained to verify the status. If the embolus is caught in the snare, the whole assembly of the snare, the microcatheter, and the guide catheter is pulled out as a unit. This is done to minimize the risk of dislodging the embolus from the snare [31, 42, 43].

Gore Neuro Thrombectomy Device

For intracranial vessel occlusion different mechanical thrombectomy devices are currently in use and include the Merci Retrieval System, the Neuronet (Guidant Corporation, Indianapolis, IN),the Microsnare (Microvena, Minneapolis, MN), the In-Time Retriever (Target, Fremont, CA), the EnSnare (Medical Device Technologies, Gainesville, FL) and the Phenox Clot Retriever (Phenox GmbH, Germany) (Fig. 15.4). The GORE neuro thrombectomy device (W. L. Gore & Associates, Inc., Flagstaff, AZ) is intended to restore blood flow in the neurovasculature by removing thrombus in patients experiencing ischemic stroke. Patients who are ineligible for intravenous tissue plasminogen activator (IV t-PA) or who fail IV t-PA therapy are candidates for treatment. The GORE neuro thrombectomy device is introduced through a previously placed microcatheter beyond the thrombus and the distal end is expanded using a proximal handle. The expanded distal end is designed to engage and remove thrombus. At the time of this writing, initiation of a clinical trial to evaluate the safety and efficacy of this device is expected during the latter part of 2008 (Fig. 15.5).

Conclusions

Cerebral embolism is still an unresolved problem of the endovascular treatment of carotid occlusive disease. Several effective techniques are now available to protect the cerebral circulation from accidental embolism, but how to rescue the brain from an embolism is still a work in progress, because of the potential for complications, failure, and the need for multiple approaches [44–51]. It should be emphasized that physicians performing CAS must be familiar with intracranial vascular anatomy, microcatheter navigation techniques, and the use of thrombolytic agents, GP-IIb/IIIa inhibitors, and mechanical thrombectomy devices, in order to provide stroke rescue treatment when embolic complications occur during the stent procedure (Fig. 15.7).

Key Points

- In a patient suffering from a neurological event during CAS, if angiography fails to show intracranial vessel occlusion, the patient will most likely develop a minor stroke or a TIA and can be treated with heparin and GP-IIb/IIIa inhibitors.
- The presence of intracranial vessel occlusion may be associated with progression to a major stroke

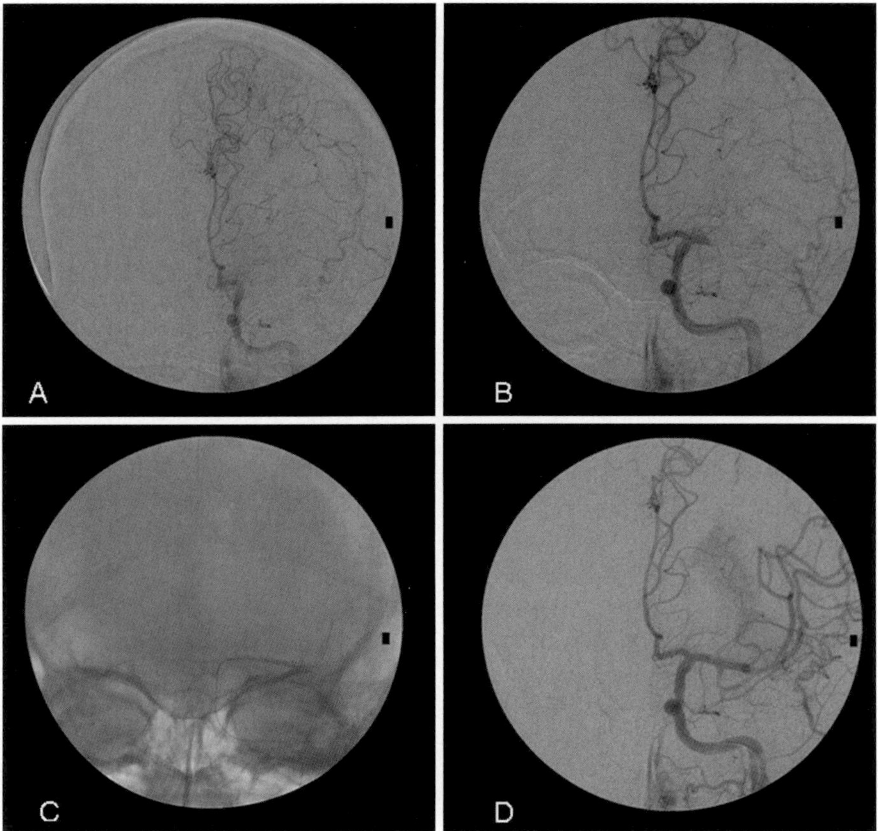

Fig. 15.7. Fifty six year old female with acute stroke treated with mechanical thrombectomy under reversal of flow. (A) Diagnostic angiogram showing complete occlusion of the left middle cerebral artery (MCA). (B) Follow up angiogram after starting flow reversal shows partial recanalization of the Left MCA (C) A 2 mm balloon was inflated at the MCA and active aspiration preformed through the guiding catheter to avoid distal embolization. (D) Final angiogram showing complete recanalization of the MCA with adequate flow to the MCA branches.

if left untreated, and aggressive recanalization strategies are therefore advocated.

- GP-IIb/IIIa inhibitors should not be used routinely in carotid stenting as the incidence of intracerebral bleeding was greater following the administration of GP-IIb/IIIa inhibitors in all series evaluating its use.
- Although the effectiveness of intraarterial thrombolytic therapy for acute intracranial vessels occlusion has been demonstrated by randomized controlled trials, the drawbacks of this therapy include an increased incidence of serious hemorrhagic complications and failure to achieve arterial recanalization in approximately one third of patients.
- In patients with embolic MCA occlusion, the embolus is often so large as to be resistant to thrombolysis, and time-consuming thrombolytic therapy with high doses of thrombolytic agents may be required, which may result in a high incidence of bleeding. Mechanical revascularization may be needed under these circumstances.
- Mechanical revascularization strategies, including direct balloon angioplasty, and the use of thrombectomy devices, may obtain rapid flow restoration without the risk of intracranial bleeding. The potential risks associated with mechanical revascularization include arterial rupture, spasm, and distal embolization.

- Intracranial flow reversal can be used during acute stroke as a means of eliminating distal embolization and to facilitate mechanical embolectomy or local drug delivery. Reversal of flow may prevent distal embolization and help retrieve particles from the cerebral vasculature.
- General anesthesia and local hypothermia are desirable to reduce oxygen demand during cerebral ischemia.

References

1. Schonholz CJ, Uflacker R, Mendaro E, Parodi JC, Guimaraes M, Hannegan C, Selby B. Techniques for carotid artery stenting under cerebral protection. J Cardiovasc Surg (Torino). 2005;46(3):201–217.
2. Parodi JC, La Mura R, Ferreira LM, Mendez M, Cersosimo H, Schonholz C, Garelli G. Initial evaluation of carotid angioplasty and stenting with three different cerebral protection devices. J Vasc Surg. 2000;32(6):1127–1136.
3. OrlandiG,FanucchiS,FiorettiC,AcerbiG,PuglioliM, Padolecchia Ret-al.,Characteristics of cerebral microembolism during carotid stenting and angioplasty alone. Arch Neurol. 2001;58:1410–1413.
4. Parodi JC, Schönholz C, Parodi FE, Sicard G, Ferreira M. Initial 200 cases of carotid artery stenting using a reversal-of-flow cerebral protection device. J Cardiovasc Surg (Torino). 2007;48(2):117–124.
5. Reimers B, Sievert H, Schuller GC, Tubler Tet-al., Proximal endovascular flow blockage for cerebral protection during carotid artery stenting: results from a prospective multicenter registry. J Endovasc Ther. 2005;12(2):156–165.
6. Ohki T, Roubin GS, Veith FJ, Iyer SS, Brady E. Efficacy of a filter device in the prevention of embolic events during carotid angioplasty and stenting: an ex vivo analysis. J Vasc Surg. 1999;30: 1034–1044.
7. Wholey MH, Wholey MH, Tan WA, Toursarkissian B, Bailey S, Eles G, Jarmolowski C. Management of neurological complications of carotid artery stenting. J Endovasc Ther. 2001;8(4):341–353.
8. Kittusamy PK, Koenigsberg RA, McCormick DJ. Abciximab for the treatment of acute distal embolization associated with internal carotid artery angioplasty. Catheter Cardiovasc Interv. 2001;54(2): 221–233.
9. Wallace RC, Furlan AJ, Moliterno DJ, Stevens GHJ, Masaryk TJ, Perl J. Basilar artery rethrombosis: successful treatment with platelet glycoprotein IIB/IIIA receptor inhibitor. Am J Neuroradiol. 1997;18:1257–1260.
10. Lefkovits J, Plow EF, Topol EJ. Platelet glycoprotein IIb/IIIa receptors in cardiovascular medicine. N Engl J Med. 1995;332:1553–1559.
11. Mascelli MA, Marciniak SJ, Weisman HF, Jordan R. In vitro characterization of dethrombosis by abciximab (Reopro). Thromb Haemost. 1997;77(suppl):PS2696.
12. Sila CA. Cerebrovascular aspects of glycoprotein IIb/IIIa inhibitors. In: Lincoff AM, Topol EJ, editors. Platelet glycoprotein IIb/IIIa inhibitors in cardiovascular disease. New Jersey: Humana; 1999. pp 315–326.
13. Ho DS, Wang Y, Chui M, Wang Y, Ho SL, Cheung RT. Intracarotid abciximab injection to abort impending ischemic stroke during carotid angioplasty. Cerebrovasc Dis. 2001;11(4):300–304.
14. Qureshi AI, Suri MFK, Khan J, Fessler RD, Guterman LR, Hopkins LN. Abciximab as an adjunct to high-risk carotid or vertebrobasilar angioplasty: preliminary experience. Neurosurgery. 2000;46:1316–1325.
15. Tong FC, Cloft HJ, Joseph GJ, Samules OB, Dion JE. Abciximab rescue in acute carotid stent thrombosis. Am J Neuroradiol. 2000;21:1750–1752.
16. Kapadia SR, Bajzer CT, Ziada KM, et al. Initial experience of platelet glycoprotein IIb/IIIa inhibition with abciximab during carotid stenting: a safe and effective adjunctive therapy. Stroke. 2001;32: 2328–2332.
17. Hofmann R, Kerschner K, Steinwender C, et al. Abciximab bolus injection does not reduce cerebral ischemic complications of elective carotid artery stenting: a randomized study. Stroke. 2002;33: 725–727.
18. Qureshi AI, Saad M, Zaidat OO, et al. Intracerebral hemorrhages associated with neurointerventional procedures using a combination of antithrombotic agents including abciximab. Stroke. 2002;33: 1916–1919.
19. Wholey MH, Wholey MH, Eles G, et al. Evaluation of glycoprotein IIb/IIIa inhibitors in carotid angioplasty and stenting. J Endovasc Ther. 2003;10: 33–41.
20. Fiorella D, Albuquerque FC, Han P, McDougall CG. Strategies for the management of intraprocedural thromboembolic complications with abciximab (ReoPro). Eurosurgery. 2004;54(5):1089–1097; discussion, 1097–1098.
21. Uflacker R. How to optimize carotid artery stenting. J Cardiovasc Surg (Torino). 2007;48(2):131–149.
22. Lutsep HL. Thrombolytic and newer mechanical device treatment for acute ischemic stroke. Expert Rev Neurother. 2006;6(7):1099–1105.
23. Qureshi AI, Luft AR, Sharma MBS, Guterman LR, Hopkins LN. Prevention and treatment of

thromboembolic and ischemic complications associated with endovascular procedures: Part II – clinical aspects and recommendations. Neurosurgery. 2000;46(6):1360–1375.

24. Barnwell SL, Clark WM, Nguyen TT, O'Neill OR, Wynn ML, Coull BM. Safety and efficacy of delayed intraarterial urokinase therapy with mechanical clot disruption for thromboembolic stroke. AJNR Am J Neuroradiol. 1994;15:1817–1822.
25. Sorimachi T, Fujii Y, Tsuchiya N, Nashimoto T, Harada A, Ito Y, Tanaka R. Recanalization by mechanical embolus disruption during intra-arterial thrombolysis in the carotid territory. AJNR Am J Neuroradiol. 2004;25(8):1391–1402.
26. del Zoppo GJ, Higashida RT, Furlan AJ, Pessin MS, Rowley HA,Gent M, et al. PROACT: a phase II randomized trial of recombinant pro-urokinase by direct arterial delivery in acute middle cerebral artery stroke. Stroke. 1998;29:4–11.
27. Furlan A, Higashida R, Wechsler L, Gent M, Rowley H, Kase C, Pessin M, Ahuja A, Gallahan F, Clark WM, Silver F, Rivera F, for the PROACT Investigators. Intra-arterial prourokinase for acute ischemic stroke. The PROACT II study: a randomized controlled trial. *JAMA*. 1999;282 :2003–2011.
28. Kesava P, Graves V, Salamat S, Rappe A. Intraarterial thrombolysis in a pig model: a preliminary note. AJNR Am J Neuroradiol. 1997;18:915–920.
29. Jungreis CA, Weschler LR, Horton JA. Intracranial thrombolysis via a catheter embedded in the clot. Stroke. 1989;20:1578–1580.
30. Green DW, Sanchez LA, Parodi JC, Geraghty PJ, Ferreira LM, Sicard GA. Acute thromboembolic events during carotid artery angioplasty and stenting: etiology and a technique of neurorescue. J Endovasc Ther. 2005;12(3):360–365.
31. Wikholm G. . Transarterial embolectomy in acute stroke. Am J Neuroradiol. 2003;24:892–894.
32. Tountopoulou A, Ahl B, Weissenborn K, Becker H, Goetz F. Intra-arterial thrombolysis using rt-PA in patients with acute stroke due to vessel occlusion of anterior and/or posterior cerebral circulation. Neuroradiology. 2008;50:75–83.
33. Arnold M, Schroth G, Nedeltchev K, Loher T, Remonda L, Stepper F, Sturzenegger M, Mattle HP. Intra-arterial thrombolysis in 100 patients with acute stroke due to middle cerebral artery occlusion. Stroke. 2002;33:1828–1833.
34. Nesbit G, Luh G, Tien R, Barnwell SL. New and future endovascular treatment strategies for acute ischemic stroke. J Vasc Interv Radiol. 2004;15 :S103–S110.
35. Lutsep HL, Clark WM, Nesbit GM, Kuether TA, Barnwell SL. Intraarterial suction thrombectomy in acute stroke. AJNR Am J Neuroradiol. 2002;23 :783–786.
36. Gobin YP, Starkman S, Duckwiler GR, Grobelny T, Kidwell CS, Jahan R, Pile-Spellman J, Segal A, Vinuela F, Saver JL. Merci 1: a phase 1 study of mechanical embolus removal in cerebral ischemia. Stroke. 2004;35:2848–2854.
37. Smith WS, Sung G, Starkman S, Saver JL, Kidwell CS, Gobin YP, Lutsep HL, Nesbit GM, Grobelny T, Rymer MM, Silverman IE, Higashida RT, Budzik RF, Marks MP. MERCI Trial Investigators. Safety and efficacy of mechanical embolectomy in acute ischemic stroke: results of the MERCI trial. Stroke. 2005;36(7):1432–148.
38. Marder V, Chute D, Starkman S, Abolian A, Kidwell C, Ovbiagele B, Vinuela F, Duckwiler G, Jahan R, Rajajee V, Selco S, Saver JL. Histology of thrombi retrieved from acute ischemic stroke patients by endovascular embolectomy. Stroke. 2005;36:516.
39. Versnick EJ, Do HM, Albers GW, Tong DC, Marks MP. Mechanical thrombectomy for acute stroke. AJNR Am J Neuroradiol. 2005;26(4):875–879.
40. Mayer TE, Hamann GF, Brueckmann HJ. Treatment of basilar artery embolism with a mechanical extraction device: necessity of flow reversal. Stroke. 2002;33(9):2232–2235.
41. Tytle TL, Prati RC,Jr , Steven T. McCormack the 'gooseneck' concept in microvascular retrieval. AJNR Am J Neuroradiol. 1995;16:1469–1471.
42. Chopko BW, Kerber C, Wong W, Georgy B. Transcatheter snare removal of acute middle cerebral artery thromboembolism: technical case report. Neurosurgery 2000;46:1529–1531.
43. Kerber CW, Barr JD, Berger RM, et al. Snare retrieval of intracranial thrombus in patients with acute stroke. J Vasc Interv Radiol. 2002;13: 1269–1274.
44. Ringer AJ, Qureshi AI, Fessler RD, Guterman LR, Hopkins LN. Angioplasty of intracranial occlusion resistant to thrombolysis in acute ischemic stroke. Neurosugery. 2001;48:1282–1288.
45. Nakano S, Yokogami K, Ohta H, Yano T, Ohnishi T. Direct percutaneous transluminal angioplasty for acute middle cerebral artery occlusion. Am J Neuroradiol. 1998;19:767–772.
46. Ueda T, Hatakeyama T, Kohno K, Kumon Y, Sakaki S. Endovascular treatment for acute thrombotic occlusion of the middle cerebral artery: local intraarterial thrombolysis combined with percutaneous transluminal angioplasty. Neuroradiology. 1997;39:99–104.
47. Tsai FY, Berberian B, Matovich V, Lavin M, Alfieri K. Percutaneous transluminal angioplasty adjunct to thrombolysis for acute middle cerebral artery rethrombosis. Am J Neuroradiol. 1994;15:1823–1829.

48. Purdy PD, Devous MD, Sr, Unwin DH, Giller CA, Batjer HH. Angioplasty of an atherosclerotic middle cerebral artery associated with improvement in regional cerebral blood flow. Am J Neuroradiol. 1990;11:878–880.
49. Higashida RT, Tsai FY, Halbach VV, Dowd CF, Smith T, Fraser K, Hieshima GB. Transluminal angioplasty for atherosclerotic disease of the vertebral and basilar arteries. J Neurosurg. 1993;78:192–198.
50. Parodi JC, Rubin BG, Azizzadeh A, Bartoli M, Sicard GA. Endovascular treatment of an internal carotid artery thrombus using reversal of flow: a case report. J Vasc Surg. 2005;41(1):146–150.
51. Van den Berg JC. Dealing with complications related to carotid artery stenting. J Cardiovasc Surg (Torino). 2007;48(2):151–159.
52. Endo S, Kuwayama N, Hirashima Y, Akai T, Nishijima M, Takaku A. Results of urgent thrombolysis in patients with major stroke and atherothrombotic occlusion of the cervical internal carotid artery. AJNR Am J Neuroradiol. 1998;19:1169–1175.
53. Nesbit GM, Clark WM, O'Neill OR, Barnwell SL. Intracranial intraarterial thrombolysis facilitated by microcatheter navigation through an occluded cervical internal carotid artery. J Neurosurg. 1996;84:387–392.

16 Surveillance: Diagnosis and Management of In-Stent Restenosis

Brajesh K. Lal, Babak Abai, and Robert W. Hobson II

Introduction

Carotid endarterectomy (CEA) is the preferred treatment for symptomatic [1–3] and asymptomatic [4, 5] patients with high-grade extracranial carotid stenosis, compared with the best medical therapy. The increase in the number of CEAs done worldwide has resulted in a number of post-CEA carotid restenosis (CR) cases. Carotid artery stenting (CAS) has recently emerged as a less-invasive alternative to CEA for cerebral revascularization. Our institution [6–10], along with others [11–14], has demonstrated that CAS is technically feasible and safe in high-risk patients. Two randomized trials [14, 15] and results from the lead-in phase of the Carotid Revascularization, Endarterectomy vs. Stent Trial (CREST) [16] reported low periprocedural complication rates with CAS, indicating clinical equipoise between the two procedures. This resulted in the approval of CAS in the United States in high-risk patients with significant carotid stenosis (≥70%) and neurological symptoms (ipsilateral stroke, transient ischemic attack, and amaurosis fugax) [17]. Two additional randomized trials were not able to demonstrate equivalence of CAS with CEA with respect to postprocedural stroke, myocardial infarction, or death. These results notwithstanding, it is clear that the number of CAS procedures will continue to progressively increase until a more definitive answer is available from larger studies powered to assess superiority of one procedure over the other (e.g., the NIH-sponsored CREST).

Current reports indicate that the incidence of post-CAS in-stent restenosis (ISR) ranges from 1–50% [6]. Therefore, it is anticipated that there will be a corresponding increase in the number of ISR cases. Considerable controversy still persists regarding the clinical significance, natural history, optimal diagnosis, threshold for management, and appropriate intervention for ISR. This review analyzes current information on this important clinical problem and presents evidence-based recommendations for the diagnosis and management of recurrent carotid stenosis.

Pathophysiology of In-Stent Restenosis

Two mechanisms can account for the restenosis that occurs after carotid stenting. Restenosis early (<24 months) after the procedure is generally attributed to intimal hyperplasia. This is a universal response seen in any vascular bed subjected to vessel wall injury. The exact mechanisms of this response are not well known and are the subject of ongoing research. Histologically, stenting is associated with the migration and proliferation of smooth muscle cells and fibroblasts and with the deposition of new extracellular matrix. The initial response to the stent is adherence of a fine film of protein on the metal surfaces and thrombus in the interstices [18]. This results in adherence of platelets and lymphocytes and their activation leads to the release of cellular mediators. These mediators stimulate proliferation

S. Macdonald and G. Stansby (eds.), *Practical Carotid Artery Stenting*,
DOI: 10.1007/978-1-84800-299-9_16, © Springer-Verlag London Limited 2009

of smooth muscle cells and collagen matrix and result in neointimal hyperplasia. The injury from stenting is prolonged and robust when compared to that from angioplasty alone, and leads to a more vigorous reaction [19, 20]. There is evidence that the reactive process after stent injury goes beyond the intima to the medial layer. Furthermore, it may cause progressive atrophy in the adventitial layers and form giant cell bodies [21].

Restenosis that occurs >24 months after carotid stenting is generally believed to be caused by progressive atherosclerosis [22, 23]. The same mechanical, chemical, and physiologic processes that led to the primary carotid stenosis are presumably present and ongoing in the patient. These processes, over time, can lead to recurrent atherosclerotic lesions in the carotid artery.

Rationale for Surveillance After Carotid Artery Stenting

Intimal hyperplastic recurrence has been observed after coronary stenting in 16–59% of cases and after iliac stenting in 13–39% of reported series [24]. A valid concern was that CAS could be associated with equivalent rates of recurrent stenosis within the stent (in-stent restenosis, ISR) during follow-up. DeGroote and associates [25] emphasized the importance of using life-table methods to determine the incidence of restenosis in the context of patients undergoing CEA. Calculation of an absolute restenosis rate (arteries with restenotic lesions/total carotid procedures) will generally underestimate the incidence of restenosis, because it is independent of the duration, frequency, and completeness of clinical follow-up. Using this principle, we have provided reliable estimates of ISR after CAS [10] (Fig. 16.1). Over a follow-up period of 1–74 months (mean, 18.8 ± 10), 22 of 122 patients demonstrated ISR ≥40%. Although restenotic lesions ranged from 40 to 99%, only five patients demonstrated high-grade ISR (≥80%). The 5-year rate for ISR ≥80% using life-table analysis was 6.4%. Cumulative 4-year rate of ISR ≥60% was 16.4%, and of ISR ≥40% was 42.7%. These observations were subsequently confirmed by other authors [26]. Although ISR does not appear to occur at the high rates associated with

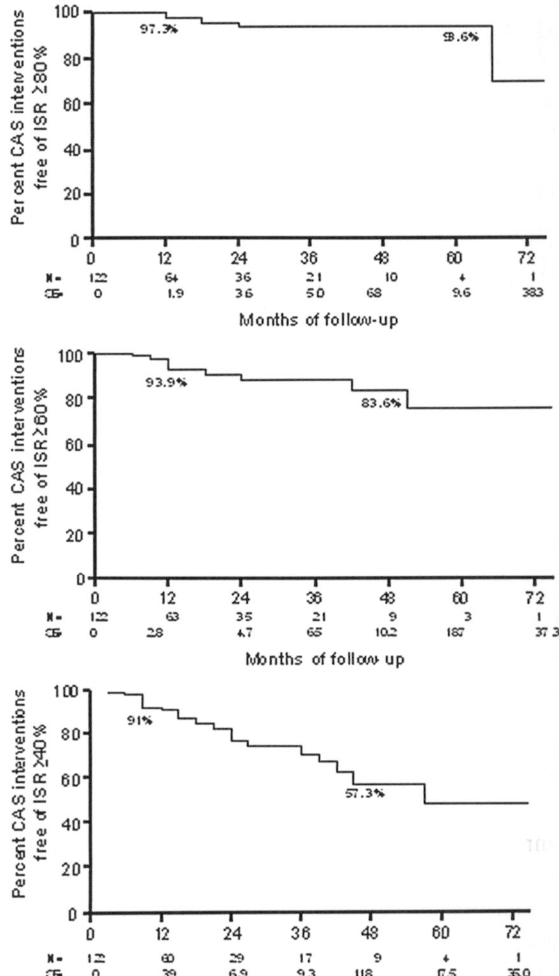

FIG. 16.1. Incidence of in-stent restenosis after carotid artery stenting. Kaplan–Meier cumulative event rates (**a**) for clinically significant ISR ≥80%, (**b**) for ISR ≥60%, and (**c**) for ISR ≥40%, after carotid artery stenting. Number of patients at the beginning of each time interval and standard error are indicated below the *X* axis of each graph. *N* number at risk, *SE* standard error [10]

coronary stenting, a substantial number of patients can be anticipated to progress. Clearly, some will advance to high-grade ISR requiring reintervention. Therefore surveillance is essential after CAS

The majority of restenoses ≥40% in our series of CAS procedures occurred within 18 months (13/22, 60%) of the procedure, and the majority of high-grade restenoses ≥80% occurred within 15 months (3/5, 60%) of their intervention [10] (Fig. 16.2). We

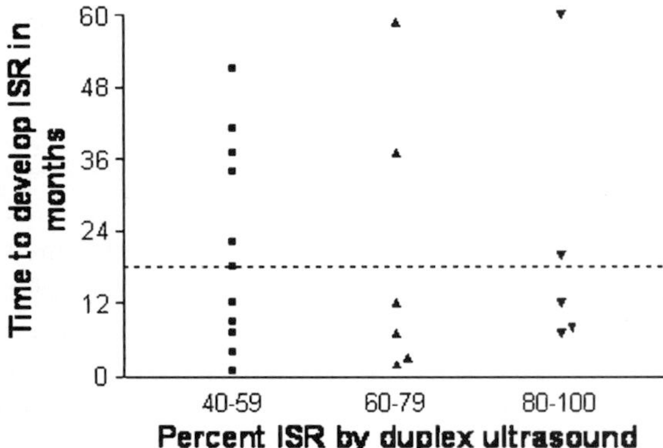

FIG. 16.2. Distribution of in-stent restenosis cases based on time of diagnosis from initial carotid artery stenting procedure. Note that the majority of restenoses occurred within 18 months of the initial carotid artery stenting procedure. The dotted line identifies the 18-month post-procedure mark. *ISR, in-stent restenosis* [10]

recommend that all patients undergoing CAS must be placed in a regular follow-up protocol with more frequent Duplex ultrasonography (DU) evaluations early after CAS. In our own practice, we evaluate patients every 6 months for the first 2 years, and annually thereafter. We also recommend early registration of baseline velocity measurements after CAS against which future results should be compared. The first follow-up DU must occur as soon after the procedure as possible, preferably during the same admission. B-mode imaging spectral waveform analysis must be used to supplement and enhance the accuracy of velocity criteria. Elevations in peak-systolic velocity (PSV) or ICA/CCA (internal carotid artery–common carotid artery) ratios or both are indicative of developing ISR, and as described in the following section, these patients must then undergo angiographic evaluation when appropriate thresholds are reached.

Diagnosis of In-Stent Restenosis

For the purposes of follow up, a diagnostic test should be able to reliably predict the true luminal diameter of the carotid artery. Furthermore, it should be inexpensive, easy to implement, and readily available. The gold standard for such measurements still remains multiplanar angiography; however, it is invasive. The attendant complications render it less useful as a screening modality; however, it can be used to confirm a recurrent lesion prior to re-treatment. In addition to being expensive, MRI and CT angiography still require additional investigation to validate their accuracy.

The standard diagnostic and screening tool used in the evaluation of primary carotid arterial stenosis and in the follow-up of patients who have undergone CEA has been DU. DU correlates well with angiographic levels of stenosis in the native carotid artery. In addition, appropriate velocity criteria using DU for determination of threshold degrees of stenosis have been well established [27–29]. However, US velocity criteria have not been well established for patients undergoing CAS. In 2004, we reported that the placement of a stent altered the biomechanical properties of the carotid territory such that compliance was reduced [9] (Fig. 16.3). We speculated that the enhanced stiffness of the stent–arterial wall complex could render the flow–pressure relationship of the carotid artery closer to that observed in a rigid tube [30]. The native artery allows some of the kinetic energy of blood to change to potential energy of the arterial wall. Since the compliance of the wall decreases with stenting, there is no transfer of this kinetic energy to the arterial wall. This could explain in part why the blood flow velocities would be increased in the presence of a stent. In this report, we compared post-CAS ultrasound velocities with angiographically measured residual in-stent stenosis after 90 CAS procedures. Mean angiographic residual stenosis after CAS was 5.4% while corresponding PSV on US was 120.4 cm s^{-1}. Receiver operating characteristic (ROC) analysis demonstrated that a combined threshold of PSV ≥150 cm s^{-1} and ICA/CCA ratio ≥2.16 were optimal for detecting residual stenosis ≥20%. We concluded that revised velocity criteria would need to be developed to identify higher grades of ISR in stented carotid arteries.

Subsequently, at least four studies have tested this hypothesis. Peterson et al. [31] compared DU velocity and angiography in three patients with high-grade ISR and proposed new criteria defining ISR ≥70% (PSV >170, EDV >120). Stanziale et al. [32] analyzed velocity/angiography observations obtained primarily from procedural angiography and angiography in patients with suspected high-grade

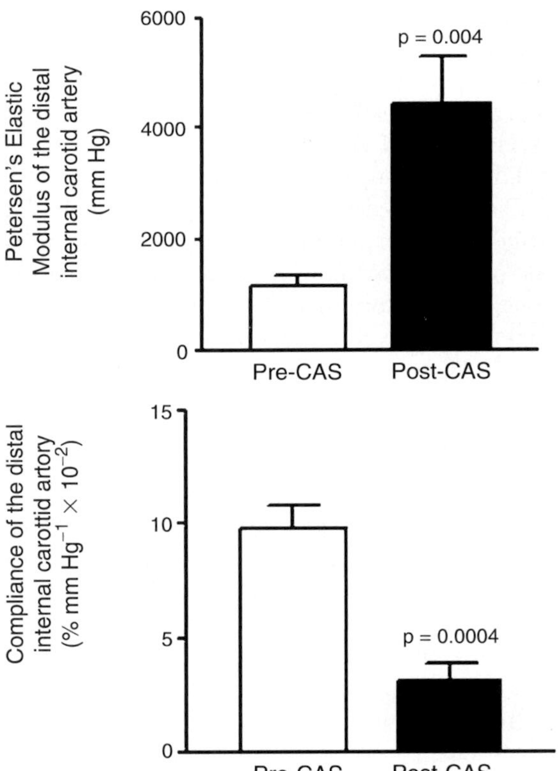

FIG. 16.3. Carotid artery stenting alters the biomechanical properties of the stent–arterial complex. Measurement of elastic modulus (**a**) and compliance (**b**) of the native internal carotid artery vs. stented internal carotid artery [9]

ISR. They proposed new criteria defining ISR ≥70% (PSV ≥350 and ICA/CCA ratio ≥4.75), and ISR ≥50% (PSV >225 and ICA/CCA ratio ≥2.5). Chi et al. [33] analyzed 13 pairs of US and angiogram observations and offered criteria to define ISR ≥70% (PSV ≥450 or ICA/CCA ratio ≥4.3) and ISR ≥50% (PSV ≥240 or ICA/CCA ratio ≥2.45). Chahwan et al. [34] analyzed six pairs of observations from patients with high-grade ISR. They concluded that larger studies would be required to determine appropriate threshold criteria for high grades of ISR. These studies confirm that ISR is overestimated in the stented artery when velocity criteria for native arteries are utilized. However, procedural risks did not allow sufficient patients to undergo angiographic follow-up, thereby limiting the number of velocity/angiography comparisons. This explains why each report proposed different threshold velocity criteria for ISR.

In a more recent report [35], we have compared DU velocity measurements with luminal stenosis measured by either angiography or CT angiography during follow-up of all our CAS patients (n = 310 observations). During DU, we measured peak-systolic (PSV) and end-diastolic velocities (EDV) in the native CCA; in the proximal, mid, and distal stent; and in the distal ICA. The accuracy of CT angiography vs. CA was confirmed (r^2 = 0.88) in a subset of patients (n = 19). Post-CAS PSV (r^2= 0.85) and ICA/CCA ratios (r^2= 0.76) correlated most with the degree of stenosis. Receiver operating characteristic (ROC) analysis showed the following optimal threshold criteria: residual stenosis ≥20% (PSV ≥150 cm s^{-1} and ICA/CCA ratio ≥2.15), ISR ≥50% (PSV ≥220 cm s^{-1} and ICA/CCA ratio ≥2.7), and ISR ≥80% (PSV ≥340 cm s^{-1} and ICA/CCA ratio ≥4.15) (Fig. 16.4). Table 16.1 summarizes the New Jersey Medical School

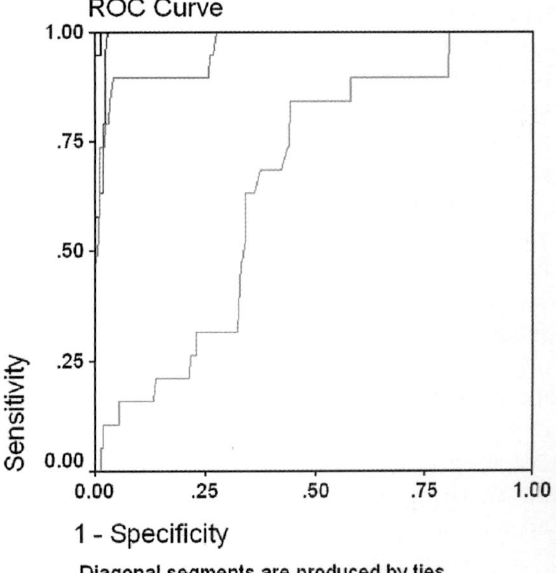

FIG. 16.4. Receiver operating characteristic (ROC) analysis to determine accuracy parameters of threshold velocities appropriate for the identification of high-grade in-stent restenosis (ISR) ≥80%; ROC curves were developed for PSV (*bold black line*), ICA/CCA ratios (*red line*), EDV (*green line*), and PSV/EDV ratios (*blue line*) for each threshold stenosis [35]

TABLE 16.1. New Jersey Medical School velocity criteria for the native and stented carotid arteries.

	Stented carotid artery		Native carotid artery
0–19%	PSV <150 cm s^{-1} and ICA/CCA ratio <2.15	0–19%	PSV <130 cm s^{-1}
20–49%	PSV 150–219 cm s^{-1}	20–49%	PSV 130–189 cm s^{-1}
50–79%	PSV 220–339 cm s^{-1} and ICA/CCA ratio ≥2.7	50–79%	PSV 190–249 cm s^{-1} and EDV <120 cm s^{-1}
80–99%	PSV ≥340 cm s^{-1} and ICA/CCA ratio ≥4.15	80–99%	PSV ≥250 cm s^{-1} and EDV ≥120 cm s^{-1}, or ICA/CCA ratio ≥3.2

PSV and EDV measurements for stented carotid arteries are taken within the stented segments *PSV* peak systolic velocity, *ICA* internal carotid artery, *CCA* common carotid artery, *EDV* end diastolic velocity

(NJMS) velocity criteria [35] for the evaluation of stented carotid arteries. While our results can be used as guidelines, individual laboratories must develop threshold criteria that are accurate for their own environment. These proposed criteria can form the basis for additional prospective validation studies.

Risk Factors for the Development of ISR

Predictors for neointimal hyperplasia are the subject of continued investigation and there is limited information on which factors constitute to the risks for carotid ISR. Diabetes is a well-known predictor of early and aggressive IH and ISR after coronary artery stenting [36, 37]. One report has observed an increased incidence of ISR in patients with uncontrolled diabetes undergoing CAS [38]. Skelly et al. [39] analyzed 109 CAS patients for risk factors that may lead to restenosis. Asymptomatic restenosis occurred in 12 patients (11%); high-grade ISR necessitating reintervention occurred in five of those patients. Using Cox proportional hazards modeling, they identified prior neurological symptoms (stroke, transient ischemic attack, amaurosis fugax) and prior cervical radiation as significant predictors of future ISR.

Primary stenting prevents carotid artery recoil and constrictive remodeling [40], and post-CAS ISR can be primarily attributed to neointimal hyperplasia (IH) [40, 41]. Therefore the patterns of developing IH lesions may reflect the aggressiveness of the intimal hyperplastic response and may also predict the future development of high-grade ISR (≥80%), necessitating reintervention. We assessed the morphologic patterns of ISR using B-mode imaging in patients after CAS [42]. ISR lesions were classified on the basis of their length and location according to the NJMS classification of patterns of post-CAS ISR [42]: type I (focal ≤10-mm end-stent lesions), II (focal ≤10 mm, intrastent), III (diffuse >10 mm, intrastent), IV (diffuse >10 mm proliferative, extending outside the stent), and V (total occlusion) (Fig. 16.5). We then entered potential risk factors, including the pattern of ISR, age, gender, hypercholesterolemia, diabetes, hypertension, coronary artery disease, etiology of primary stenosis, prior symptomatic status, prior history of ISR, type of stent used, number of stents used, length of stent, and residual stenosis after CAS, into a multivariate regression model to determine independent predictors of future high-grade ISR and the need for reintervention. Eighty-five ISR lesions developed after 255 CAS procedures. Their distribution was 40% (type I), 25.9% (type II), 12.9% (type III), 20% (type IV), and 1.2% (type V). Thirteen lesions were ≥80% diameter-reducing, and underwent endovascular reintervention. A univariate analysis showed that the need for reintervention was highest in type IV lesions ($p = 0.001$). A history of prior ISR ($p = 0.003$) and of diabetes ($p = 0.02$) occurred more frequently with type IV ISR lesions. On multivariate analysis, it was found that only the type of ISR (odds ratio [OR], 5.1) and a history of diabetes (OR, 9.7) were independent predictors of high-grade recurrent ISR and reintervention [42].

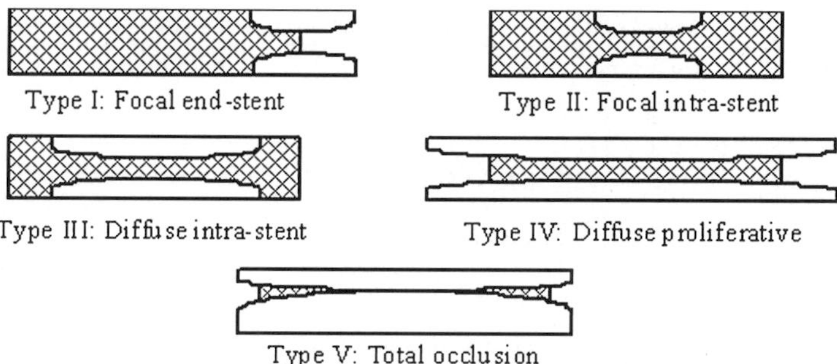

FIG. 16.5. New Jersey Medical School (NJMS) classification of post-CAS instent restenosis. Type I is a focal end stent lesion. Type II is a focal intrastent lesion. Type III is a diffuse intrastent lesion. Type IV is a diffuse proliferative lesion extending outside the stent. Type V is an occlusive lesion

Follow-up duplex US evaluations after CAS must therefore include an assessment of the morphologic pattern of ISR so that patients with type IV lesions can be placed on a more intensive monitoring program (perhaps every 6 months for life). Similarly, intensive monitoring is also warranted in diabetic patients, in those with a history of cervical radiation, and in those who have been treated for ISR. Additional data are needed to validate these recommendations in prospectively implemented studies at multiple centers.

Management of Carotid Restenosis

The clinical significance of ISR is still debated. Owing to the small number of patients who develop significant ISR after CAS, and the lack of clinical trials following up these patients for extended periods of time, it is a difficult issue to address. The incidence of symptomatic CR after CEA ranges from 0–8.2%, while asymptomatic CR occurs in 1.3–37% [43]. Consensus exists regarding the need for treatment of symptomatic CR. In asymptomatic CR, however, authors have acknowledged that the risk of stroke or progression to total occlusion is uncommon [22, 44]. On the basis of the low incidence of symptoms in this cohort of patients, these authors have proposed careful surveillance alone for asymptomatic patients. This recommendation was made in the absence of randomized trial data, with the belief that neointimal hyperplasia carries a low risk for embolization, and that reoperation may carry an increased risk of perioperative neurological events and cranial nerve palsies.

Conversely, other surgeons have taken a more aggressive approach toward asymptomatic CR, and elect to operate on high-grade (≥80%) asymptomatic lesions. In the report of O'Hara et al. [45] on 206 redo-CEAs, only 43% had symptoms. Mansour et al. [46] operated on 82 CRs of which 66% were symptomatic and the remaining had high-grade asymptomatic stenoses ≥80%. The rationale for this approach is that it is extremely difficult to predict which high-grade (>80%) lesions will progress to occlusion. Our group subscribes to this view, and we have reported our low complication rate with redo-CEAs for asymptomatic high-grade (>80%) and symptomatic (>50%) CR [6]. Our recommendations for the management of ISR after CAS are based on the published experience with CR after CEA. Therefore, we recommend that symptomatic patients with ISR >50% and asymptomatic patients with ISR >80% should be considered for reintervention.

Endovascular Treatment of Carotid Restenosis

Most patients currently treated with CAS usually harbor one of more high-risk features for CEA. These risk factors will persist in the eventuality that the patients develop ISR during follow-up. In our program, patients developing ≥80% diameter-reducing ISR undergo angiographic confirmation of the lesion and preferential endovascular treatment [10, 24, 47]. As Table 16.2 demonstrates, there are several available techniques for reintervention. The fact that these multiple techniques were used in a single cohort also implies that there is currently limited consensus regarding the most efficacious approach. Angioplasty alone is perhaps the simplest means of intervention; however, the hyperplastic lesions may recoil, resulting in incomplete restoration of luminal diameters. In these situations, a cutting balloon may restore patency; however, on occasion restenting may become necessary. Research continues in the fields of systemic or local pharmaceutical agents and local brachytherapy to prevent the neointimal hyperplasia.

There is limited long-term follow-up on these patients, and further studies are needed to evaluate durability of the results. Setacci et al. [48] reported on 372 patients who had follow-up after CAS. Fifteen patients underwent reintervention for ISR >80%. Three patients were treated with angioplasty alone; eight underwent restenting after angioplasty; and four were treated with cutting balloon angioplasty. The reinterventions were successful in all patients and resulted in no morbidity or mortality. Over a median follow-up of 12.4 months, there were no recurrent restenoses. Zhou et al. [49] have recently reported on the successful treatment of seven ISR lesions. In our most recent publication [42], endovascular re-treatment was required in 3 of 11 instances of type III ISR and 10 of 17 instances of type IV ISR (Table 16.2). The mean interval between CAS and reintervention was 18.2 months. We observed a significant increase in reintervention in association with increasing levels of ISR classification (0, 0, 27.3, and 58.8% for types I–IV, respectively; χ^2 trend = 29.4; $p = 0.001$). Procedural success was achieved in all these cases, without evidence of any abrupt arterial closure or neurological events. Endovascular treatment of ISR resulted in similar percent diameter residual stenoses in all instances and was not influenced by ISR class. Three of the patients have required repeat interventions. One patient has required two repeated interventions over a follow-up period of 3 years. Increasing experience with the treatment of these lesions will enable formulation of standardized approaches and establish potential limitations of repeated treatments. However, we currently recommend angioplasty as the primary approach to these intimal hyperplastic lesions, with restenting in those cases with suboptimal results.

Surgical Management of Recurrent Stenosis

Recurrent ISR after endovascular management of ISR has been reported in our series as well as by others [10, 24, 48, 49]. They tend to occur in a small percentage of cases and respond well to repeated angioplasty or stenting or both. Individual instances of stent explantation and repeated endarterectomy have been reported by our group [47]

TABLE 16.2. Details of endovascular reinterventions done for in-stent restenosis after carotid artery stenting [35].

	Patterns of ISR			
	Focal end-stent I (n = 34)	Focal intrastent II (n = 22)	Diffuse intrastent III (n = 11)	Diffuse proliferative IV (n = 17)
Incidence of TLR*	0	0	27.3	58.8
Devices used for treatment of ISR (n)				
Balloon angioplasty	0	0	1	3
Stent	0	0	1	5
Cutting balloon	0	0	0	1
Cutting balloon + stent	0	0	1	1
Posttreatment result (% residual stenosis)	NA	NA	10.4 ± 6.9	11.9 ± 6.1

Values are expressed as percents
ISR in-stent restenosis,
TLR target lesion revascularization
*p =0.001

and others [50, 51]. They are reserved for heavily calcified lesions with suboptimal primary stenting results [47], for preocclusive lesions no longer responsive or approachable by angioplasty [50, 51], for technical failure of stent material [52], or for primary stent thrombosis [53]. As we gain experience in using endovascular approaches toward recurrent lesions, and as technological advances in catheters, guidewires, and stents occur, we anticipate a decreasing need for explantation operations.

Conclusions

We have restricted the majority of our clinical experience with CAS to post-CEA restenoses, surgically inaccessible lesions, radiation-induced stenoses, and patients presenting with prohibitively high medical risks. CAS done for these indications appears to be safe and associated with low recurrence rates. Duplex ultrasonography is the preferred method of monitoring the carotid artery after CAS. However, revised velocity criteria must be utilized to determine the degree of restenosis. Most restenoses occur early after CAS and the morphologic patterns of the lesions predict the aggressiveness of the hyperplastic reaction. Type IV patterns and diabetes predict a higher risk of progression to >80% restenosis and need for reintervention. Subsequent endovascular reinterventions for ISR are technically feasible and are associated with low morbidity.

Key Points

- Current reports indicate that the incidence of post-CAS in-stent restenosis (ISR) ranges from 1–50%.
- Considerable controversy still persists regarding the clinical significance, natural history, optimal diagnosis, threshold for management, and appropriate intervention for ISR.
- Two mechanisms can account for the restenosis that occurs after carotid stenting.
  a. Restenosis early (<24 months) after the procedure is generally attributed to intimal hyperplasia.
  b. Restenosis that occurs >24 months after carotid stenting is generally believed to be caused by progressive atherosclerosis.
- Calculation of an absolute restenosis rate (arteries with restenotic lesions/total carotid procedures) will generally underestimate the incidence of restenosis, because it does not account for the duration, frequency, and completeness of clinical follow-up.
- Patients who undergo CAS should have routine surveillance ultrasonography at baseline and every 6 months for 2 years, and then annually thereafter.
- US velocity criteria have not been well established for patients undergoing CAS, and placement of a stent alters the biomechanical properties of the carotid territory such that compliance is reduced.
- Modified duplex US criteria for stented carotid arteries should be used for the follow-up evaluation of CAS patients.
- Follow-up duplex US evaluations after CAS must include an assessment of the morphologic pattern of ISR so that patients with type IV lesions can be placed on a more intensive monitoring program. Additional candidates for more intensive follow-up surveillance may include diabetic patients and those with a history of prior cervical radiation.
- Symptomatic patients with ISR >50% and asymptomatic patients with ISR of >80% are candidates for reintervention.
- The reintervention could take the form of angioplasty, cutting balloon angioplasty, restenting, or a combination.
- In cases where endovascular reintervention is not possible or contraindicated, open surgical correction should be undertaken.

References

1. North American Symptomatic Carotid Endarterectomy Trial Collaborators, Beneficial effect of carotid endarterectomy in symptomatic patients with high-grade carotid stenosis. N Engl J Med, 1991. 325(7): pp. 445–53.
2. Randomised trial of endarterectomy for recently symptomatic carotid stenosis: final results of the MRC European Carotid Surgery Trial (ECST). Lancet, 1998. 351(9113): pp. 1379–87.
3. Barnett, H.J., et al., North American Symptomatic Carotid Endarterectomy Trial Collaborators, Benefit of carotid endarterectomy in patients with symptomatic

moderate or severe stenosis. N Engl J Med, 1998. 339(20): pp. 1415–25.
4. Executive Committee for the Asymptomatic Carotid Atherosclerosis Study, Endarterectomy for asymptomatic carotid artery stenosis. JAMA, 1995. 273(18): pp. 1421–8.
5. Hobson, R.W., II, et al., The Veterans Affairs Cooperative Study Group, Efficacy of carotid endarterectomy for asymptomatic carotid stenosis. N Engl J Med, 1993. 328(4): pp. 221–7.
6. Hobson, R.W., II, et al., Carotid restenosis: operative and endovascular management. J Vasc Surg, 1999. 29(2): pp. 228–35; discussion 235–8.
7. Hobson, R.W., II, et al., Carotid artery stenting: analysis of data for 105 patients at high risk. J Vasc Surg, 2003. 37(6): pp. 1234–9.
8. Hobson, R.W., II, et al., Carotid artery closure for endarterectomy does not influence results of angioplasty-stenting for restenosis. *J Vasc Surg,* 2002. 35(3): pp. 435–8.
9. Lal, B.K., et al., Carotid artery stenting: is there a need to revise ultrasound velocity criteria? J Vasc Surg, 2004. 39(1): pp. 58–66.
10. Lal, B.K., et al., In-stent recurrent stenosis after carotid artery stenting: life table analysis and clinical relevance. J Vasc Surg, 2003. 38(6): pp. 1162–8; discussion 1169.
11. Ohki, T., and F.J. Veith, Carotid artery stenting: utility of cerebral protection devices. J Invasive Cardiol, 2001. 13(1): pp. 47–55.
12. Roubin, G.S., et al., Immediate and late clinical outcomes of carotid artery stenting in patients with symptomatic and asymptomatic carotid artery stenosis: a 5-year prospective analysis. Circulation, 2001. 103(4): pp. 532–7.
13. Vitek, J.J., et al., Carotid angioplasty with stenting in post-carotid endarterectomy restenosis. J Invasive Cardiol, 2001. 13(2): pp. 123–5; discussion 158–70.
14. Yadav, J.S., et al., Protected carotid-artery stenting versus endarterectomy in high-risk patients. N Engl J Med, 2004. 351(15): pp. 1493–501.
15. NACPTAR Investigators, Update of the immediate angiographic results and in-hospital central nervous system complications of cerebral percutaneous transluminal angioplasty. Circulation, 1995. 92(1): p. 383.
16. Hobson, R.W., II, Carotid artery stenting. Surg Clin North Am, 2004. 84(5): pp. 1281–94, vi.
17. FDA, FDA Approves New Stent System to Help Prevent Stroke. FDA News, 2004. http://www.fda.gov/bbs/topics/news/2004/NEW01111.html.
18. Baier, R.E. and R.C. Dutton, Initial events in interactions of blood with a foreign surface. J Biomed Mater Res, 1969. 3(1): pp. 191–206.
19. Schwartz, R.S., et al., Restenosis and the proportional neointimal response to coronary artery injury: results in a porcine model. J Am Coll Cardiol, 1992. 19(2): pp. 267–74.
20. Kornowski, R., et al., In-stent restenosis: contributions of inflammatory responses and arterial injury to neointimal hyperplasia. J Am Coll Cardiol, 1998. 31(1): pp. 224–30.
21. Sanada, J.I., et al., An experimental study of endovascular stenting with special reference to the effects on the aortic vasa vasorum. Cardiovasc Intervent Radiol, 1998. 21(1): pp. 45–9.
22. Lattimer, C.R. and K.G. Burnand, Recurrent carotid stenosis after carotid endarterectomy. Br J Surg, 1997. 84(9): pp. 1206–19.
23. Sterpetti, A.V., et al. Natural history of recurrent carotid artery disease. Surg Gynecol Obstet, 1989. 168(3): pp. 217–23.
24. Chakhtoura, E.Y., et al., In-stent restenosis after carotid angioplasty-stenting: incidence and management. J Vasc Surg, 2001. 33(2): pp. 220–5; discussion 225–6.
25. DeGroote, R.D., et al., Carotid restenosis: long-term noninvasive follow-up after carotid endarterectomy. Stroke, 1987. 18(6): pp. 1031–6.
26. Bosiers, M., et al., Does carotid artery stenting work on the long run: 5-year results in high-volume centers (ELOCAS Registry). J Cardiovasc Surg (Torino), 2005. 46(3): pp. 241–7.
27. Faught, W.E., et al., Color-flow duplex scanning of carotid arteries: new velocity criteria based on receiver operator characteristic analysis for threshold stenoses used in the symptomatic and asymptomatic carotid trials. J Vasc Surg, *1994.* 19(5): pp. 818–27; discussion 827–8.
28. Lal, B.K. and I.R. Hobson, Carotid artery occlusive disease. Curr Treat Options Cardiovasc Med, 2000. 2(3): pp. 243–54.
29. Mintz, B.L. and R.W. Hobson, II, Diagnosis and treatment of carotid artery stenosis. J Am Osteopath Assoc, 2000. 100(11 suppl): pp. S22–6.
30. Green, J.F., Mechanical concepts in cardiovascular and pulmonary physiology. 1977, Philadelphia: Lea & Febiger, pp. 47–53.
31. Peterson, B.G., et al., Duplex ultrasound remains a reliable test even after carotid stenting. Ann Vasc Surg, 2005. 19(6): pp. 793–7.
32. Stanziale, S.F., et al., Determining in-stent stenosis of carotid arteries by duplex ultrasound criteria. J Endovasc Ther, 2005. 12(3): pp. 346–53.

33. Chi, Y.W., et al., Ultrasound velocity criteria for carotid in-stent restenosis. Catheter Cardiovasc Interv, 2007. 69(3): pp. 349–54.
34. Chahwan, S., et-al., Carotid artery velocity characteristics after carotid artery angioplasty and stenting. J Vasc Surg, 2007. 45(3): pp. 523–6.
35. Lal, B.K., et al., Duplex ultrasound velocity criteria for the stented carotid artery. J Vasc Surg, 2008. 47(1): pp. 63–73.
36. Mehran, R., et al., Angiographic patterns of in-stent restenosis: classification and implications for long-term outcome. Circulation, 1999. 100(18): pp. 1872–8.
37. Abizaid, A., et al., The influence of diabetes mellitus on acute and late clinical outcomes following coronary stent implantation. J Am Coll Cardiol, 1998. 32(3): pp. 584–9.
38. Willfort-Ehringer, A., et al., Neointimal proliferation within carotid stents is more pronounced in diabetic patients with initial poor glycaemic state. Diabetologia, 2004. 47(3): pp. 400–6.
39. Skelly, C.L., et al., Risk factors for restenosis after carotid artery angioplasty and stenting. J Vasc Surg, 2006. 44(5): pp. 1010–15.
40. Willfort-Ehringer, A., et al., Arterial remodeling and hemodynamics in carotid stents: a prospective duplex ultrasound study over 2 years. J Vasc Surg, 2004. 39(4): pp. 728–34.
41. Piamsomboon, C., et al., Relationship between oversizing of self-expanding stents and late loss index in carotid stenting. Cathet Cardiovasc Diagn, 1998. 45(2): pp. 139–43.
42. Lal, B.K., et al., Patterns of in-stent restenosis after carotid artery stenting: Classification and implications for long-term outcome. J Vasc Surg, 2007. 46(5): pp. 833–40.
43. Beebe, H.G., Scientific evidence demonstrating the safety of carotid angioplasty and stenting: do we have enough to draw conclusions yet? J Vasc Surg, 1998. 27(4): pp. 788–90.
44. Healy, D.A., et al., Long-term follow-up and clinical outcome of carotid restenosis. J Vasc Surg, 1989. 10(6): pp. 662–8; discussion 668–9.
45. O'Hara, P.J., et al., Reoperation for recurrent carotid stenosis: early results and late outcome in 199 patients. J Vasc Surg, 2001. 34(1): pp. 5–12.
46. Mansour, M.A., et al., Carotid endarterectomy for recurrent stenosis. J Vasc Surg, 1997. 25(5): pp. 877–83.
47. Choi, H.M., et al., Technical challenges in a program of carotid artery stenting. J Vasc Surg, 2004. 40(4): pp. 746–51; discussion 751.
48. Setacci, C., et al., In-stent restenosis after carotid angioplasty and stenting: a challenge for the vascular surgeon. Eur J Vasc Endovasc Surg, 2005. 29(6): pp. 601–7.
49. Zhou, W., et al., Management of in-sent restenosis after carotid artery stenting in high-risk patients. J Vasc Surg, 2006. 43(2): pp. 305–12.
50. Akin, E., et al., Instent restenosis after carotid stenting necessitating open carotid surgical repair. Eur J Cardiothorac Surg, 2004. 26(2): pp. 442–3.
51. Gray, W.A., et al., Carotid stenting and endarterectomy: a clinical and cost comparison of revascularization strategies. Stroke, 2002. 33(4): pp. 1063–70.
52. de Vries, J.P., et al., Stent fracture after endoluminal repair of a carotid artery pseudoaneurysm. J Endovasc Ther, 2005. 12(5): pp. 612–15.
53. Setacci, C., et al., Surgical management of acute carotid thrombosis after carotid stenting: a report of three cases. J Vasc Surg, 2005. 42(5): pp. 993–6.

17 Optimizing Outcomes

David Beckett and Peter A. Gaines

Introduction

Carotid angioplasty and stenting (CAS) is increasingly used in the treatment of symptomatic severely stenotic carotid disease. Since the introduction of CAS, many technical and pharmacological advances have been made to optimize the outcome of the intervention. These factors have largely addressed the risk of embolic stroke and include patient selection, material choices, and ultimately, the skill of the operator. In addition, to further improve outcomes of CAS, there should be recognition of the nonembolic causes of stroke. This chapter focuses upon what can be done to optimize the outcome for the patient treated by CAS.

Patient Selection

Time to Intervention

In symptomatic patients (transient ischemic attack (TIA), amaurosis fugax, and recovered stroke) intervention upon the carotid stenosis is intended to reduce the risk of stroke and death after the index event. Any benefit gained is highly dependent on the delay from presenting symptoms to intervention. Since half of the 90-day events after the index symptom occur in the first 48 h, greatest benefit is seen in patients treated within the first 2 weeks [1]. As an example of how effective this policy would be, for patients with a high-grade stenosis (50% stenosis or more) the number needed to undergo surgery to prevent one ipsilateral stroke at 5 years is 5 for those treated less than 2 weeks from their TIA vs 125 for those treated outside 12 weeks. No similar data are available for CAS but it is reasonable to assume that the same improved benefit would apply.

Specific Selection Criteria

Decision-making as to the relative suitability of CAS or CEA for a patient with carotid disease is complex. It is likely that several factors will impact upon the risk of complications for both the modalities in the same way (e.g., general medical fitness of the patient and age). Certain considerations, however, are specific for CAS and will be considered further.

Vessel Anatomy

Because the morphology of the arch branch vessels will determine whether the case is suitable for CAS and the choice of materials used, it is important that such information is available before intervention is begun. In addition, morphological contraindications are related to the experience of the operator. Such morphological information can reasonably be obtained quickly with helical CT, MR angiography, or catheter angiography. Preprocedural imaging should at least assess the severity of the lesion, and the anatomy of the arch and the common carotid and internal carotid vessels. Origin disease of the branch vessels should be avoided for routine CAS since catheterization of these vessels will put the

S. Macdonald and G. Stansby (eds.), *Practical Carotid Artery Stenting*,
DOI: 10.1007/978-1-84800-299-9_17,

patient at risk of stroke. Alternative strategies can be considered (e.g., combining CAS with CEA by a surgical approach to the common carotid artery (CCA)). Tortuosity of the CCA makes access to the ICA difficult. With experience this can usually be overcome, but the inexperienced operator should avoid such cases. Tortuosity of the ICA makes placement of a filter protection device difficult and increases the risk that a stent will cause a kink and occlude the vessel. Although alternative strategies can be devised (e.g., reverse flow cerebral protection, flexible stent) where there is marked tortuosity, CEA, probably as an eversion technique, should be strongly considered.

Hammer et al. described a relationship between embolic load as defined by DW-MRI and difficult anatomical variations [2]. Arch angle <45° or tortuosity of the CCA were associated with a higher embolic load within the anterior circulation (36% vs. 5%).

A further study by Faggioli et al. [3] set out to establish the risk of CAS complications in patients with aortic arch anomalies. Of 214 consecutive patients undergoing CAS, 189 (88.3%) had normal arch anatomy and 25 (11.7%) had arch anomalies. The arch abnormalities included common origin of brachiocephalic trunk and left CCA, separate origin of right subclavian and common carotid, and left common carotid agenesis with separate arch origin of internal and external carotid. Technical failure was higher in the arch anomaly group; however, the difference did not reach statistical significance (89.6% vs. 76.4%). Neurological complications occurred more frequently in the arch anomaly group (20% vs. 5.3%, $p = 0.039$).

These studies support the concept that focused manipulation within the arch and careful patient selection based on evaluation of the arch and tortuosity of the extracranial carotid circulation will reduce the number of embolic events. Direct cannulation of the symptomatic carotid vessel should be attempted only during CAS and not during preprocedural imaging.

Plaque Analysis

The indication for CAS is mostly based on the percentage of stenosis and the presence or absence of preprocedural neurological symptoms. Plaque analysis informs the clinician not only on the decision to intervene but may predict the outcome following an intervention. Whether prior knowledge may help us decide between CEA and CAS is currently under debate and as yet this question remains unanswered.

The echogenicity of plaque is determined by its composition. Areas of intraplaque hemorrhage and lipid-rich plaques are homogenously echopoor. There has been much discussion regarding the ICAROS study [4]. Biasi et al. showed that carotid plaque echolucency as defined by a grey scale medium (GSM) of <25 increases the risk of stroke in CAS. Complication rate was 5.3% for symptomatic vs. 2.8% for asymptomatic patients. Within the GSM > 25 subset, rates fell to 3.3% vs. 0.6% respectively. This study failed to demonstrate that these patients were better treated with CEA than with CAS. In addition, a later study by Reiter et al. [5] demonstrated that plaque echolucency measured by objective and subjective grading did not identify patients with an increased risk of peri-interventional neurological events in patients undergoing elective CAS from a prospective single-center registry database.

High-resolution MRI provides a more detailed analysis of plaque than echography. MRI identification of ruptured plaque correlates with a history of TIA/Stroke. Plaque composition may be determined in vivo. Qualitative assessment of plaque components according to a high-resolution MRI classification is possible. Tissue quantification is accurate and reproducible. In a study by Saam et al. [6], 31 subjects scheduled for carotid endarterectomy were imaged with a 1.5T scanner using time-of-flight-, T1-, proton-density-, and T2-weighted images. A total of 214 MR imaging locations were matched to corresponding histology sections. For MRI and histology, area measurements of the major plaque components such as lipid-rich/necrotic core, calcification, loose matrix, and dense (fibrous) tissue were recorded as percentages of the total wall area. MRI measurements of plaque composition were statistically equivalent to those of histology for the lipid-rich/necrotic core, loose matrix, and dense (fibrous) tissue. Calcification differed significantly when measured as a percentage of wall area.

Ultimately, plaque analysis may help us to define and stratify disease subsets (active vs. inactive) and successfully aid in clinical decision-making. To this end, there have been several studies published.

Bosiers et al. [7] sought to identify whether carotid stent design, especially free cell area, impacts on the 30-day rates for stroke, death, and TIA after CAS. In a procedure heavily dependant on well-designed medical devices, it is to be expected that questions will be asked as to whether all stents are equal. This study was not without its limitations; CAS was done within each unit's existing standards of care. Given that stent selection was tailored towards individual patients, the allocation of stent design was not random. In addition, a stent with a small cell area (NexStent) had the second worse outcome in asymptomatic patients [8]. To date there is no good evidence to indicate whether any one stent has better outcomes over another. Nevertheless, device characteristics most likely affect outcome and this represents an area for future research.

Patient-Based Training vs. Simulation-Assisted Training Pathways

Of late there has been a shift away from the traditional time-based learning methods towards competency-based assessment and training. Mentor assessment and the so-called apprenticeship model of training have been criticized for lacking objectivity, while logbook experience may correlate poorly with ability [9]. While few patients suffer adverse outcomes following CAS, this makes evaluation and assessment of an individual's skills difficult when based on clinical outcome alone.

In addition to technical proficiency, a sound range of cognitive skills are required. A successful blend of clinical management skills and knowledge of pathology, natural history, neuroanatomy, and physiology is required. Such a skills base would be best achieved by the formation of a clinical management team.

Within the UK, current recommendations for training in CAS [10] include the following:

- An interventionalist should not enter CAS until basic endovascular experience is achieved.
- A program with 3 stages.
  - A structured day of lectures with live cases. The lectures will cover clinical, surgical, and pharmacological management of CAS. The whole multidisciplinary team should attend.
  - A visit to observe cases within an established center.
  - A proctor attends the hospital to train the interventionalist to the satisfaction of the proctor.

To date, one of the most compelling trials to support the need for adequate training and experience is the EVA-3S trial, a randomized noninferiority trial of CAS vs. CEA [11]. At 6 months, the incidence of any stroke or death was 6.1% after endarterectomy and 11.7% after stenting ($p = 0.02$). The natural conclusion from the trial was that CEA had better outcomes at 30 days and 6 months. But is the answer that simple? Possibly not. Some insight into the hugely different outcomes lies in the respective skills of the operators undertaking CEA and CAS. To undertake CEA, the surgeon needed to have done at least 25 endarterectomies before entering the trial. To undertake CAS little or no experience was required. Not only was training severely limited but so was experience. A total of 30 centers participated. Half the work was done within 5 centers and the other half within 25 centers. The average enrolment per center was therefore only 1.7 patients per year. Such limitation in training and experience explains the high crossover from CAS to CEA and probably some of the high 30-day complication rates in the CAS arm.

But how much experience is required to undertake CAS? Data from CAVATAS suggest that the more cases that are performed, the better the results [12]. The exact number of cases that should be undertaken per year to ensure maintenance of clinical skills is unclear, but published data suggest around 25. In a recent single-center study it was only after the first 195 cases that the yearly major stroke rate remained stable at less than 2% [13].

The Role of Virtual Reality

Issues relating to patient safety when training for complex procedures, which carry substantial risk, have fuelled an interest in simulation training. Satava first described virtual reality (VR) as a method for surgical procedural skills training in 1991 [14]. In 2002 level-1 evidence was published that demonstrated the efficacy of simulation for improving intraoperative performance in minimally invasive surgery [15]. Within the USA the Food and Drug Administrations approval of an

TABLE 17.1.

Trial	Inclusion criteria	Primary end point
Carotid Revascularization Endarterectomy vs. Stent Trial (CREST)	≥60% Stenosis	30 day stroke/death/MI 4 year ipsilateral stroke
Transatlantic Asymptomatic Carotid Intervention Trial (TACIT)	≥70% Stenosis	30 day stroke/death/MI 3 year ipsilateral stroke
Asymptomatic Carotid Surgery Trial 2 (ACST-2)		30 day stroke/death/MI 5 year ipsilateral stroke
Carotid Angioplasty and Stenting vs. Endarterectomy in Asymptomatic Subjects with Significant Extracranial Carotid Occlusive Disease Trial (ACT 1)	≥80% Stenosis	30 day stroke/death/MI 1 year ipsilateral stroke

TABLE 17.2. Commercially available simulators now in use for CAS training.

Simulator	Manufacturer
ANGIO Mentor	Simbionix USA, Cleveland, OH
Endovascular AccuTouch System	Immersion Medical, Gaithersburg, MD
SimSuite	Medical Simulation, Denver, CO
VIST: Procedicus vascular intervention system training simulator	Mentice AB, Göteborg, Sweden

endovascular device for CAS included, for the first time, a requirement for training, which included procedural steps on a VR simulator. Several commercially available simulators now exist for use in CAS training (Table 17.2).

Simulation offers the possibility of reducing the learning curve, enabling the trainee to gain both cognitive and procedural experience without risk to the patient. Patel and colleagues instructed 20 interventional cardiologists in angiography and had the subjects perform 5 serial simulations [16]. There were measurable improvements between the first and the fifth intervention, based on procedure time, contrast used, fluoroscopy time, and catheter handling errors. This suggests that some reduction in the learning curve can occur on the simulation. Performance on an endovascular simulator has also been shown to discriminate between novices and experienced endovascular clinicians.

Van Herzeele et al. [17] set out to objectively assess psychomotor skills acquisition of experienced interventionalists attending a 2-day CAS course, using a VR simulator. Significant differences were noted between pre- and postcourse performance for procedure (36 vs. 20 min), X-ray (20 vs. 11 min), delivery-retrieval time of the embolic protection device (12 vs. 9 min), inappropriate advancement of the guiding catheter, without a leading wire occurred to a greater extent pre- vs. postcourse, and degree of spasm of the internal carotid. This study has objectively proven a benefit for experienced interventionalists to attend CAS courses for skills acquisition measured by a VR simulator. These data can be used to offer participants an insight into their skills and objectively audit course efficacy.

Future directions for VR simulation are likely to concentrate on procedural competency. It has the potential to be used as a method of cognitive and technical assessment. As an educational tool, it has the promise to make training safer and more efficient. It is clear from the literature that VR simulators are likely to accelerate the learning curve but do not replace clinical experience.

Medical Therapy

Atherosclerosis is a systemic disease. Clinical manifestation of disease in one arterial territory is highly suggestive of disease elsewhere within either the carotid or the peripheral vascular tree. In our aims to optimize outcomes particular attention should be paid to both the peri- and postprocedural periods.

Antiplatelet Therapy

There is level-1 evidence for the use of aspirin in the secondary prevention of stroke. In addition to aspirin all patients should receive 75 mg clopidogrel 5 days prior to the procedure (where this is not possible an oral loading dose of 300–600 mg can be given the day before) and continued for at least 30 days following CAS. The benefit of combined aspirin and clopidogrel in CAS was demonstrated in a trial that randomized patients between either aspirin and 24-h heparin or aspirin and clopidogrel [18]. The neurological complication rate in the 24-h heparin group was 25%, compared with 0% in the clopidogrel group ($p = 0.02$). The 30-day 50–100% stenosis rates were 26% in the heparin group and 5% in the clopidogrel group. It was concluded that the dual antiplatelet regime had a significant impact on reducing adverse neurological outcomes without an additional increase in bleeding complications. This study was terminated prematurely because of an unacceptable level of complications in the heparin arm of the trial.

The CARESS (clopidogrel and aspirin for reduction of emboli in symptomatic carotid stenosis) trial proved the effectiveness of the combination of clopidogrel and aspirin, compared with aspirin alone, in reducing the presence and number of microembolic signals (MES) in patients with recently symptomatic carotid stenosis [19]. Patients were screened with TCD, and if MES were detected, they were randomized to clopidogrel and aspirin or aspirin monotherapy. Intention-to-treat analysis revealed a significant reduction in the primary end point: 43.8% of dual-therapy patients were MES-positive on day 7, compared with 72.7% of monotherapy patients. The secondary end point of MES frequency per hour was reduced in the dual-therapy group at day 7 and by 61.6% on day 2.

These studies add to the literature on the use of combined antiplatelet regimes in CAS and support the evidence that platelet aggregation plays a critical role in stent occlusion and embolic complication. There is not any level-1 evidence to suggest the optimum period of treatment. Stent endothelialization is slow and may take up to 96 days. Use of clopidogrel outside this period is therefore not advocated. Current expert opinion suggests the use of clopidogrel for 28 days following CAS.

Statin Therapy

Cholesterol-lowering regimes have been well established in the management of stroke patients. Statins exert their effect by stabilizing the plaque. Crisby et al. [20] set out to investigate the effect of 3 months of pravastatin treatment on the composition of human carotid plaques removed during carotid endarterectomy. He concluded that pravastatin decreased lipids, lipid oxidation, inflammation, MMP-2, and cell death and increased TIMP-1 and collagen content in human carotid plaques, confirming its plaque-stabilizing effect in humans. To what extent this could be translated into clinical benefit was observed by Gröschel and colleagues [21].

Gröschel et al. [21] set out to retrospectively determine whether preprocedural statin treatment was associated with a reduction of cardiovascular events after carotid angioplasty and stent placement (CAS) in patients with symptomatic carotid stenosis. Consecutive patients ($n = 180$) from the prospective database underwent CAS for high-grade symptomatic carotid disease. The frequency of cardiovascular complications between 127 patients without preprocedural statin treatment and that of 53 patients with preprocedural statin treatment at CAS were compared. The overall 30-day myocardial infarction rate was 2/180 (1%) patients, the minor stroke rate was 16/180 (9%) patients, the major stroke rate was 1/180 (0.5%) patients, and the death rate was 2/180 (1%) patients. The incidence of cardiovascular events (composite of stroke, myocardial infarction, and death within 30 days after CAS) was significantly different between patients with preprocedural treatment (4%) and those without preprocedural statin treatment (15%) ($p < 0.05$). They concluded that preprocedural statin therapy appears to reduce the incidence of stroke, myocardial infarction, and death within 30 days after CAS. Future prospective randomized trials are warranted to further assess this potential protective effect of statin drugs during carotid interventions.

Procedural Heparin

Anticoagulation is mandatory because of long catheter dwelling times, selective catheterization of the carotid vessels, and reduced flow. Zaman et al. [22] demonstrated that on average 3,000 units of heparin provides 30 min of anticoagulation while 5,000 units will achieve anticoagulation for 45 min. Procedure length will be dependant on both operator experience and the complexity of the case. It is currently our practice to give 7,500 units of heparin once arterial access has been achieved in the safe knowledge that it will adequately cover a procedure that on average takes 45 min.

Procedural Glycoprotein IIb/IIIa Antagonists

Glycoprotein IIb/IIIa antagonists work by reducing thrombus propagation and stabilization after stenting. The neurological sequel in carotid stent patients receiving glycoprotein IIb/IIIa inhibitors has been shown to be more numerous and consequential and hence the use of GP IIb/IIIa inhibitors in carotid stenting should be discouraged. Their use may be warranted in the event of acute stent thrombus or distal embolization but the data to support this are poor [23].

Procedural Considerations

Cerebral Protection Devices

Stroke is the most feared risk of CAS and in the majority of cases this probably results from the liberation of embolic material. In more than 90% of treatment episodes emboli are detected by transcranial Doppler. To reduce the rate of procedural complications, strategies to avoid cerebral embolization in the form of embolic protection devices (EPD) have been used. EPD can be divided into 3 principal types (Table 17.3).

1. Distal Occlusion Balloons
2. Filters
3. Proximal protection (flow arrest vs. flow reversal)

While their use would appear to be intuitive, they do have complications of their own. What data are there to demonstrate that the use of EPDs conferred benefit?

Observational Data

Kastrup et al. [24] conducted a systematic review of studies reporting on the incidence of minor stroke, major stroke, or death within 30 days after CAS for studies published between January 1990 and June 2002. In 2,357 patients a total of 2,537 CAS procedures had been done without protection devices, and in 839 patients 896 CAS procedures had been done with protection devices. The combined stroke and death rate within 30 days in both symptomatic and asymptomatic patients was 1.8% in patients treated with cerebral protection devices, compared with 5.5% in patients treated without.

TABLE 17.3. Examples of the 3 principal types of embolic protection devices.

	Size (mm)	Pore size (μm)
Distal filtration		
Angioguard XP (Cordis)	4–8	100
FilterWire EZ (Boston Scientific)	3.5–5.5	80
SpiderRχ™ (EV3)	3–7	50–200
AccuNet Rχ (Guidant)	4.5–7.5	115
Rubicon filter (Rubicon)	4–6	100
EmboShield (Abbot)	3–6	140
Interceptor (Medtronic)	4.5–6.5	100
TRAP (Microvena)	2.5–7	65–200
Distal balloon occlusion	Elastomeric balloon mounted on a 0.014-in. hypotube. This is in turn attached to a floppy-tipped angioplasty wire.	
PercuSurge™ GuardWire (Medtronic)		
Proximal flow arrest	Protects the brain from embolization by two highly compliant atraumatic balloons, blocking antegrade blood flow from the common carotid artery and retrograde blood flow from the ECA.	
Moma™ (Invatec)		
Flow reversal	Occludes both IC and ECA. Blood is shunted into the femoral vein.	
ArteriA™ (Gore)		

This effect was mainly due to a decrease in the occurrence of minor strokes (3.7% without cerebral protection vs. 0.5% with cerebral protection) and major strokes (1.1% without cerebral protection vs. 0.3% with cerebral protection), whereas death rates were almost identical.

The Wholey Registry comprised data from major interventional centers in Europe, North and South America, and Asia [25]. The survey addressed the relevant issues of the patients enrolled, procedure techniques, and results of carotid stenting, including complications and restenosis. The combined minor and major strokes and procedure-related death rate was 3.98%, based on procedure number. Subsets of questions were directed at the new use of distal embolic protection devices. There were 6,753 cases performed without protection, which incurred a 5.29% rate of strokes and procedure-related deaths. In the 4,221 cases with cerebral protection, there was a 2.23% rate of stroke and procedure-related death.

From July 1996 to March 2003, 1,483 patients from 26 hospitals were included in the prospective CAS Registry of the ALKK study group [26]. A protection device was used in 668 of 1,483 patients (45%). The use of a PD led to a 10-min longer intervention. Patients treated with a PD had a lower rate of ipsilateral stroke (1.7% vs. 4.1%, $p = 0.007$) and a lower rate of all nonfatal strokes and all deaths (2.1% vs. 4.9%, $p = 0.004$) during the hospital stay. A similar reduction could be found for symptomatic as well as asymptomatic carotid artery stenosis.

In 2004 Reimers et al. [27] published data from the Italian registry. Two hundred and seventy-five consecutive patients underwent percutaneous angioplasty and/or stenting of the extracranial carotid artery between June 1997 and July 2001. In the first 125 (45.4%) patients, the procedures were done without cerebral protection. After January 2000, protection devices were routinely used. In the unprotected group, 5 (4.0%) complications occurred: 3 minor strokes, 1 TIA, and 1 subarachnoid hemorrhage. In the patients treated under cerebral protection, there were 2 complications: 1 minor stroke and 1 subarachnoid hemorrhage. There were 4 periprocedural embolic complications in the unprotected group, vs. 1 in the protected patients. The authors concluded that the use of the cerebral protection systems reduced the acute neurological event rate related to embolic complications by 79% within the registry population, although the overall event rate was low.

Boltuch et al. [28] examined procedure-related complications and neurological adverse events of unprotected over-the-wire (OTW) and protected rapid exchange (RX) carotid artery stenting (CAS) in a single-center patient series during an 8-year period. Procedure-related complications occurred in 86 (18.3%) of 471 unprotected OTW CAS procedures vs. 18 (10.0%) of 180 protected RX CAS procedures ($p = 0.010$). Transient ischemic attacks (3.2% vs. 2.8%), minor stroke (1.7% vs. 0.6%), and major stroke (2.1% vs. 0.6%) showed a trend toward a difference between unprotected OTW and protected RX CAS ($p = 0.076$); combined 30-day stroke/death rates were 3.8% for OTW vs. 1.2% for RX CAS ($p = 0.073$).

In contrast, the German Pro-CAS registry published data from 2000 to 2003. There was no difference in permanent neurological deficit between unprotected and protected groups [29].

Despite the high volumes of literature published surrounding the use of EPD, these studies, at best, represent level-III/IV evidence. Protected patients have been compared with historical controls and the growing technological advances are all too easy to overlook. Technical advances in the form of dedicated carotid stents have significantly improved the outcome in comparison to adapted stents. CAVATAS has demonstrated the impact of the learning curve, and pharmacological support has increased in the form of dual antiplatelet regimes consisting of aspirin and clopidogrel.

Randomized Trial Data

There are no adequately powered RCT to assess protected vs. unprotected CAS. If all the stroke and death rates in the systematic review for studies reporting after 2002 were analyzed to prove noninferiority of unprotected CAS more than 2,000 patients would be required. This number would further increase in any superiority trial. Data pertaining to RCT focus around the EVA-3S and SPACE trials [11, 30]. The Safety Committee of the EVA-3S trial, published in 2004, recommended stopping unprotected CAS because the 30-day rate of stroke was 3.9 (0.9–16.7) times higher than that of CAS with cerebral protection (4/15 vs. 5/58). The 30-day results from the randomized SPACE trial, comparing CAS and carotid endarterectomy, indicated that the ipsilateral stroke and death rate was 7.3% in those patients in whom protection had been used and 6.7% in unprotected patients. That is to say there was no significant difference between the two groups. The data are conflicting and although the benefits of routine use of cerebral protection have not been confirmed by level-1 evidence, a consensus supports such use.

Predilation

Predilatation is recommended for all patients. A suggestion that predilatation may be of benefit prior to stent placement came from the stopped "Leicester Trial" when the protocol mandated primary stent placement without prior balloon dilatation [31]. The outcomes were dreadful. Bosiers et al. subsequently noted a significant difference in the amount of neurological complications in patients treated with primary stenting, compared with the subgroup receiving PTA before stent implantation (3-year stroke/death rates of 11.8% and 5% respectively) [32]. They hypothesized that predilatation premodels the plaque, causing a reduction in plaque protrusion through the stent material.

Stent Selection and Design

The number of carotid stents on the market has risen. The use of a specific stent design in relation to lesion characteristics has brought about the concept of "tailored" CAS. Knowledge of the vascular anatomy, plaque characteristics, and complexity of the case is essential. The currently available devices differ in relation to their conformity, scaffolding/free cell area, radial strength, and degree of foreshortening, and they can be summarized as being one of the following:

- Cobalt alloy structure – e.g., The Carotid Wallstent (Boston Scientific)
- Nitinol open cell – e.g., Acculink (Guidant), Exponent (Medtronic), Protegè (EV3), Precise (Cordis)
- Nitinol closed cell – e.g., Xact (Abbott)

It remains unclear as to whether, for the same patient, one stent system is better than another. Experience has shown that the open cells do not straighten the ICA as much as closed cell designs or the Wallstent does and it is therefore reasonable to use these when there is tortuosity of the ICA so that this tortuosity is not converted to an occlusive kink. In addition, it is reasonable to use a stent with high radial force in heavily calcified lesions.

Strategies for Avoidance of Nonembolic Stroke

Hemodynamic Depression

Hemodynamic disturbances following carotid intervention are common. The physiological mechanisms relating to this phenomenon are complex. The removal of atheromatous plaque during CEA reduces pressure wave dampening with a resultant increase in baroreceptor stimulation. A more sustained fall in blood pressure in those undergoing CAS has been shown to relate in part to the distension of the carotid sinus from compressed plaque during angioplasty and from additional pressures exerted from the stent. A more sustained effect on blood pressure has been seen during the postprocedural period in those patients in which a stent is used over angioplasty alone. Subset analysis has shown a significant difference in blood pressure response in the balloon-expandable group, with a more marked lowering of systolic blood pressure over the first 24 h. The additional radial force seen in balloon-mounted stents may explain this.

It is clear that hemodynamic instability is common, but to what extent is it clinically significant? Gupta et al. [33] at the Cleveland clinic retrospectively analyzed data on 500 consecutive CAS procedures over a 5-year period. Hemodynamic depression was defined as periprocedural hypotension (systolic blood pressure, <90 mmHg) or bradycardia (heart rate, <60 beats per second). Hemodynamic depression occurred during 210 procedures (42%), whereas persistent HD developed in 84 procedures (17%). Features that independently predicted HD included lesions involving the carotid bulb or the presence of a calcified plaque. Prior ipsilateral CEA was associated with reduced risk of HD. Although HD is common following CAS, it is easily managed. Patients who developed persistent HD were at a significantly increased risk of a periprocedural major adverse clinical complications. Indeed further studies have shown a correlation between the magnitude of change in systolic pressure and the severity of neurological events.

In a recent study by Tan et al. [34] symptomatic hypotension occurred in 7 of 204 patients. In the 7 patients with symptomatic hypotensive events postprocedure, the mean difference in systolic pressure before and immediately after stenting was 42.9 mmHg and the mean difference in diastolic pressure was 22.0 mmHg. In comparison, in the 197 patients with no symptomatic hypotensive events, the mean difference in systolic pressure before and after stenting was 13.3 mmHg and that in diastolic pressure was 3.3 mmHg. Subanalysis of hemodynamic changes showed that patients with significant reduction in diastolic pressure (15 mmHg or more) immediately after CAS are at higher risk for symptomatic hypotension.

Avoidance of Hemodynamic Instability

Appropriately timed administration of atropine (1.2 mg) or glycopyrrolate (600 μg) prior to predilatation helps to prevent baroreceptor stimulation leading to bradycardia. Administration of isoprenaline has been shown to reduce the occurrence of both bradycardia and periprocedural hypotension [35]. There is however a dilemma here. It is likely that keeping systolic pressure low may protect against reperfusion injury (see below). It is not our practice therefore to attend to any hypotension in the majority of patients. The associated increase in baroreceptor activity is thought to be a short-term phenomenon and there is evidence to suggest that they may reset early with prompt mobilization of the patient.

Hyperperfusion Syndrome

Cerebral hyperperfusion syndrome is characterized by headache, hypertension, seizures, and focal neurological deficits. Following restoration of flow during either CAS or CEA, there is transient loss of cerebral autoregulation with areas of hyperperfusion in previous areas of underperfusion. One study with perfusion MRI reported 4 patients with symptoms suggestive of cerebral hyperperfusion syndrome but with only moderate increases in perfusion [36]. Recent data on CAS have highlighted an overall incidence of up to 5% [37]. Many conditions may predispose to cerebral hyperperfusion syndrome. The evidence is somewhat clouded by confounding factors for atherosclerosis. Nevertheless, acknowledgment of predisposing factors for hyperperfusion syndrome is essential for prompt recognition and treatment: hypertension, diabetes, recent contralateral CEA, high-grade carotid artery stenosis, contralateral carotid occlusion, incomplete Circle of Willis, preoperative hypoperfusion, and periprocedural infarction. Factors aimed at avoidance of cerebral hyperperfusion include the following:

- Aggressive monitoring of blood pressure within the periprocedural period and up to 2 weeks following CAS
- Limiting the duration of balloon inflation
- Educating the support teams (nurses, junior doctors, general practioners)

Contrast Encephalopathy

Contrast encephalopathy following CAS is rare. Transient neurotoxicity after carotid interventions must be differentiated from massive cerebral infarction and hyperperfusion syndrome, but the prognosis is excellent. The volume of contrast should be kept to a minimum and hence the complexity of the procedure should correlate with the operator experience.

Stent Thrombosis

The available literature suggests that the incidence of acute stent thrombosis is 0.5–2%. As previously alluded to within this chapter, there is level-1 evidence to support the use of aspirin and clopidogrel during CAS [18]. Mechanisms of antiplatelet drug resistance include poor compliance, interactions with other drugs, genetic polymorphism, and increased platelet turnover. More research is needed to assess the clinical significance and prognostic value of antiplatelet drug resistance detected by laboratory tests in patients undergoing CAS. Future work may help identify a subgroup of patients at high risk for CAS.

The inappropriate choice of stent in the setting of a tortuous ICA may result in subacute thrombosis. A closed cell, nonconforming stent may propagate a kink which if left untreated could have significant hemodynamic consequences. In this situation the placement of an additional open cell, conforming stent is indicated. The choice of stent design in relation to the lesion being treated is discussed elsewhere in this chapter.

Key Points

- Patient selection: Decision-making as to the relative suitability of CAS is complex. Studies support that careful patient selection, based on evaluation of the arch and tortuosity of the extracranial circulation will reduce embolic events. Device characteristics most likely affect outcome. To what extent represents an area for future research. As to whether prior knowledge of plaque characteristics can help us to decide between CEA or CAS is currently under debate. There are no data to support the use of CAS routinely in asymptomatic patients.
- Training: Data from RCTs, in particular the EVA-3S trial, have shown us that training and experience matter. The exact number of cases that should be undertaken per year to ensure maintenance of clinical skills is unclear and appears self-serving. There is growing interest in the role of virtual reality but it remains as yet to be validated.
- Adjunctive pharmaceuticals: There exists level-1 evidence for the routine use of aspirin and clopidogrel in the periprocedural period. Retrospective analysis of registry data suggests that benefit is conveyed through statin therapy. The synergistic nature of peripheral and cardiac disease should warrant their use. Routine use of glycoprotein IIb/IIIa is not recommended. Preprocedural statin therapy appears to reduce the incidence of stroke, myocardial infarction, and death within 30 days after CAS. This at best represents level-3 evidence.
- Cerebral protection and procedural considerations: Observational data and those from RCT are conflicting. There are no adequately powered RCT to assess protected vs. unprotected CAS and although the benefits of routine use of cerebral protection have not been confirmed by level-1 evidence, a consensus supports their use. It remains unclear as to whether, for the same patient, one stent system is better than another. Experience has shown that the open cells do not straighten the ICA as much as closed cell designs or the Wallstent does. In addition, it is reasonable to use a stent with high radial force in heavily calcified lesions.
- Ultimately, if the clinicians follow the above guidelines, know how to resolve common complications, plan carefully around their limitations, and have a good understanding of the available technology they can optimize their outcomes from CAS.

References

1. Fiarhead JF, Mehta Z, Rothwell PM. Population-based study of delays in carotid imaging and surgery and the risk of recurrent stroke. Neurology. 2005;65:371–5.
2. Hammer FD, Lacroix V, Duprez T, et al. Cerebral microembolization after protected carotid artery stenting in surgical high-risk patients: results of a 2-year prospective study. J Vasc Surg. 2005;42(5):847–53.
3. Faggioli GL, Ferri M, Freyrie A, et al. Aortic arch anomalies are associated with increased risk of neurological events in carotid stent procedures. Eur J Vasc Endovasc Surg. 2007;33(4):436–41.
4. Biasi GM, Froio A, Diethrich EB et al., Carotid plaque echolucency increases the risk of stroke in carotid stenting: The Imaging in Carotid Angioplasty and Risk of Stroke (ICAROS) Study. Circulation. 2004;110:756–62.
5. Reiter M, Bucek RA, Effenberger I, et al. Plaque echolucency is not associated with the risk of stroke in carotid stenting. Stroke. 2006;37(9):2378–80.
6. Saam T, Ferguson MS, Yarnykh VL, et al. Quantitative evaluation of carotid plaque composition by in vivo MRI. Arterioscler Thromb Vasc Biol. 2005;25(1):234–9.
7. Bosiers M, de Donato G, Deloose K, et al. Does free cell area influence the outcome in carotid artery stenting? Eur J Vasc Endovasc Surg. 2007;33:135–41.
8. Gaines PA. Re: Does free cell area influence the outcome in carotid artery stenting? Eur J Vasc Endovasc Surg. 2007;33:142–3.
9. Beard JD, Jolly BC, Newble DI, etal. Assessing the technical skills of surgical trainees. Br J Surg. 2005;92(6):778–82.
10. Gaines P, Nicholson T. A suggested training programme for carotid artery stenting (CAS). Eur J Radiol. 2006:60;37–9.
11. Mas JL, Chatellier G, Beyssen B, et al. Endarterectomy versus stenting in patients with symptomatic severe carotid stenosis. N Engl J Med. 2006 19;355(16): 1660–71.

12. Endovascular versus surgical treatment in patients with carotid stenosis in the Carotid and Vertebral Artery Transluminal Angioplasty Study (CAVATAS): a randomised trial. Lancet. 2001;357(9270):1729–37.
13. Verzioi F, Cao P, De Rango P, et al. Appropriateness of learning curve for carotid artery stenting: an analysis of periprocedural complications. J Vasc Surg. 2006;44:1205–12.
14. Satava RM. Virtual reality surgical simulator: the first steps–1993. Clin Orthop Relat Res. 2006;442:2–4.
15. Seymour N, Gallagher AG, O'Brian M, et al. Virtual reality training improves operating room performance: results of a randomised, double-blinded study. Ann Surg. 2002;236(4):458–63.
16. Patel AD, Gallagher AG, Nicholson WJ, et al. Learning curves and reliability measures for virtual reality simulation in the performance of carotid angiography. J Am Coll Cardiol. 2006;47:1796–802.
17. Van Herzeele I, Aggarwal R, Neequaye S, et al. Experienced endovascular interventionalists objectively improve their skills by attending carotid artery stent training courses. Eur J Vasc Endovasc Surg. 2008;35(5):541–50.
18. McKevitt FM, Randall MS, Cleveland TJ, et al. The benefits of combined anti-platelet treatment in carotid artery stenting. Eur J Vasc Endovasc Surg. 2005;29(5):522–7.
19. Dittrich R, Ritter MA, Kaps M, et al. The use of embolic signal detection in multicenter trials to evaluate antiplatelet efficacy: signal analysis and quality control mechanisms in the CARESS (clopidogrel and aspirin for reduction of emboli in symptomatic carotid stenosis) trial. Stroke. 2006;37(4):1065–9.
20. Crisby M, Nordin-Fredriksson G, Shah PK, et al. Pravastatin treatment increases collagen content and decreases lipid content, inflammation, metalloproteinases, and cell death in human carotid plaques: implications for plaque stabilization. Circulation. 2001;103(7):926–33.
21. Gröschel K, Ernemann U, Shulz JB, et al. Statin therapy at carotid angioplasty and stent placement: effect on procedure-related stroke, myocardial infarction, and death. Radiology. 2006;240(1):145–51.
22. Zaman SM, de Vroos Meiring P, Gandhi MR, et al. The pharmacokinetics and UK usage of heparin in vascular intervention. *Clin Radiol.* 1996;51(2):113–6.
23. Ho DS, Wang Y, Chui M, et al. Intracarotid abciximab injection to abort impending ischemic stroke during carotid angioplasty. Cerebrovasc Dis. 2001;11(4):300–4.
24. Kastrup A, Groschel K, Krapf H, et al. Early outcome of carotid angioplasty and stenting with and without cerebral protection devices: a systematic review of the literature. Stroke. 2003;34(3):813–9.
25. Wholey MH, Al-Mubarak N, Wholey MH. Updated review of the global carotid artery stent registry. Catheter Cardiovasc Interv. 2003;60(2):259–66.
26. Zahn R, Mark B, Niedermaier N, et al. Embolic protection devices for carotid artery stenting: better results than stenting without protection? Eur Heart J. 2004;25(17):1550–8.
27. Reimers B, Schuler M, Castriota F, et al. Routine use of cerebral protection during carotid artery stenting: results of a multicenter registry of 753 patients. Am J Med. 2004;116(4):217–22.
28. Boltuch J, Sabeti S, Amight J, et al. Procedure-related complications and early neurological adverse events of unprotected and protected carotid stenting: temporal trends in a consecutive patient series. J Endovasc Ther. 2005;12(5):538–47.
29. Theiss W, Hermanek P, Mathias K, et al. Pro-CAS: A prospective registry of carotid angioplasty and stenting. Stroke. 2004;35:2134–9.
30. SPACE Collaborative Group. 30 day results from the SPACE trial of stent-protected angioplasty versus carotid endarterectomy in symptomatic patients: a randomised non-inferiority trial. Lancet. 2006;368(9543):1239–47.
31. Naylor AR, Bolia A, Abbott RJ, et al. Randomized study of carotid angioplasty and stenting versus carotid endarterectomy: a stopped trial. J Vasc Surg. 1998;28(2):326–34.
32. Bosiers M, Peeters P, Deloose K, et al. Does carotid artery stenting work on the long run: 5-year results in high-volume centers (ELOCAS Registry). J Cardiovasc Surg (Torino). 2005;46(3):241–7.
33. Gupta R, Abou-Chebl A, Bajzer CT, et al. Rate, predictors, and consequences of hemodynamic depression after carotid artery stenting. J Am Coll Cardiol. 2006;47(8):1538–43.
34. Tan KT, Cleveland TJ, Berczi V, McKevitt FM, Venables GS, Gaines PA. Timing and frequency of complications after carotid artery stenting: what is the optimal period of observation? J Vasc Surg. 2003;38:236–43.
35. Van Sambeck M, Hendriles JM, van Dijk LC, et al. Hemodynamic changes during CAS cause half of the complications: how can they be prevented? The 32nd Annual Meeting on Vascular and Endovascular Issues, Techniques and Horizons, Veith Synopsium, New York, November 17–20, 2005.
36. Karapanayiotides T, Meuli R, Devuyst G, et al. Postcarotid endarterectomy hyperperfusion or reperfusion syndrome. Stroke. 2005;36(1):21–6.
37. Morrish W, Grahovac S, Douen A, et al. Intracranial hemorrhage after stenting and angioplasty of extracranial carotid stenosis. AJNR Am J Neuroradiol. 2000;21:1911–6.

Index